Exosomes - Recent Advances From Bench to Bedside

Edited by Sherin Saheera

Published in London, United Kingdom

Exosomes - Recent Advances From Bench to Bedside
http://dx.doi.org/10.5772/intechopen.106308
Edited by Sherin Saheera

Contributors
Leisheng Zhang, Yuanguang Zhao, Shuang Chen, Xiaowei Gao, Shixun Ma, Miao Yu, Xianghong Xu, Yonghong Li, Xiaonan Yang, Tiankang Guo, Hui Cai, Bhawana Bissa, Naveen Soni, Jitender Jangra, Gargi Nandi, Megha Chaudhary, Sushanta Kumar Barik, Jyotirmayee Turuk, Kundave Rajendran Venkataswamy, Diane Irvine Duncan, Byong Seung Cho, Yankun Liu, Mengyuan Hou, Jingwu Li, Zhiwu Wang, Yuelin Zhang, Huifeng Zheng, Yimei Hong, Bei Hu, Xin Li, Alisa Petkevich, Aleksandr Abramov, Vadim Pospelov, Gözde Atila Uslu, Hamit Uslu

First published in London, United Kingdom, 2022 by IntechOpen
IntechOpen is the global imprint of INTECHOPEN LIMITED, registered in England and Wales, registration number: 11086078, 5 Princes Gate Court, London, SW7 2QJ, United Kingdom
Printed in Croatia

British Library Cataloguing-in-Publication Data
A catalogue record for this book is available from the British Library

Additional hard and PDF copies can be obtained from orders@intechopen.com

Exosomes - Recent Advances From Bench to Bedside
Edited by Sherin Saheera
p. cm.

This title is part of the Physiology Book Series, Volume 20
Topic: Cell Physiology
Series Editor: Tomasz Brzozowski
Topic Editor: Angel Catala

Print ISBN 978-1-83768-949-1
Online ISBN 978-1-83768-950-7
eBook (PDF) ISBN 978-1-83768-951-4
ISSN 2631-8261

IntechOpen Book Series
Physiology
Volume 20

Aims and Scope of the Series

Modern physiology requires a comprehensive understanding of the integration of tissues and organs throughout the mammalian body, including the cooperation between structure and function at the cellular and molecular levels governed by gene and protein expression. While a daunting task, learning is facilitated by identifying common and effective signaling pathways mediated by a variety of factors employed by nature to preserve and sustain homeostatic life. As a leading example, the cellular interaction between intracellular concentration of Ca+2 increases, and changes in plasma membrane potential is integral for coordinating blood flow, governing the exocytosis of neurotransmitters, and modulating gene expression and cell effector secretory functions. Furthermore, in this manner, understanding the systemic interaction between the cardiovascular and nervous systems has become more important than ever as human populations' life prolongation, aging and mechanisms of cellular oxidative signaling are utilised for sustaining life. Altogether, physiological research enables our identification of distinct and precise points of transition from health to the development of multimorbidity throughout the inevitable aging disorders (e.g., diabetes, hypertension, chronic kidney disease, heart failure, peptic ulcer, inflammatory bowel disease, age-related macular degeneration, cancer). With consideration of all organ systems (e.g., brain, heart, lung, gut, skeletal and smooth muscle, liver, pancreas, kidney, eye) and the interactions thereof, this Physiology Series will address the goals of resolving (1) Aging physiology and chronic disease progression (2) Examination of key cellular pathways as they relate to calcium, oxidative stress, and electrical signaling, and (3) how changes in plasma membrane produced by lipid peroxidation products can affect aging physiology, covering new research in the area of cell, human, plant and animal physiology.

Meet the Series Editor

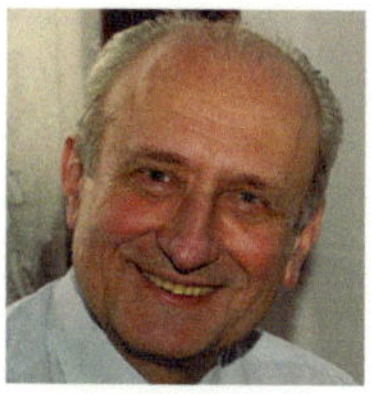

Prof. Dr. Thomas Brzozowski works as a professor of Human Physiology and is currently a Chairman at the Department of Physiology and is V-Dean of the Medical Faculty at Jagiellonian University Medical College, Cracow, Poland. His primary area of interest is physiology and pathophysiology of the gastrointestinal (GI) tract, with a major focus on the mechanism of GI mucosal defense, protection, and ulcer healing. He was a postdoctoral NIH fellow at the University of California and the Gastroenterology VA Medical Center, Irvine, Long Beach, CA, USA, and at the Gastroenterology Clinics Erlangen-Nuremberg and Munster in Germany. He has published 290 original articles in some of the most prestigious scientific journals and seven book chapters on the pathophysiology of the GI tract, gastroprotection, ulcer healing, drug therapy of peptic ulcers, hormonal regulation of the gut, and inflammatory bowel disease.

Meet the Volume Editor

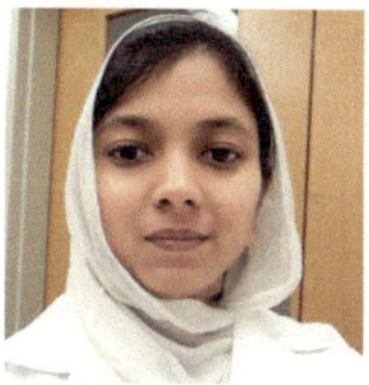

Sherin Saheera pursued both her undergraduate and graduate studies in Biotechnology at the University of Kerala, India. She completed her Ph.D. in Cellular and Molecular Cardiology at the Sree Chitra Tirunal Institute for Medical Sciences and Technology, Kerala, India. During her doctoral research, she worked under Dr. Renuka Nair, focusing on the study of cardiac stem cell aging in hypertensive rat models. Following her Ph.D., Dr. Saheera joined the lab of Dr. Prasanna Krishnamurthy at the University of Alabama, USA, and investigated the molecular mechanisms through which exosomes enhance the recovery process after myocardial infarction. Currently, she is pursuing postdoctoral training at the University of Massachusetts Chan Medical School, USA, focusing on deciphering the role of epigenetics in cardiovascular development.

Contents

Preface

Exosomes – Recent Advances from Bench to Bedside provides comprehensive insights into the fascinating field of exosomes, which are nanosized extracellular vesicles. These extracellular vesicles have been recognized as critical mediators and regulators of both physiological and pathological processes. The book is organized into three sections, each exploring different aspects of exosomes.

Section 1, "Stem Cell-derived Exosomes", focuses on the uses of exosomes derived from mesenchymal stem cells (MSCs). It includes two chapters. Chapter 1 details the application of these exosomes in treating cardiovascular diseases, with a particular emphasis on myocardial infarction (heart attack). Chapter 2 explores the potential use of exosomes in tissue engineering and how they can be utilized for disease diagnosis.

Section 2, "Exosomes and Infectious Diseases", delves into the involvement of exosomes in various infectious diseases. It includes 3 chapters that collectively provide an overview of the role played by exosomes in the immune system. Chapter 3 offers general information on the role of exosomes in immune reactions, while Chapter 4 focuses on the transmission of pathogens through exosomes. Chapter 5 specifically examines the role of exosomes in tuberculosis.

Section 3, "Application of Exosomes", includes four chapters that discuss the diverse applications of exosomes. Chapter 6 explores the use of exosomes as drug delivery systems, highlighting their potential in targeted therapy. Chapters 7 and 8 explore the signaling mechanisms employed by exosomes and provide detailed insights into the contents of exosomes. Finally, Chapter 9 reviews the use of exosomes for aesthetic purposes, potentially indicating their application in cosmetic procedures.

Overall, *Exosomes – Recent Advances from Bench to Bedside* offers a comprehensive exploration of the current understanding and potential applications of exosomes. The book covers various fields, including stem cell-derived exosomes, infectious diseases, and the broader applications of exosomes in diagnostics, therapeutics, and aesthetic practices.

Sherin Saheera
Postdoctoral Associate,
University of Massachusetts Chan Medical School,
Worcester, Massachusetts, USA

Section 1

Stem Cell-Derived Exosomes

Chapter 1

Mesenchymal Stem Cell-Derived Exosomes for Myocardial Infarction Treatment

Huifeng Zheng, Yimei Hong, Bei Hu, Xin Li and Yuelin Zhang

Abstract

Myocardial infarction (MI) is a major cause of morbidity and mortality in modern society. Over the past decades, mesenchymal stem cell (MSCs)-based therapy has shown promising results in the treatment of MI due to their unique properties of multi-differentiation ability, immune-privileged phenotype and paracrine activity. Recently, MSC-derived exosomes (MSC-EXO) have been proposed as a promising therapeutic strategy for MI with their ability to inhibit cardiomyocyte apoptosis and stimulate vascular angiogenesis. They also aid immunoregulation and rejuvenation of cardiomyocyte senescence by transporting their unique content such as proteins, lipids, and miRNAs. Compared with MSC transplantation, MSC-EXO administration has shown several advantages, including lower toxicity and immunogenicity and no risk of tumor formation. Nonetheless the potential mechanisms underlying MSC-EXO-based therapy for MI are not fully understood. In addition, lack of modification of MSC-EXOs can impact therapeutic efficacy. It is vital to optimize MSC-EXO and enhance their therapeutic efficacy for MI. We summarize the recent advances regarding biological characteristics, therapeutic potential and mechanisms, and optimal approaches to the use of MSC-EXOs in the treatment of MI.

Keywords: mesenchymal stem cells, exosome, myocardial infarction, treatment, therapeutic effect

1. Introduction

Myocardial infarction (MI) results in irreversible loss of cardiomyocytes due to a restricted blood supply and is the major cause of morbidity and mortality worldwide. It has been estimated to account for 80% of deaths in patients with ischemic heart disease worldwide, and its prevalence continues to increase every year leading to a significant medical, social, and financial burden [1]. Despite the availability of advanced surgical interventions and medications including primary percutaneous coronary intervention, angiotensin-converting enzyme drugs and β-blockers, there remains no effective means to prevent cardiomyocyte loss due to myocardial ischemia [2]. The only cure for this devastating disease is heart transplantation but this is restricted by its high cost, a shortage of donor hearts, and the occurrence of immune rejection following transplantation [3]. Exploration of novel therapies for left ventricle remodeling and dysfunction following infarction is urgently needed.

Over the past decades, stem cell-based therapy has become a promising strategy to treat MI with significant progress made in animal studies and clinical trials [4–6]. Among all types of stem cell under investigation, mesenchymal stem cells (MSCs) have garnered huge interest due to their easy isolation, high reproductive activity, differentiation capability and immunomodulatory properties [7, 8]. MSCs can be isolated from multiple tissues or cells including bone marrow, adipose tissue, umbilical cord blood and even pluripotent stem cells [9–12]. There is accumulating evidence that MSCs are promising candidates for MI treatment [13–15]. More importantly, it is now widely accepted that the cardioprotective effects of MSC-based therapy in MI are due to their strong paracrine effects, rather than trans-differentiation ability [7, 16–18]. Therefore, researchers are increasingly huge interested in the therapeutic efficacy of MSC-derived bioactive molecules, especially exosome (EXO), that are considered major components of the paracrine effect in MSC-based therapy [19, 20]. EXO, a subgroup of extracellular vesicles (EVs), are 40–160 nm diameter membrane-bound vesicles that can be found in almost all biological fluids. It has been well documented that MSC-EXO exert their cardioprotective effects in MI by delivering diverse biological molecules, including non-coding RNA, DNA, lipids and proteins [21–24]. More importantly, compared with MSC transplantation, MSC-EXO have several advantages such as easier storage and transplantation, less immune rejection, minimum risk of immunogenicity and no risk of tumor formation [25]. We discuss the current understanding of the biological characteristics, therapeutic effects and potential mechanisms of MSC-based therapy in MI. We also highlight the current challenges and potential approaches to improve the efficacy and production of MSC-EXO in regenerative medicine to guide their future clinical application.

2. Characterization and Isolation of MSC-EXO

EVs are bilayer lipid membrane-bound subcellular vesicles released by all types of cells and present in all body fluids. According to MISEV2018, EVs are divided into "small EVs" (sEVs, <100 nm or <200 nm) and "medium/large EVs"(m/lEVs, >200 nm) respectively [26]. EXO are sEVs approximately 40–160 nm in diameter (100 nm on average) and the main subclass of EVs [27]. The biogenesis of EXO begins with inward budding to form an early endosome. Finally, EXO are built when multi vesicular bodies (MVBs, late endosomes) fuse with plasma membrane and are secreted into the extracellular space [28, 29]. MSC-EXO express EXO-specific markers CD9, CD63, CD81, Alix and Tsg101 as well as MSC surface markers including CD29, CD44, CD90 and CD73. Among these, CD29 and CD44 have been identified previously as the specific biomarkers for MSC-EXO [30, 31]. The size and concentration of EXO can be characterized by nanoparticle tracking analysis (NTA) and transmission electron microscopy (TEM) [32]. Recently, plasmonic scattering microscopy has been applied to image exosomes and analyze biomarkers [33].

It is difficult to show whole landscape of EXO dispersed in solution. Therefore, purification of EXO is of importance for EXO definition. EXO are distributed throughout body fluids and this represents a challenge to their isolation. EXO are secreted into body fluids such as blood, urine, saliva, lymph, breast milk, cerebrospinal fluid and pericardial fluid etc. [34]. EXO components reflects the state of the original cell. Different methods of isolation of EXO varies from various body fluids. Meanwhile, the extraction result differs from types of biological fluid. Which was optimal remains controversial [35]. Isolation of abundant EXO can help in the assessment of their biological functions [36]. Several recent alternative methods ranging from conventional to newly developed techniques to isolate and purify EXO are summarized in **Table 1**. Different methods for EXO isolation have different advantages and disadvantages. During isolation, ultracentrifugation and density gradient centrifugation are the most commonly used techniques [47]. Currently, several new methods have been established to facilitate high-throughput and high-purity manufacture of EXO. The characterization and isolation of MSC-EXO are summarized in **Figure 1**.

No.	Methods of EXO isolation	Advantages and disadvantages	Ref.
1	Ultracentrifugation	1. Most widely used 2. Gold standard for exosome separation 3. A series of speed centrifugation 4. Time consuming	[37]
2	Density gradient centrifugation	1. Sorts: Sucrose density gradient Iodixanol density gradient Optiprep density gradient 2. Improve purity of exosomes 3. Sucrose density gradient cannot effectively separate EXO and retroviruses 4. Time consuming and complex procedure	[38]
3	Chromatography (size-based isolation techniques)	1. Sorts: Mini-size exclusion chromatography (mini-SEC) Size exclusion chromatography 2. Quick, easy, small material consumption 3. May be applied with other particles of similar size	[39]
4	Ultrafiltration (size-based isolation techniques)	1. Uses ultrafiltration membranes with different molecular weight cutoffs (MWCO) 2. Low cost and high enrichment efficiency 3. Low purity and non-specific binding of EXO	[40]
5	Tangential flow filtration (size-based isolation techniques)	1. Using a cutoff TFF cartridge 2. Fluid flows tangentially across the surface, avoiding filter cake formation 3. Fast and efficient 4. Volume is limited by the instrument dead volume	[41]
6	Polymer-based precipitation separation	1. Uses polyethylene glycol (PEG) as a medium 2. Easy to operate with short analysis time 3. Polymer is difficult to remove	[42]
7	Immunoaffinity chromatography (IAC)	1. Based on the specific binding of antibodies and ligands 2. Storage conditions of EXO are relatively harsh and are not suitable for large-scale separation of EXO	[43]

No.	Methods of EXO isolation	Advantages and disadvantages	Ref.
8	Microfluidic technologies	1. Sorts Physical-property-based microfluidics Immunoaffinity-based microfluidics 2. Miniaturization, integration, high-throughput capacity, low-time consumption 3. Specialized equipment needed	[44]
9	Deterministic lateral displacement separation	1. Uses tilted pillar arrays that generate a fluid bifurcation and a unique number of streamlines between the gaps 2. Low separation throughput; particle adhesion and clogging; complex and bulky experimental setup	[45]
10	Acoustic fluid separation	1. Uses ultrasound waves to exert radiation forces on particles 2. Highly controllable, and versatile 3. The device is relatively low in a single channel microfluidic device	[46]

Table 1.
Methods of MSC-EXO isolation.

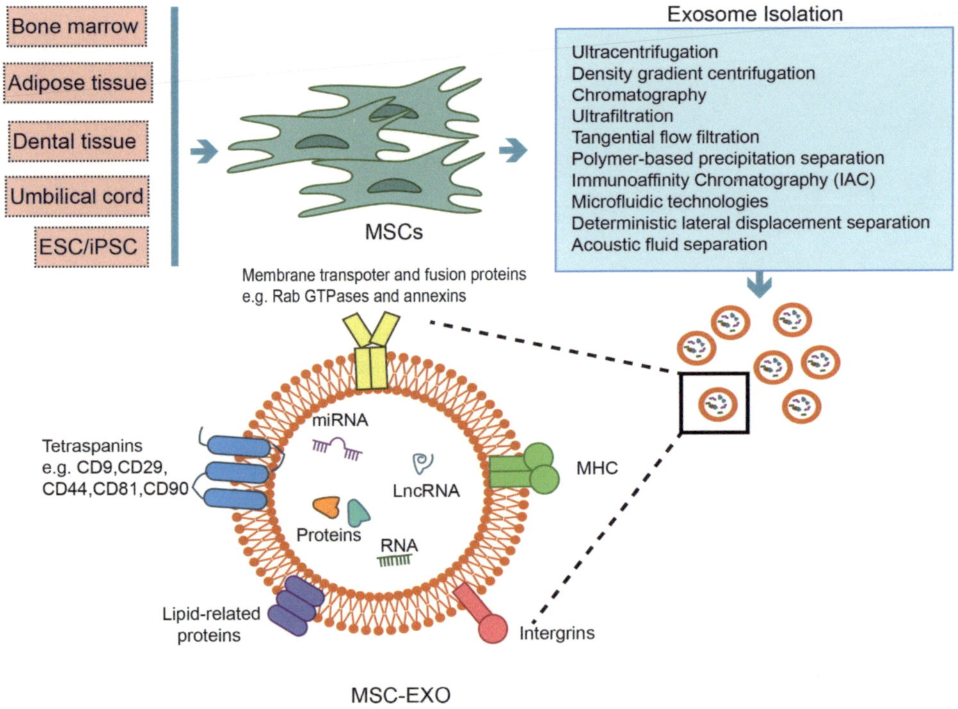

Figure 1.
Characterization and isolation of MSC-EXO.

3. The bioactive constituents of MSC-EXO for MI treatment

MSC-EXO exert their benefits in various diseases by enclosing and transporting a vast array of molecules [48]. It has been demonstrated that exosomal components are almost dependent on the source cell and cellular conditions [25, 49, 50]. Generally, EXO contain multiple characteristic molecules with typical physiological functions [51–53]. MSC-EXO comprise a variety of substances, including many kinds of proteins and a lot of noncoding RNA, including microRNAs (miRNAs) and long noncoding RNAs (lncRNA) [54]. These components can act as paracrine factors, mediating cell-to-cell signaling and communication. More importantly, they can be used as prognostic and diagnostic markers [55, 56].

3.1 Exosomal miRNAs in MSC-EXO for MI treatment

miRNAs are endogenous and 19–25 nucleotides in size. They can be isolated from cells, tissues and body fluids [57]. By pairing to the mRNAs of protein-coding genes, miRNAs play an important role in regulating post-transcriptional silencing of target genes [58, 59]. There is accumulating evidence that miRNAs are enriched in MSC-EXO and are the major bioactive constituents [60–62]. In the last few decades, the cardioprotective role of MSC-derived exosomal miRNAs has attracted huge attention [63]. It has been well documented that many MSC-derived exosomal miRNAs have beneficial functions in MI treatment [64]. Importantly, several potential mechanisms have been identified such as promotion of angiogenesis, reduction of cell death and an antifibrotic effect [65]. Enhanced angiogenesis is one of the important repair mechanisms underlying MSC-EXO-based therapy for MI [66–68]. Through direct miRNAs transfer, MSC-EXO convey their proangiogenic signals to injured cardiomyocytes [69]. Previous study has shown that silenced MSC-derived exosomal miR-210 largely lost its proangiogenic effect. Further experimental study revealed that exosomal miR-210 improves angiogenesis of MSC-EXO via targeting of Efna3 [70]. Zhu et al. demonstrated that macrophage migration inhibitory factor (MIF) could enhance the pro-angiogenic effect of MSC-EXO by enhancing the level of miR-133a-3p via regulation of the AKT signaling pathway [71]. miR-221 is one of the most studied miRNAs. A recent study reported that up-regulated exosomal miR-221-3p derived from senescent MSCs improved their ability of angiogenesis, migration and proliferation, and suppressed apoptosis by regulating the PTEN/AKT pathway [72]. Ma et al. revealed that miR-132-electroporated MSC-EXO could promote angiogenesis both *in vitro* and *in vivo* by downregulating RASA1 [23]. These studies show that MSC-EXO improve angiogenesis by transmitting miRNAs via various biological signaling pathway following MI.

There is increasing evidence that ameliorating cardiomyocyte death is another major mechanism by which EXO restore cardiac function following MI. MSC-EXO reduce myocardial cell death via multiple mechanisms including an anti-apoptosis action, inhibition of pyroptosis and an anti-inflammatory effect [73]. Apoptosis is programmed cell death that is strongly associated with myocardial ischemia [74]. Previous studies have proved that MSCs have an anti-apoptotic effect through secretion of exosomes enriched in miRNAs [75]. Hypoxia-elicited MSC-EXO (Hypo-EXO) facilitates cardiac repair by preventing cell death in MI via delivery of miR-125b.

Mechanistically, miR-125b-5p suppresses apoptosis of cardiomyocytes by down-regulating the expression of apoptotic genes p53 and BAK1 [63]. Another study demonstrated that EXO derived from miR-146a-modified adipose-MSCs attenuated MI via inhibition of apoptosis, the inflammatory response, and fibrosis in a rat model of AMI by targeting early growth response factor 1(EGR1) [76]. Wang et al. reported that adipose-MSC-EXO carrying miR-671 reduced the apoptosis of cardiomyocytes and alleviated myocardial fibrosis and inflammation via inactivation of the TGFBR2/Smad2 Axis [77]. miR-153-3p plays an important role in modulating cell proliferation, apoptosis and angiogenesis. It has been illustrated that EXO-miR-153-3p significantly reduces apoptosis of endothelial cells and cardiomyocytes and promotes their viability. By targeting ANGPT1, miR-153-3p can regulate the VEGF/VEGFR2/PI3K/AKT/eNOS pathways to prevent hypoxic damage to endothelial cells and cardiomyocytes [78]. Furthermore, a growing number of studies have shown that stem cell-derived exosomal miRNAs, such as miR-150-5p, miR-126, and miR-486-5p, demonstrate antiapoptotic activity in MI treatment [79–81]. These findings indicate that the anti-apoptotic effect of MSC-EXO can be partly ascribed to the delivery of some anti-apoptotic miRNAs.

Autophagy is a self-destructive process during which a cell degrades and recycles unnecessary or dysfunctional cellular components [82]. Autophagy is involved in promoting cell death and exacerbates myocardial dysfunction following severe ischemic stress. There is accumulating evidence that MSC-EXO reduce cell death by mediating autophagy. Xiao et al. determined that MSC-EXO reduced autophagic flux in infarcted hearts via exosomal transfer of miR-125b by interfering with p53/Bnip3 signaling and protected cardiomyocytes against damage [83]. Liu et al. showed that miR-93-5p-enhanced ADSC-EXO had a greater cardioprotective effect by suppressing hypoxia-induced autophagy and inflammatory cytokine expression via targeting of Atg7 and Toll-like receptor 4 (TLR4), respectively [84]. Furthermore, Li et al. reported that exosomal miR-301 derived from MSCs protected against MI by inhibiting myocardial autophagy [85]. In addition, MSC-exosomal miRNAs exerted a cardioprotective effect in MI by attenuating cardiac fibrosis. Inflammation and subsequent fibrosis are important pathological reactions that result in scar formation post-MI. Human umbilical cord MSCs-EXO containing miR-29b have been shown to prevent cardiac fibrosis following MI, leading to a reduction in infarct size and improved cardiac function in a mouse model of MI [86]. Moreover, miR-671 carried by adipose-derived MSC-EXO has been proven to also reduce myocardial fibrosis and inflammation both *in vitro* and *in vivo* [77]. The roles of MSC-exosomal miRNA and the potential mechanism for MI treatment are summarized in **Table 2**.

3.2 Exosomal lncRNAs in MSC-EXO for MI treatment

LncRNAs are defined as RNA transcripts >200 nucleotides without protein-coding potential. lncRNAs play important roles in regulating a variety of biological processes. Recent studies have shown that they participate in the initiation and progression of MI through regulation of gene expression at the epigenetic, transcriptional and post-transcriptional levels [87]. Moreover, MSC-derived exosomal lncRNAs have been shown to have cardioprotective effects for MI. LncRNA KLF3-AS1 in human MSC-EXO ameliorated pyroptosis of cardiomyocytes in a rat model of MI via regulation of the miR-138-5p/Sirt1 axis [88]. A recent study has illustrated that hypoxia promoted MSCs to secret lncRNA-UCA1-enriched EXO

Model	Sources of EXO	Related-effectors	Biological effects	Involved pathway	Ref.
MI mouse with LAD ligation	BM-MSCs	miR-210	Angiogenesis	Efna3	[65]
MI rat with LAD ligation	UC-MSCs	miR-133-3p	Angiogenesis Anti-apoptosis Anti-fibrosis	P-AKT	[66]
MI rat with LAD ligation	BM-MSCs	miR-221-3p	Angiogenesis Anti-apoptosis	PTEN/AKT pathway	[67]
MI mouse with LAD ligation	BM-MSCs	miR-132	Angiogenesis increase tube formation enhance neovascularization	RASA1	[18]
MI mouse with LAD ligation	BM-MSCs	miR-125b	Anti-apoptosis	P53 and BAK1	[58]
MI rat with LAD ligation	AD-MSCs	miR-146	Anti-apoptosis Anti-inflammation Anti-fibrosis	EGR1/TLR4/NFκB	[71]
MI rat with LAD ligation	AD-MSCs	miR-671	Anti-fibrosis Anti-inflammation	TGFBR2/Smad2	[72]
Vitro model	BM-MSCs	miR-153-3p	Anti-apoptosis Angiogenesis	ANGPT1-VEGF/PI3k/AKT/eNOS	[73]
MI mouse with LAD ligation	BM-MSCs	miR-150-5p	Anti-apoptosis	Bax	[74]
MI rat with LAD ligation	AD-MSCs	miR-126	Anti-apoptosis Anti-inflammation Anti-fibrosis Angiogenesis	_	[75]
MI rat with LAD ligation	BM-MSCs	miR-486-5p	Anti-apoptosis	PTEN/PI3K/AKT	[76]
MI mouse with LAD ligation	BM-MSCs	miR-125b	Decreasing autophagic flux	p53/Bnip3	[78]
MI rat with LAD ligation	BM-MSCs	miR-301	Inhibiting myocardial autophagy	—	[80]
MI mouse with LAD ligation	UC-MSCs	miR-29b	Anti-fibrosis	—	[81]

Table 2.
MSC-exosomal miRNAs for MI treatment.

that had a cardioprotective effect via the lncRNA-UCA1/miR-873-5p/XIAP axis. Furthermore, exosomal lncRNA-UCA1 in human plasma may be considered a potential noninvasive biomarker for the diagnosis of AMI [89]. Similarly, Huang et al. showed that Atorvastatin pretreatment enhanced the therapeutic efficacy of MSC-EXO in a rat MI model via up-regulation of LncRNA H19 by promoting endothelial cell function [90]. The roles of MSC-exosomal LncRNA and their potential mechanism in MI treatment are summarized in **Table 3**.

Model	Sources of EXO	Related-effectors	Biological effects	Involved pathway	Ref.
MI rats with LAD ligation	hMSCs	LncRNA KLF3-AS1	Amelioration of pyroptosis	miR-138-5p/Sirt1	[83]
MI rats with LAD ligation	hMSCs	LncRNA-UCA1	Anti-apoptosis	miR-873-5p/ XIAP	[84]
MI rats with LAD ligation	BM-MSCs	LncRNA H19	Anti-apoptosis Angiogenesis Anti-inflammation Anti-fibrosis	miR-675, VEGF and ICAM-1	[85]

Table 3.
MSC-exosomal LncRNAs for MI treatment.

3.3 Exosomal proteins in MSC-EXO for MI treatment

MSC-EXOs further elicit benefit by delivering their cargo of potentially therapeutic proteins to recipient cells [91]. To date, nearly two thousand proteins in MSC-EXO have been identified [92–96]. Like miRNAs and lncRNAs, proteins in MSC-EXO have the potential to protect cardiomyocytes against injury following MI. Proteins in MSC-EXO whose role is basic cellular function, include common proteins, enzymes and signaling molecules [97]. One study suggested that hucMSC-EXO protected myocardial cells against apoptosis and promoted cell proliferation and angiogenesis by improving the expression of Bcl-2 family [98]. EXO secreted from CXCR4 overexpressing MSCs have been shown to promote cardiomyocyte survival and angiogenesis in ischemic hearts following MI via the AKT signaling pathway [99]. Deng et al. reported that EXO from AD-MSCs could ameliorate cardiac damage following MI by activating S1P/SK1/S1PR1 signaling and promoting macrophage M2 polarization [100]. The roles of MSC-exosomal proteins and their potential mechanism for MI treatment are summarized in **Table 4**.

Taken together, although current knowledge is limited, it can be inferred that various proteins carried by MSC-EXO protect ischemic cardiomyocytes through different mechanisms.

Model	Sources of EXO	Related-effectors	Biological effects	Involved pathway	Ref.
MI rats with LAD ligation	UC-MSCs	Bcl-2 family, Ki67	Anti-fibrosis angiogenesis	—	[98]
MI rat with LAD ligation	BM-MSCs	DMBT1	Promotes angiogenesis	PI3K-AKT/ GSK3β/β-catenin/ VEGF	[99]
MI rat with LAD ligation	AD-MSCs	S1P, SK1, S1PR1	Anti-apoptosis anti-fibrosis anti-inflammation promotes macrophage M2 polarization	S1P/SK1/S1PR1	[100]

Table 4.
MSC-Exosomal proteins for MI treatment.

4. Potential strategies to improve the therapeutic efficacy of MSC-EXO for MI

Although MSC-EXO-based therapy has shown promising results in MI, their therapeutic efficacy is heavily restricted by the low production and concentration of biological molecules released by EXO derived from MSCs under routine culture conditions. The production and biological components of MSC-EXO vary depending on the different external stimuli surrounding MSCs and MSC status. Therefore, modifying and optimizing exosomal content in MSC-EXO *in vitro* prior to transplantation to enhance their therapeutic efficacy for MI is vital. Over the past decades, several novel strategies, including altering culture conditions and pretreatment with pharmacological compounds and molecules, have been explored to generate modified MSC-EXO with greater benefits for MI treatment [56, 101]. More importantly, genetic modification of MSCs has had a great impact on the release of MSC-EXO, directly modulating their therapeutic efficacy. The influence of these factors on production and function of MSC-EXO will be discussed in the following sections. Different strategies to improve the therapeutic effects of MSC-EXO in MI are summarized in **Figure 2**.

4.1 MSC-EXO generated from different culture conditions

The status of MSCs is largely dependent on culture conditions. Changes to culture conditions may influence MSC-EXO content and its biological functions. As a key impact on MSC culture, oxygen concentration plays a critical role in the regulation of gene expression, exon splicing, and phenotype of MSCs [102]. Therefore, oxygen gradients control MSC functions and generate different biological functions of MSC-EXO. MSCs survive under hypoxic conditions after transplantation into the ischemic heart and then release EXO to exert their benefit. Nonetheless MSCs are usually cultured under normoxic conditions *in vitro*. Therefore, the EXO released from MSCs under normoxic conditions *in vitro* and under hypoxic conditions *in vivo* carry different biological molecules with correspondingly different therapeutic effects. It has been reported that transplantation of MSCs under hypoxic conditions results in an enhanced therapeutic effect for MI [103, 104], indicating that hypoxic preconditioning may be a potential approach to prime MSC-EXO for MI treatment. Accumulating

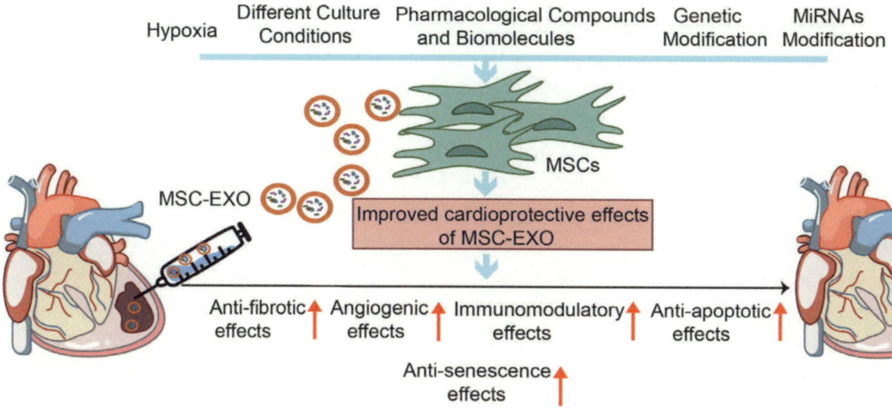

Figure 2.
Different strategies to improve the therapeutic effects of MSC-EXO in MI.

evidence shows that EXO from hypoxia-primed MSCs used to treat MI are superior to EXO from MSCs cultured under normoxic conditions [63, 105, 106]. Hypoxic preconditioning can enrich some specific miRNAs in the MSC-EXO that protect against MI by promoting angiogenic potential, attenuating inflammation and ameliorating apoptosis of cardiomyocytes [101]. It has been documented that hypoxic preconditioning of MSC-EXO elicits better therapeutic efficacy for MI by reducing the apoptosis of cardiomyocytes via upregulation of miR-210 that targets AIFM3 protein [75]. Zhang et al. showed that EXO isolated from hypoxic MSCs improved myocardial function in a rat model of myocardial ischemia-reperfusion injury by suppressing oxidative stress and the inflammatory response via delivery of miR-98-5p [107]. More importantly, EXO derived from MSCs stably overexpressing hypoxia inducible factor (HIF)-1α displayed an increased angiogenic capacity, partially due to the high level of Jagged1. This may have potential applications for MI treatment [108]. Indeed, transplantation of EXO collected from HIF-1α overexpressing MSCs improved heart function by promoting angiogenic formation in a rat model of MI [109]. Apart from hypoxic conditions, culture medium with different types of serum influence the characteristics of MSCs, modulating the efficacy of MSC-EXO-based therapies. Compared with normal serum, MSCs cultured with serum collected from the blood of mice with middle cerebral artery occlusion robustly demonstrated an upregulated level of miR-20a in their EXO [110]. Whether culturing MSCs with special serum can improve the efficacy of MSC-EXO for MI remains to be determined. Recently, it has been reported that the production of MSC-EXO can be augmented using a 3D porous scaffold structure instead of the traditional 2D culture in plastic plates, providing a novel strategy to optimize MSC-EXO for MI treatment [111]. Therefore, exploring suitable culture conditions for MSCs will not only improve the yield of EXO but also modify the therapeutic components of the EXO, ultimately enhancing their efficacy for MI treatment.

4.2 MSC-EXO generated following preconditioning with pharmacological compounds and biomolecules of MSCs

There is accumulating evidence that preconditioning with pharmacological agents and biomolecules robustly improves the therapeutic efficacy of MSCs in MI by enhancing MSC survival and paracrine effects [112–115]. These results prompted us to determine whether pharmacological preconditioning could be a novel approach to enhance the cardioprotective effects of MSC-EXO. Our group has shown that compared with MSC-EXO, EXO isolated from MSCs pretreated with hemin, a potent heme oxygenase-1 (HO-1) inducer, exhibited better cardioprotection for MI via inhibition of cardiomyocyte senescence by elevating the level of miR-183-5p [116]. Huang et al. demonstrated that EXO obtained from atorvastatin-pretreated MSCs had greatly enhanced therapeutic efficacy for MI treatment in terms of promoting angiogenesis and inhibiting inflammation [90]. In addition to pharmacological agents, preconditioning with specific biomolecules can contribute to the secretion of MSC-EXO. EXO derived from interferon-gamma (IFN-γ)-treated MSCs exhibited more potent cardioprotective function in a rat model of MI by increasing angiogenesis and inhibiting cardiomyocyte apoptosis through upregulation of miR-21 [117]. Interestingly, Xiao et al. found that compared with MSC-EXO, EXO derived from MSCs pretreated with ischemic rat heart extracts enriched with IL-22 promoted the angiogenic capacity of human umbilical vein endothelial cells, indicating a novel preconditioning approach to optimize MSC-EXO for MI treatment [99]. These reports confirm that preconditioning with pharmacological compounds or biomolecules can alter the surrounding microenvironment of the culture conditions of MSCs and influence their paracrine effects, ultimately affecting the action of their derived EXO.

4.3 MSC-EXO isolated from genetically modified MSCs

Genetic modification of MSCs via knockdown or overexpression of some RNAs or proteins is another efficient approach to improve the therapeutic effect of MSC-EXO. Our previous study showed that compared with MSC-EXO, administration of EXO secreted by MSCs transduced with macrophage migration inhibitory factor, a proinflammatory cytokine, exhibited a better therapeutic efficacy for MI by downregulating cardiomyocyte mitochondrial fragmentation, reactive oxygen species generation, and apoptosis [118]. A recent report revealed that EXO collected from stromal-derived factor 1-overexpressing MSCs intravenously administered in a mouse model displayed enhanced heart protection by inhibiting apoptosis and autophagy of myocardial cells and increasing angiogenesis by the regulating PI3K signaling pathway [119]. In another study, EXO from MSCs transduced with lentiviral CXCR4 promoted restoration of cardiac function in a rat model of MI by ameliorating cardiomyocyte apoptosis and increasing angiogenesis via upregulation of IGF-1α and p-AKT levels and downregulation of active caspase 3 level [120]. As discussed above, miRNAs are important biological components that play a pivotal role in the cardioprotective effect of MSC-EXO in MI [121–123]. Therefore, overexpression of miRNAs in MSCs can enhance the efficacy of MSC-EXO for MI treatment. Direct injection of MSC-EXO with miR-183-5p overexpression has been shown to result in better cardiac function via suppression of apoptosis and oxidative stress of cardiomyocytes by targeting FOXO1 [124]. Administration of EXO derived from miR-129-5p-modified MSCs displayed enhanced cardiac function following MI in mice by downregulating apoptosis of cardiomyocytes and production of inflammatory cytokines via targeting of HMGB1 [125]. Moreover, EXO derived from miR-126-overexpressing adipose-MSCs demonstrated better beneficial effects by inhibiting cardiac fibrosis and inflammatory cytokine expression and increasing angiogenesis [80]. Thus, genetically modified MSC-EXO have been considered an effective means by which to enhance their cardioprotective effects in MI.

5. Limitations and challenges of MSC-EXO-based therapy for MI

Despite several significant advantages over MSCs, there remain some limitations and challenges to the clinical application of MSC-EXO for MI treatment. First, the rapid clearance of MSC-EXO from ischemic heart tissue after transplantation limits the beneficial effects for MI. An optimum delivery route for administration of MSC-EXO is unavailable. Currently, intramyocardial transplantation is the most efficacious. Exploration of alternative approaches to optimize retention and engraftment of MSC-EXO in the ischemic heart is urgently needed. Second, although the biological components in MSC-EXO, including miRNAs, lncRNA, recombinant proteins, and cytokines, have been intensively investigated, the exact mechanisms underlying MSC-EXO-based therapy for MI require further investigation. Third, MSC-EXO are currently isolated mainly depending on their vesicle size. Different sizes of MSC-EXO may contain different components with corresponding different therapeutic outcomes for MI. A more accurate isolation and purification method for MSC-EXO should be adopted. Fourth, multiple harmful and unwanted biological components in MSC-EXO may restrict their efficiency. Several strategies to modify and remove unwanted components are under investigation. Finally, although classic high-speed centrifugation is the most common method used for MSC-EXO isolation, it is limited by the disadvantages of low production of EXO, high heterogeneity and non-scalability. A scalable isolation protocol for mass production of homogenous MSC-EXO for clinical application is needed.

6. Conclusion

Over the past decades, administration of MSC-EXO has been shown to attenuate cardiac remodeling and improve heart function recovery following MI by inhibiting cardiomyocyte apoptosis, stimulating vascular angiogenesis, immunoregulation and rejuvenating cardiomyocyte senescence. Although the great potential of MSC-EXO therapy for heart function recovery has been clearly demonstrated, the therapeutic role of MSC-EXO in MI is extremely complex. Many issues remain to be carefully addressed and evaluated including the need for a high quality isolation protocol, delivery routes, and optimum EXO dose. In addition, potential risks must be carefully evaluated prior to translation into clinical trials. MSC-EXO-based therapy is still in its infancy and most experimental studies have been in a small animal model. The therapeutic efficacy of MSC-EXO should be evaluated in a porcine model or pre-clinical large animal model. This may provide further evidence to support clinical translation of MSC-EXO-based therapy to humans. Despite the unresolved issues, with the advanced development and technical breakthroughs in EXO research, it is hoped that clinical translation of MSC-EXO to promote cardiac regeneration and repair will soon be a reality for patients with MI.

Acknowledgements

This research was in part supported by the Natural Science Foundation for Distinguished Scholarship of Guangdong Province of China (2022B1515020104 to Y. Zhang), the Distinguished Scholarship of Guangdong Provincial People's Hospital (KY0120220132 to Y. Zhang), National Natural Science Grant of China (No. 82270253 to Y. Zhang, No. 82072225 to X. Li), Natural Science Foundation of Chongqing (No. cstc2020jycj-msxmX0301 to H. Zheng) and NSFC Incubation Program of GDPH (KY012021167 to Y. Hong).

Conflict of interest

The authors confirm that they have no conflicts of interest.

Other declarations

The authors thank Ms. S Aglionby for editing the manuscript.

Author details

Huifeng Zheng[1,2†], Yimei Hong[1†], Bei Hu[1], Xin Li[1*] and Yuelin Zhang[1*]

1 Department of Emergency Medicine, Guangdong Provincial People's Hospital (Guangdong Academy of Medical Sciences), Southern Medical University, Guangzhou, Guangdong, China

2 Department of Intensive Care Unit, Chongqing General Hospital, Chongqing, China

*Address all correspondence to: xlidoct@qq.com; zhangyuelin1999@163.com

† Huifeng Zheng and Yimei Hong contributed equally to this study.

References

[1] GBD 2016 Mortality Collaborators. Global, regional, and national under-5 mortality, adult mortality, age-specific mortality, and life expectancy, 1970-2016: A systematic analysis for the global burden of disease study 2016. Lancet. 2017;**390**:1084-1150. DOI: 10.1016/s0140 6736(17)31833-0

[2] Heusch G, Gersh BJ. The pathophysiology of acute myocardial infarction and strategies of protection beyond reperfusion: A continual challenge. European Heart Journal. 2017;**38**:774-784. DOI: 10.1093/eurheartj/ehw224

[3] Kittleson MM, Kobashigawa JA. Cardiac transplantation: Current outcomes and contemporary controversies. JACC Heart Failure. 2017;**5**:857-868. DOI: 10.1016/j.jchf.2017.08.021

[4] Feric NT, Radisic M. Strategies and challenges to myocardial replacement therapy. Stem Cells Translational Medicine. 2016;**5**:410-416. DOI: 10.5966/sctm.2015-0288

[5] Raziyeva K, Smagulova A, Kim Y, Smagul S, Nurkesh A, Saparov A. Preconditioned and genetically modified stem cells for myocardial infarction treatment. International Journal of Molecular Sciences. 2020;**21**:7301. DOI: 10.3390/ijms21197301

[6] Parizadeh SM, Jafarzadeh-Esfehani R, Ghandehari M, Parizadeh MR, Ferns GA, Avan A, et al. Stem cell therapy: A novel approach for myocardial infarction. Journal of Cellular Physiology. 2019;**234**:16904-16912. DOI: 10.1002/jcp.28381

[7] Sid-Otmane C, Perrault LP, Ly HQ. Mesenchymal stem cell mediates cardiac repair through autocrine, paracrine and endocrine axes. Journal of Translation Medecine. 2020;**18**:336. DOI: 10.1186/s12967-020-02504-8

[8] Sun SJ, Lai WH, Jiang Y, Zhen Z, Wei R, Lian Q, et al. Immunomodulation by systemic administration of human-induced pluripotent stem cell-derived mesenchymal stromal cells to enhance the therapeutic efficacy of cell-based therapy for treatment of myocardial infarction. Theranostics. 2021;**11**:1641-1654. DOI: 10.7150/thno.46119

[9] Pittenger MF, Mackay AM, Beck SC, Jaiswal RK, Douglas R, Mosca JD, et al. Multilineage potential of adult human mesenchymal stem cells. Science. 1999;**284**:143-147. DOI: 10.1126/science.284.5411.143

[10] Caplan AI. Mesenchymal stem cells. Journal of Orthopaetic Research. 1991;**9**:641-650. DOI: 10.1002/jor.1100090504

[11] Lian QZ, Lye E, Yeo KS, Tan EKW, Salto-Tellez M, Liu TM, et al. Derivation of clinically compliant mscs from CD105+, CD24- differentiated human escs. Stem Cells. 2007;**25**:425-436. DOI: 10.1634/stemcells.2006-0420

[12] Lian QZ, Zhang YL, Zhang J, Zhang HK, Wu X, Zhang Y, et al. Functional mesenchymal stem cells derived from human induced pluripotent stem cells attenuate limb ischemia in mice. Circulation. 2010;**121**:1113-1123. DOI: 10.1161/circulationaha.109.898312

[13] Chen Z, Chen L, Zeng C, Wang WE. Functionally improved mesenchymal stem cells to better treat myocardial infarction. Stem Cells International. 2018;**2018**:7045245. DOI: 10.1155/2018/7045245

[14] Liang P, Ye F, Hou CC, Pi L, Chen F. Mesenchymal stem cell therapy for patients with ischemic heart failure-past, present, and future. Current Stem Cell Research & Therapy. 2021;**16**: 608-621. DOI: 10.2174/1574888x15666200309144906

[15] Yong KW, Choi JR, Mohammadi M, Mitha AP, Sanati-Nezhad A, Sen A. Mesenchymal stem cell therapy for ischemic tissues. Stem Cells International. 2018;**2018**:8179075. DOI: 10.1155/2018/8179075

[16] Yan W, Abu-El-Rub E, Saravanan S, Kirshenbaum LA, Arora RC, Dhingra S. Inflammation in myocardial injury: Mesenchymal stem cells as potential immunomodulators. American Journal of Physiology Heart and Circulatory Physiology. 2019;**317**:H213-H225. DOI: 10.1152/ajpheart.00065.2019

[17] Zhu F, Chen YH, Li JJ, Yang ZY, Lin Y, Jiang BX, et al. Human umbilical cord mesenchymal stem cell-derived exosomes attenuate myocardial infarction injury via mir-24-3p-promoted m2 macrophage polarization. Advanced Biology (Weinh). 2022;**6**:e2200074. DOI: 10.1002/adbi.202200074

[18] Suzuki E, Fujita D, Takahashi M, Oba S, Nishimatsu H. Therapeutic effects of mesenchymal stem cell-derived exosomes in cardiovascular disease. Advances in Experimental Medicine and Biology. 2017;**998**:179-185. DOI: 10.1007/978-981-10-4397-0_12

[19] Ferreira JR, Teixeira GQ, Santos SG, Barbosa MA, Almeida-Porada G, Gonçalves RM. Mesenchymal stromal cell secretome: Influencing therapeutic potential by cellular pre-conditioning. Frontiers in Immunology. 2018;**9**:2837. DOI: 10.3389/fimmu.2018.02837

[20] Chen LJ, Qu JJ, Mei QH, Chen X, Fang YX, Chen L, et al. Small extracellular vesicles from menstrual blood-derived mesenchymal stem cells (menscs) as a novel therapeutic impetus in regenerative medicine. Stem Cell Research & Therapy. 2021;**12**:433. DOI: 10.1186/s13287-021-02511-6

[21] Meng H, Cheng WT, Wang L, Chen SQ, Teng Y, Lu ZW, et al. Mesenchymal stem cell exosomes in the treatment of myocardial infarction: A systematic review of preclinical in vivo studies. Journal of Cardiovascular Translational Research. 2022;**15**:317-339. DOI: 10.1007/s12265-021-10168-y

[22] Pu L, Kong X, Li H, He X. Exosomes released from mesenchymal stem cells overexpressing microrna-30e ameliorate heart failure in rats with myocardial infarction. American Journal of Translational Research. 2021;**13**:4007-4025

[23] Ma T, Chen Y, Chen Y, Meng Q, Sun J, Shao L, et al. Microrna-132, delivered by mesenchymal stem cell-derived exosomes, promote angiogenesis in myocardial infarction. Stem Cells International. 2018;**2018**:3290372. DOI: 10.1155/2018/3290372

[24] Lazar E, Benedek T, Korodi S, Rat N, Lo J, Benedek I. Stem cell-derived exosomes-an emerging tool for myocardial regeneration. World Journal of Stem Cells. 2018;**10**:106-115. DOI: 10.4252/wjsc.v10.i8.106

[25] Shao L, Zhang Y, Lan B, Wang J, Zhang Z, Zhang L, et al. Mirna-sequence indicates that mesenchymal stem cells and exosomes have similar mechanism to enhance cardiac repair. BioMed Research International. 2017;**2017**:4150705. DOI: 10.1155/2017/4150705

[26] ISEV 2018 Collaborators. Minimal information for studies of extracellular

vesicles 2018 (MISEV2018): A position statement of the International Society for Extracellular Vesicles and update of the MISEV2014 guidelines. Journal of Extracellular Vesicles. 2018;(7):1535750. DOI: 10.1080/20013078.2018.1535750

[27] Kalluri R, Lebleu VS. The biology, function, and biomedical applications of exosomes. Science. 2020;**367**:eaau6977. DOI: 10.1126/science.aau6977

[28] Abbaszadeh H, Ghorbani F, Derakhshani M, Movassaghpour A, Yousefi M. Human umbilical cord mesenchymal stem cell-derived extracellular vesicles: A novel therapeutic paradigm. Journal of Cellular Physiology. 2020;**235**:706-717. DOI: 10.1002/jcp.29004

[29] Chen S, Sun F, Qian H, Xu W, Jiang J. Preconditioning and engineering strategies for improving the efficacy of mesenchymal stem cell-derived exosomes in cell-free therapy. Stem Cells International. 2022;**2022**:1779346. DOI: 10.1155/2022/1779346

[30] Cheng L, Zhang K, Wu S, Cui M, Xu T. Focus on mesenchymal stem cell-derived exosomes: Opportunities and challenges in cell-free therapy. Stem Cells International. 2017;**2017**:6305295. DOI: 10.1155/2017/6305295

[31] Zou L, Ma X, Lin S, Wu B, Chen Y, Peng C. Bone marrow mesenchymal stem cell-derived exosomes protect against myocardial infarction by promoting autophagy. Experimental and Therapeutic Medicine. 2019;**18**:2574-2582. DOI: 10.3892/etm.2019.7874

[32] Ferguson SW, Wang J, Lee CJ, Liu M, Neelamegham S, Canty JM, et al. The microrna regulatory landscape of msc-derived exosomes: A systems view. Scientific Reports. 2018;**8**:1419. DOI: 10.1038/s41598-018-19581-x

[33] Zhang P, Jiang J, Zhou X, Kolay J, Wang R, Wan Z, et al. Label-free imaging and biomarker analysis of exosomes with plasmonic scattering microscopy. Chemical Science. 2022;**13**:12760-12768. DOI: 10.1039/d2sc05191e

[34] Yakubovicha EI, Polischouka AG, Evtushenkoa VI. Principles and problems of exosome isolation from biological fluids. Biochemistry (Moscow), Supplement Series A: Membrane and Cell Biology. 2022;**16**:115-126. DOI: 10.1134/S1990747822030096

[35] Skalnikova HK, Bohuslavova B, Turnovcova K, Juhasova J, Juhas S, Rodinova M, et al. Isolation and characterization of small extracellular vesicles from porcine blood plasma, cerebrospinal fluid, and seminal plasma. Proteomes. 2019;**7**:17. DOI: 10.3390/proteomes7020017

[36] Chen J, Li P, Zhang T, Xu Z, Huang X, Wang R, et al. Review on strategies and technologies for exosome isolation and purification. Frontiers in Bioengineering and Biotechnology. 2021;**9**:811971. DOI: 10.3389/fbioe.2021.811971

[37] Klymiuk MC, Balz N, Elashry MI, Heimann M, Wenisch S, Arnhold S. Exosomes isolation and identification from equine mesenchymal stem cells. BMC Veterinary Research. 2019;**15**:42. DOI: 10.1186/s12917-019-1789-9

[38] Ramasubramanian L, Jyothi H, Goldbloom-Helzner L, Light BM, Kumar P, Carney RP, et al. Development and characterization of bioinspired lipid raft nanovesicles for therapeutic applications. ACS Applied Materials Interfaces. 2022;**14**:54458-54477. DOI: 10.1021/acsami.2c13868

[39] Zhang Y, Bi J, Huang J, Tang Y, Du S, Li P. Exosome: A review of its

classification, isolation techniques, storage, diagnostic and targeted therapy applications. International Journal of Nanomedicine. 2020;**15**:6917-6934. DOI: 10.2147/IJN.S264498

[40] Sridharan B, Lim HG. Exosomes and ultrasound: The future of theranostic applications. Materials Today Bio. 2023;**19**:100556. DOI: 10.1016/j.mtbio.2023.100556

[41] Busatto S, Vilanilam G, Ticer T, Lin WL, Dickson DW, Shapiro S, et al. Tangential flow filtration for highly efficient concentration of extracellular vesicles from large volumes of fluid. Cell. 2018;7:273. DOI: 10.3390/cells7120273

[42] Brown PN, Yin H. Polymer-based purification of extracellular vesicles. Methods in Molecular Biology. 2017;**1660**:91-103. DOI: 10.1007/978-1-4939-7253-1_8

[43] Sidhom K, Obi PO, Saleem A. A review of exosomal isolation methods: Is size exclusion chromatography the best option? International Journal of Molecular Science. 2020;**21**:6466. DOI: 10.3390/ijms21186466

[44] Gholizadeh S, Shehata Draz M, Zarghooni M, Sanati-Nezhad A, Ghavami S, Shafiee H, et al. Microfluidic approaches for isolation, detection, and characterization of extracellular vesicles: Current status and future directions. Biosensors & Bioelectronics. 2017;**91**:588-605. DOI: 10.1016/j.bios.2016.12.062

[45] Salafi T, Zhang Y, Zhang Y. A review on deterministic lateral displacement for particle separation and detection. Nanomicro Letters. 2019;**11**:77. DOI: 10.1007/s40820-019-0308-7

[46] Lee K, Shao H, Weissleder R, Lee H. Acoustic purification of extracellular microvesicles. ACS Nano. 2015;**9**:2321-2327. DOI: 10.1021/nn506538f

[47] Song J, Song B, Yuan L, Yang G. Multiplexed strategies toward clinical translation of extracellular vesicles. Theranostics. 2022;**12**:6740-6761. DOI: 10.7150/thno.75899

[48] Tenchov R, Sasso JM, Wang XM, Liaw WS, Chen CA, Zhou QA. Exosomes-nature's lipid nanoparticles, a rising star in drug delivery and diagnostics. ACS Nano. 2022;**16**:17802-17846. DOI: 10.1021/acsnano.2c08774

[49] Ferguson SW, Nguyen J. Exosomes as therapeutics: The implications of molecular composition and exosomal heterogeneity. Journal of Controlled Release. 2016;**228**:179-190. DOI: 10.1016/j.jconrel.2016.02.037

[50] Takeuchi R, Katagiri W, Endo S, Kobayashi T. Exosomes from conditioned media of bone marrow-derived mesenchymal stem cells promote bone regeneration by enhancing angiogenesis. PLoS One. 2019;**14**:e0225472. DOI: 10.1371/journal.pone.0225472

[51] Saheera S, Jani VP, Witwer KW, Kutty S. Extracellular vesicle interplay in cardiovascular pathophysiology. American Journal of Physiology-Heart and Circulatory Physiology. 2021;**320**:H1749-H1H61. DOI: 10.1152/ajpheart.00925.2020

[52] Saheera S, Potnuri AG, Krishnamurthy P. Nano-vesicle (mis) communication in senescence-related pathologies. Cell. 2020;**9**:1974. DOI: 10.3390/cells9091974

[53] Patil M, Saheera S, Dubey PK, Kahn-Krell A, Kumar GP, Singh S, et al. Novel mechanisms of exosome-mediated phagocytosis of dead cells in injured heart. Circulation Research.

2021;**129**:1006-1020. DOI: 10.1161/CIRCRESAHA.120.317900

[54] Lee BC, Kang I, Yu KR. Therapeutic features and updated clinical trials of mesenchymal stem cell (msc)-derived exosomes. Journal of Clinical Medicine. 2021;**10**:711. DOI: 10.3390/jcm10040711

[55] Giebel B, Kordelas L, Borger V. Clinical potential of mesenchymal stem/stromal cell-derived extracellular vesicles. Stem Cell Investigation. 2017;**4**:84. DOI: 10.21037/sci.2017.09.06

[56] Wang X, Tang Y, Liu Z, Yin Y, Li Q, Liu G, et al. The application potential and advance of mesenchymal stem cell-derived exosomes in myocardial infarction. Stem Cells International. 2021;**2021**:5579904. DOI: 10.1155/2021/5579904

[57] Lu TX, Rothenberg ME. Microrna. The Journal of Allergy Clinical Immunology. 2018;**141**:1202-1207. DOI: 10.1016/j.jaci.2017.08.034

[58] Cai Y, Yu X, Hu S, Yu J. A brief review on the mechanisms of mirna regulation. Genomics, Proteomics & Bioinformatics. 2009;**7**:147-154. DOI: 10.1016/S1672-0229(08)60044-3

[59] Fabian MR, Sonenberg N. The mechanics of mirna-mediated gene silencing: A look under the hood of mirisc. Nature Structural & Molecular Biology. 2012;**19**:586-593. DOI: 10.1038/nsmb.2296

[60] Jahangiri B, Khalaj-Kondori M, Asadollahi E, Purrafee Dizaj L, Sadeghizadeh M. Msc-derived exosomes suppress colorectal cancer cell proliferation and metastasis via mir-100/mtor/mir-143 pathway. International Journal of Pharmaceutics. 2022;**627**:122214. DOI: 10.1016/j.ijpharm.2022.122214

[61] Cheng C, Chen X, Wang Y, Cheng W, Zuo X, Tang W, et al. MSCs-derived exosomes attenuate ischemia-reperfusion brain injury and inhibit microglia apoptosis might via exosomal mir-26a-5p mediated suppression of cdk6. Molecular Medicine. 2021;**27**:67. DOI: 10.1186/s10020-021-00324-0

[62] Xu J, Chen P, Yu C, Shi Q, Wei S, Li Y, et al. Hypoxic bone marrow mesenchymal stromal cells-derived exosomal mir-182-5p promotes liver regeneration via foxo1-mediated macrophage polarization. FASEB Journal. 2022;**36**:e22553. DOI: 10.1096/fj.202101868RRR

[63] Zhu LP, Tian T, Wang JY, He JN, Chen T, Pan M, et al. Hypoxia-elicited mesenchymal stem cell-derived exosomes facilitates cardiac repair through mir-125b-mediated prevention of cell death in myocardial infarction. Theranostics. 2018;**8**:6163-6177. DOI: 10.7150/thno.28021

[64] Zhang Z, Yang J, Yan W, Li Y, Shen Z, Asahara T. Pretreatment of cardiac stem cells with exosomes derived from mesenchymal stem cells enhances myocardial repair. Journal of the American Heart Association. 2016;**5**:e002856. DOI: 10.1161/JAHA.115.002856

[65] Tan SJO, Floriano JF, Nicastro L, Emanueli C, Catapano F. Novel applications of mesenchymal stem cell-derived exosomes for myocardial infarction therapeutics. Biomolecules. 2020;**10**:707. DOI: 10.3390/biom10050707

[66] Chen B, Luo L, Wei X, Gong D, Li Z, Li S, et al. M1 bone marrow-derived macrophage-derived extracellular vesicles inhibit angiogenesis and myocardial regeneration following myocardial infarction via the malat1/microrna-25-3p/cdc42 axis.

Oxidative Medicine and Cellular Longevity. 2021;**2021**:9959746. DOI: 10.1155/2021/9959746

[67] Zheng Y, Lin J, Liu D, Wan G, Gu X, Ma J. Nogo-b promotes angiogenesis and improves cardiac repair after myocardial infarction via activating notch1 signaling. Cell Death & Disease. 2022;**13**:306. DOI: 10.1038/s41419-022-04754-4

[68] Zhou XL, Zhu RR, Liu S, Xu H, Xu X, Wu QC, et al. Notch signaling promotes angiogenesis and improves cardiac function after myocardial infarction. Journal of Cellular Biochemistry. 2018;**119**:7105-7112. DOI: 10.1002/jcb.27032

[69] Liu HB, Zhang YM, Yuan J, Gao J, Zhong X, Yao K, et al. Bdendritic cell-derived exosomal mir-494-3p promotes angiogenesis following myocardial infarction. International Journal of Molecular Medicine. 2021;**47**:315-325. DOI: 10.3892/ijmm.2020.4776

[70] Wang N, Chen C, Yang D, Liao Q, Luo H, Wang X, et al. Mesenchymal stem cells-derived extracellular vesicles, via mir-210, improve infarcted cardiac function by promotion of angiogenesis. Biochimica et Biophysica Acta Molecular Basis of Disease. 2017;**1863**:2085-2092. DOI: 10.1016/j.bbadis.2017.02.023

[71] Zhu W, Sun L, Zhao P, Liu Y, Zhang J, Zhang Y, et al. Macrophage migration inhibitory factor facilitates the therapeutic efficacy of mesenchymal stem cells derived exosomes in acute myocardial infarction through upregulating mir-133a-3p. Journal of Nanobiotechnology. 2021;**19**:61. DOI: 10.1186/s12951-021-00808-5

[72] Sun L, Zhu W, Zhao P, Zhang J, Lu Y, Zhu Y, et al. Down-regulated exosomal microrna-221 - 3p derived from senescent mesenchymal stem cells impairs heart repair. Frontiers in Cell and Developmental Biology. 2020;**8**:263. DOI: 10.3389/fcell.2020.00263

[73] Fang J, Zhang Y, Chen D, Zheng Y, Jiang J. Exosomes and exosomal cargos: A promising world for ventricular remodeling following myocardial infarction. International Journal of Nanomedicine. 2022;**17**:4699-4719. DOI: 10.2147/IJN.S377479

[74] Anversa P, Cheng W, Liu Y, Leri A, Redaelli G, Kajstura J. Apoptosis and myocardial infarction. Basic Research in Cardiology. 1998;**93**:8-12

[75] Cheng H, Chang S, Xu R, Chen L, Song X, Wu J, et al. Hypoxia-challenged msc-derived exosomes deliver mir-210 to attenuate post-infarction cardiac apoptosis. Stem Cell Research & Therapy. 2020;**11**:224. DOI: 10.1186/s13287-020-01737-0

[76] Pan J, Alimujiang M, Chen Q, Shi H, Luo X. Exosomes derived from mir-146a-modified adipose-derived stem cells attenuate acute myocardial infarction-induced myocardial damage via downregulation of early growth response factor 1. Journal of Cellular Biochemistry. 2019;**120**:4433-4443. DOI: 10.1002/jcb.27731

[77] Wang X, Zhu Y, Wu C, Liu W, He Y, Yang Q. Adipose-derived mesenchymal stem cells-derived exosomes carry microrna-671 to alleviate myocardial infarction through inactivating the tgfbr2/smad2 axis. Inflammation. 2021;**44**:1815-1830. DOI: 10.1007/s10753-021-01460-9

[78] Ning W, Li S, Yang W, Yang B, Xin C, Ping X, et al. Blocking exosomal mirna-153-3p derived from bone marrow mesenchymal stem cells ameliorates hypoxia-induced myocardial and microvascular damage by targeting

the angpt1-mediated vegf/pi3k/akt/enos pathway. Cellular Signalling. 2021;**77**:109812. DOI: 10.1016/j.cellsig.2020.109812

[79] Wu Z, Cheng S, Wang S, Li W, Liu J. Bmscs-derived exosomal microrna-150-5p attenuates myocardial infarction in mice. International Immunopharmacology. 2021;**93**:107389. DOI: 10.1016/j.intimp.2021.107389

[80] Luo Q, Guo D, Liu G, Chen G, Hang M, Jin M. Exosomes from mir-126-overexpressing adscs are therapeutic in relieving acute myocardial ischaemic injury. Cellular Physiology and Biochemistry. 2017;**44**:2105-2116. DOI: 10.1159/000485949

[81] Sun XH, Wang X, Zhang Y, Hui J. Exosomes of bone-marrow stromal cells inhibit cardiomyocyte apoptosis under ischemic and hypoxic conditions via mir-486-5p targeting the pten/pi3k/akt signaling pathway. Thrombosis Research. 2019;**177**:23-32. DOI: 10.1016/j.thromres.2019.02.002

[82] Wang X, Dai Y, Ding Z, Khaidakov M, Mercanti F, Mehta JL. Regulation of autophagy and apoptosis in response to angiotensin ii in hl-1 cardiomyocytes. Biochemical and Biophysical Research Communications. 2013;**440**:696-700. DOI: 10.1016/j.bbrc.2013.09.131

[83] Xiao C, Wang K, Xu Y, Hu H, Zhang N, Wang Y, et al. Transplanted mesenchymal stem cells reduce autophagic flux in infarcted hearts via the exosomal transfer of mir-125b. Circulation Research. 2018;**123**:564-578. DOI: 10.1161/CIRCRESAHA.118.312758

[84] Liu J, Jiang M, Deng S, Lu J, Huang H, Zhang Y, et al. Mir-93-5p-containing exosomes treatment attenuates acute myocardial infarction-induced myocardial damage. Molecular Therapy Nucleic Acids. 2018;**11**:103-115. DOI: 10.1016/j.omtn.2018.01.010

[85] Li Y, Yang R, Guo B, Zhang H, Zhang H, Liu S, et al. Exosomal mir-301 derived from mesenchymal stem cells protects myocardial infarction by inhibiting myocardial autophagy. Biochemical Biophysical Research Communications. 2019;**514**:323-328. DOI: 10.1016/j.bbrc.2019.04.138

[86] Yuan J, Yang H, Liu C, Shao L, Zhang H, Lu K, et al. Microneedle patch loaded with exosomes containing microrna-29b prevents cardiac fibrosis after myocardial infarction. Advanced Healthcare Materials. 2023:e2202959. DOI: 10.1002/adhm.202202959

[87] Zheng X, Hermann DM, Bahr M, Doeppner TR. The role of small extracellular vesicles in cerebral and myocardial ischemia-molecular signals, treatment targets, and future clinical translation. Stem Cells. 2021;**39**:403-413. DOI: 10.1002/stem.3329

[88] Mao Q, Liang XL, Zhang CL, Pang YH, Lu YX. Lncrna klf3-as1 in human mesenchymal stem cell-derived exosomes ameliorates pyroptosis of cardiomyocytes and myocardial infarction through mir-138-5p/sirt1 axis. Stem Cell Research & Therapy. 2019;**10**:393. DOI: 10.1186/s13287-019-1522-4

[89] Sun L, Zhu W, Zhao P, Wang Q, Fan B, Zhu Y, et al. Long noncoding rna uca1 from hypoxia-conditioned hmsc-derived exosomes: A novel molecular target for cardioprotection through mir-873-5p/xiap axis. Cell Death & Disease. 2020;**11**:696. DOI: 10.1038/s41419-020-02783-5

[90] Huang P, Wang L, Li Q, Tian X, Xu J, Xu J, et al. Atorvastatin enhances

the therapeutic efficacy of mesenchymal stem cells-derived exosomes in acute myocardial infarction via up-regulating long non-coding rna h19. Cardiovascular Research. 2020;**116**:353-367. DOI: 10.1093/cvr/cvz139

[91] Toh WS, Lai RC, Zhang B, Lim SK. MSC exosome works through a protein-based mechanism of action. Biochemical Society Transactions. 2018;**46**:843-853. DOI: 10.1042/BST20180079

[92] Anderson JD, Johansson HJ, Graham CS, Vesterlund M, Pham MT, Bramlett CS, et al. Comprehensive proteomic analysis of mesenchymal stem cell exosomes reveals modulation of angiogenesis via nuclear factor-kappab signaling. Stem Cells. 2016;**34**:601-613. DOI: 10.1002/stem.2298

[93] Kim HS, Choi DY, Yun SJ, Choi SM, Kang JW, Jung JW, et al. Proteomic analysis of microvesicles derived from human mesenchymal stem cells. Journal of Proteome Research. 2012;**11**:839-849. DOI: 10.1021/pr200682z

[94] Tan SS, Chen TS, Tan KH, Lim SK. An overview of the proteomic and mirna cargo in msc-derived exosomes. Mesenchymal Stem Cell Derived Exosomes. 2015:21-36. DOI: 10.1016/B978-0-12-800164-6.00002-2

[95] Collino F, Pomatto M, Bruno S, Lindoso RS, Tapparo M, Sicheng W, et al. Exosome and microvesicle-enriched fractions isolated from mesenchymal stem cells by gradient separation showed different molecular signatures and functions on renal tubular epithelial cells. Stem Cell Reviews and Reports. 2017;**13**:226-243. DOI: 10.1007/s12015-016-9713-1

[96] Lai RC, Tan SS, Teh BJ, Sze SK, Arslan F, De Kleijn DP, et al. Proteolytic potential of the msc exosome proteome: Implications for an exosome-mediated delivery of therapeutic proteasome. International Journal of Proteomics. 2012;**2012**:971907. DOI: 10.1155/2012/971907

[97] Deng H, Sun C, Sun Y, Li H, Yang L, Wu D, et al. Lipid, protein, and microrna composition within mesenchymal stem cell-derived exosomes. Cellular Reprogramming. 2018;**20**:178-186. DOI: 10.1089/cell.2017.0047

[98] Zhao Y, Sun X, Cao W, Ma J, Sun L, Qian H, et al. Exosomes derived from human umbilical cord mesenchymal stem cells relieve acute myocardial ischemic injury. Stem Cells International. 2015;**2015**:761643. DOI: 10.1155/2015/761643

[99] Xiao Y, Zhang Y, Li Y, Peng N, Liu Q, Qiu D, et al. Exosomes derived from mesenchymal stem cells pretreated with ischemic rat heart extracts promote angiogenesis via the delivery of dmbt1. Cell Transplantation. 2022;**31**:9636897221102898. DOI: 10.1177/09636897221102898

[100] Deng S, Zhou X, Ge Z, Song Y, Wang H, Liu X, et al. Exosomes from adipose-derived mesenchymal stem cells ameliorate cardiac damage after myocardial infarction by activating s1p/sk1/s1pr1 signaling and promoting macrophage m2 polarization. The International Journal of Biochemestry & Cell Biology. 2019;**114**:105564. DOI: 10.1016/j.biocel.2019.105564

[101] Ahmed L, Al-Massri K. New approaches for enhancement of the efficacy of mesenchymal stem cell-derived exosomes in cardiovascular diseases. Tissue Engineering and Regenerative Medicine. 2022;**19**:1129-1146. DOI: 10.1007/s13770-022-00469-x

[102] Hu X, Wu R, Shehadeh LA, Zhou Q, Jiang C, Huang X, et al. Severe hypoxia

exerts parallel and cell-specific regulation of gene expression and alternative splicing in human mesenchymal stem cells. BMC Genomics. 2014;**15**:303. DOI: 10.1186/1471-2164-15-303

[103] Ahmad B, Skorska A, Wolfien M, Sadraddin H, Lemcke H, Vasudevan P, et al. The effects of hypoxic preconditioned murine mesenchymal stem cells on post-infarct arrhythmias in the mouse model. International Journal of Molecular Sciences. 2022;**23**:8843. DOI: 10.3390/ijms23168843

[104] Song HF, Li B, Guo R, He S, Peng ZX, Qu JY, et al. Hypoxic preconditioned aged bmscs accelerates mi injury repair by modulating inflammation, oxidative stress and apoptosis. Biochemical and Biophysical Research Communication. 2022;**627**:45-51. DOI: 10.1016/j.bbrc.2022.08.039

[105] Zhang CS, Shao K, Liu CW, Li CJ, Yu BT. Hypoxic preconditioning bmscs-exosomes inhibit cardiomyocyte apoptosis after acute myocardial infarction by upregulating microrna-24. European Review for Medical and Pharmacological Sciences. 2019;**23**:6691-6699. DOI: 10.26355/eurrev_201908_18560

[106] Zhu JY, Lu K, Zhang N, Zhao Y, Ma QC, Shen J, et al. Myocardial reparative functions of exosomes from mesenchymal stem cells are enhanced by hypoxia treatment of the cells via transferring microrna-210 in an nsmase2-dependent way. Artificial Cells, Nanomedicine, and Biotechnology. 2018;**46**:1659-1670. DOI: 10.1080/21691401.2017.1388249

[107] Zhang LY, Wei QX, Liu XM, Zhang T, Wang SY, Zhou LL, et al. Exosomal microrna-98-5p from hypoxic bone marrow mesenchymal stem cells inhibits myocardial ischemia-reperfusion injury by reducing tlr4 and activating the pi3k/akt signaling pathway. International Immunopharmacology. 2021;**101**:107592. DOI: 10.1016/j.intimp.2021.107592

[108] Gonzalez-King H, García NA, Ontoria-Oviedo I, Ciria M, Montero JA, Sepúlveda P. Hypoxia inducible factor-1α potentiates jagged 1-mediated angiogenesis by mesenchymal stem cell-derived exosomes. Stem Cells. 2017;**35**:1747-1759. DOI: 10.1002/stem.2618

[109] Sun JC, Shen H, Shao LB, Teng XM, Chen YQ, Liu X, et al. Hif-1α overexpression in mesenchymal stem cell-derived exosomes mediates cardioprotection in myocardial infarction by enhanced angiogenesis. Stem Cell Research and Therapy. 2020;**11**:373. DOI: 10.1186/s13287-020-01881-7

[110] Kim EH, Kim DH, Kim HR, Kim SY, Kim HH, Bang OY. Stroke serum priming modulates characteristics of mesenchymal stromal cells by controlling the expression mirna-20a. Cell Transplantation. 2016;**25**:1489-1499. DOI: 10.3727/096368916x690430

[111] Phan J, Kumar P, Hao D, Gao K, Farmer D, Wang AJ. Engineering mesenchymal stem cells to improve their exosome efficacy and yield for cell-free therapy. Journal of Extracellular Vesicles. 2018;**7**:1522236. DOI: 10.1080/20013078.2018.1522236

[112] Chen GN, Liang XT, Han Q, Mai C, Shi LL, Shao Z, et al. Apelin-13 pretreatment promotes the cardioprotective effect of mesenchymal stem cells against myocardial infarction by improving their survival. Stem Cells International. 2022;**2022**:3742678. DOI: 10.1155/2022/3742678

[113] Deng R, Liu YM, He HW, Zhang H, Zhao CL, Cui Z, et al. Haemin

pre-treatment augments the cardiac protection of mesenchymal stem cells by inhibiting mitochondrial fission and improving survival. Journal of Cellular and Molecular Medicine. 2020;**24**:431-440. DOI: 10.1111/jcmm.14747

[114] Xiong YY, Tang RJ, Xu JY, Jiang WY, Gong ZT, Zhang LL, et al. Tongxinluo-pretreated mesenchymal stem cells facilitate cardiac repair via exosomal transfer of mir-146a-5p targeting irak1/nf-κb p65 pathway. Stem Cell Research and Therapy. 2022;**13**:289. DOI: 10.1186/s13287-022-02969-y

[115] Pittenger MF, Eghtesad S, Sanchez PG, Liu XY, Wu ZJ, Chen L, et al. Msc pretreatment for improved transplantation viability results in improved ventricular function in infarcted hearts. International Journal of Molecular Science. 2022;**23**:694. DOI: 10.3390/ijms23020694

[116] Zheng HF, Liang XT, Han Q, Shao Z, Zhang YX, Shi LL, et al. Hemin enhances the cardioprotective effects of mesenchymal stem cell-derived exosomes against infarction via amelioration of cardiomyocyte senescence. Journal of Nanobiotechnology. 2021;**19**:332. DOI: 10.1186/s12951-021-01077-y

[117] Zhang J, Lu Y, Mao YM, Yu Y, Wu TY, Zhao W, et al. Ifn-γ enhances the efficacy of mesenchymal stromal cell-derived exosomes via mir-21 in myocardial infarction rats. Stem Cell Research and Therapy. 2022;**13**:333. DOI: 10.1186/s13287-022-02984-z

[118] Liu XL, Li X, Zhu WW, Zhang YL, Hong YM, Liang XT, et al. Exosomes from mesenchymal stem cells overexpressing mif enhance myocardial repair. Journal of Cellular Physiology. 2020;**235**:8010-8022. DOI: 10.1002/jcp.29456

[119] Gong XH, Liu H, Wang SJ, Liang SW, Wang GG. Exosomes derived from sdf1-overexpressing mesenchymal stem cells inhibit ischemic myocardial cell apoptosis and promote cardiac endothelial microvascular regeneration in mice with myocardial infarction. Journal of Cellular Physiology. 2019;**234**:13878-13893. DOI: 10.1002/jcp.28070

[120] Kang K, Ma R, Cai W, Huang W, Paul C, Liang J, et al. Exosomes secreted from cxcr4 overexpressing mesenchymal stem cells promote cardioprotection via akt signaling pathway following myocardial infarction. Stem Cells International. 2015;**2015**:659890. DOI: 10.1155/2015/659890

[121] Small EM, Olson EN. Pervasive roles of micrornas in cardiovascular biology. Nature. 2011;**469**:336-342. DOI: 10.1038/nature09783

[122] Liu N, Olson EN. Microrna regulatory networks in cardiovascular development. Developmental Cell. 2010;**18**:510-525. DOI: 10.1016/j.devcel.2010.03.010

[123] Bridges MC, Daulagala AC, Kourtidis A. Lnccation: Lncrna localization and function. Journal of Cell Biology. 2021;**220**:e202009045. DOI: 10.1083/jcb.202009045

[124] Mao S, Zhao J, Zhang ZJ, Zhao Q. Mir-183-5p overexpression in bone mesenchymal stem cell-derived exosomes protects against myocardial ischemia/reperfusion injury by targeting foxo1. Immunobiology. 2022;**227**:152204. DOI: 10.1016/j.imbio.2022.152204

[125] Wang S, Dong J, Li L, Wu R, Xu L, Ren Y, et al. Exosomes derived from mir-129-5p modified bone marrow mesenchymal stem cells represses ventricular remolding of mice with myocardial infarction. Journal of Tissue Engineering and Regenerative Medicine. 2022;**16**:177-187. DOI: 10.1002/term.3268

Chapter 2

MSC-Derived Exosomes for Tissue Engineering and Disease Intervention

Leisheng Zhang, Xiaowei Gao, Shixun Ma, Miao Yu, Xianghong Xu, Yuanguang Zhao, Shuang Chen, Yonghong Li, Xiaonan Yang, Tiankang Guo and Hui Cai

Abstract

Mesenchymal stem cells (MSCs), also known as mesenchymal stromal cells or medicinal signaling cells or multipotent stem cells, are heterogeneous cell populations with unique immunomodulatory feature and hematopoietic-supporting capacity. MSCs function through a variety of approaches including paracrine and autocrine, direct- or trans-differentiation, bidirectional immunomodulation, and serving as constitutive microenvironment. Of them, exosomes and microvesicles function as the pivotal vehicle for mediating the ameliorative and therapeutic effect of MSCs toward various recurrent and refractory diseases, such as xerophthalmia, radioactive nasal mucosa injury, acute-on-chronic liver failure (ACLF), dermal chronic ulcers, and intrauterine adhesions. State-of-the-art renewal has also highlighted the promising prospective of MSC-derived exosomes (MSC-exo) and diverse biomaterial composites in regenerative medicine. In this book chapter, we mainly focus on the concept, biological phenotypes, preclinical research, and clinical practice of MSC-derived exosomes (MSC-Exos) and/or biomaterials, which will collectively supply overwhelming new references for the further development of MSC-Exos-based biotherapy and disease diagnosis in future.

Keywords: exosomes, tissue engineering, mesenchymal stem cells, disease intervention, immunomodulation

1. Introduction

Exosomes have been considered as cell-derived nanovesicles, which are indicated in disease diagnosis and treatment via the intercellular transportation of cellular constituents, such as proteins, mRNAs, microRNAs, lipids, and cytokines [1–3]. Longitudinal studies have indicated the secretion of exosome by mammalian cells and the wide distribution in cellular systems [1]. For instance, Heo et al. reported the effect of exosomes upon atherosclerosis by inducing or inhibiting progression of disease through cell-to-cell communication, which suggested the application in disease diagnosis and treatment [4]. State-of-the-art literatures also highlighted the marked technological advances of exosome-based nanotechnology to bloom the further exploitation of exosome-associated biology, pathology, chemistry, and therapeutics [5]. Despite the small membrane vesicles can be released and generated by a variety of eukaryotic cells, yet one of the major obstacles for potential application of exosomes is the strategies for high-efficient and robust enrichment of large-scale preparation with high quantity [1, 6].

Of the numerous parental cells for exosome enrichment, mesenchymal stem/stromal cells (MSCs) are considered with robust immunomodulatory property and therapeutic potential [7–9]. Differ from the relative cell types, MSCs are advantaged stem cells with high percentage of mesenchymal-associated biomarker expression (e.g., CD44, CD73, CD90, CD105), whereas with minimal expression of type II major histocompatibility complex (MHC-II) or hematopoietic-related surface marker expression (e.g., CD31, CD34, CD43, CD45) [10–12]. In this chapter, we summarize the basic and clinical research of MSC-derived exosomes (MSC-exo), including the definition, biological phenotypes and significance, preclinical and clinical investigations, and the concomitant molecular mechanism. Taken together, the contents in this chapter will benefit the further development of MSC-exo-based therapeutic regimens for refractory and recurrent disorder administration in future.

2. MSCs and exosomes

Mesenchymal stem/stromal cells (MSCs), also known as medicinal signaling cells, are unique multipotent stem cells with multi-lineage differentiation capacity and bidirectional immunomodulatory property [13]. Meanwhile, enormous literatures have demonstrated the hematopoietic-supporting effect of MSCs upon the self-renewal and lineage differentiation potential of hematopoietic stem cells (HSCs), which thus play a critical role in physiologic hematopoiesis and hematologic malignancies [14]. Since the first identification from clinical samples in 1968 [15], MSCs of different origins have been consecutively isolated from adult tissues (e.g., bone marrow, adipose tissue, dental pulp) and perinatal tissues (e.g., placenta tissue, amniotic membrane, umbilical cord, amniotic fluid) [16, 17]. Of them, bone marrow-derived MSCs (BM-MSCs) have been considered with the widest range of application, while umbilical cord-derived MSCs (UC-MSCs) have been recognized with the most robust long-term proliferation and immunoregulatory capacity, respectively [13, 18]. As shown by the ClinicalTrials.gov website, over 1400 trials have been registered for a variety of refractory and recurrent disease administration (**Figure 1**).

To date, MSCs have been considered with various origins, including mesoderm, endoderm, ectoderm, trophoblasts, and neural crest cells (NCCs) [19, 20]. Therewith, MSCs have been recognized as heterogeneous stem cells and show variations in multitudinous biofunctions. Since the year of 2005, pioneering investigators in the field have employed pluripotent stem cells (PSCs) including induced PSCs (iPSCs) and embryonic stem cells (ESCs) for the preparation of MSCs for large-scale application. For instance, Zhang et al. reported the high-efficiency MSC generation from human PSCs (hPSCs) within two weeks by a cell programming strategy, which was accomplished by the combination of a master transcription factor named MSX2 (Msh Homeobox 2) and small molecule cocktails (TGF-β, bFGF, decitabine) [19]. Subsequently, Wei et al. took advantage of two chemical compounds including OICR-9429 (a JAK signal and histone methyltransferase inhibitor) and decitabine

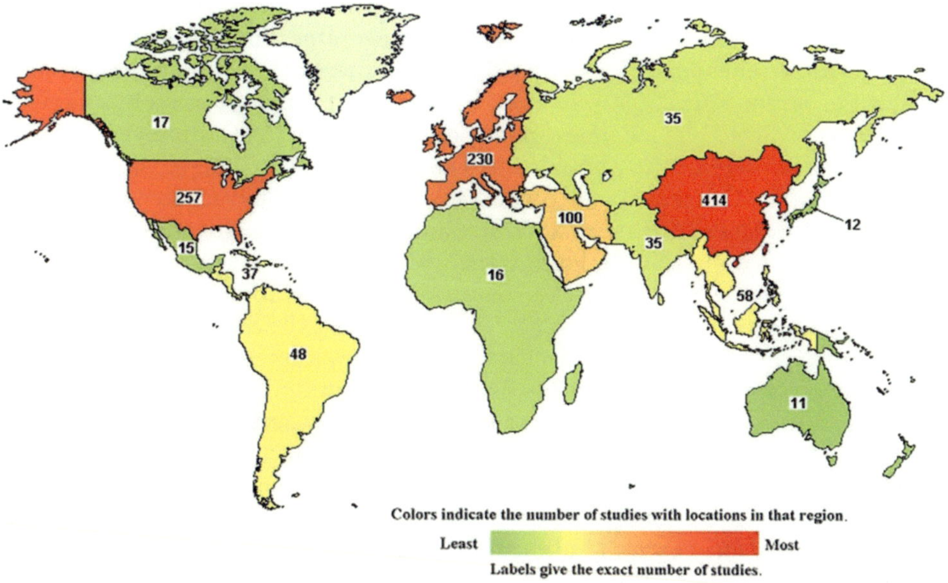

Figure 1.
Illustration of MSC-based clinical trials.

(DAC) for the enhanced induction of MSCs from hESCs [21]. Very recently, we reported the high-efficiency MSC induction from hESCs within two weeks via the non-gene-editing cell programming with LLY-507 (a JAK/STAT or BRD4 inhibitor) and AZD5153 (an epigenetic reader domain inhibitor) [10]. Similar to UC-MSCs, hPSC-MSCs revealed superiority in ex vivo proliferation and immunomodulation over the counterparts from diverse adult tissues.

MSCs function via diverse modes of action, including differentiation, immunomodulation, and secretion. Of them, exosomes and small extracellular vesicles (sEVs) are considered as the two major forms of derivatives of MSCs, which thus play a pivotal role in mediating disease diagnosis and treatment [22, 23]. Exosomes are nano-sized sEVs secreted by the parent cells and play a pivotal role in diverse physiological and pathological processes [24]. To date, a variety of components have been identified from exosomes, such as nucleic acids (e.g., mRNAs, microRNAs, tRNAs, circRNAs), proteins (e.g., cytokines, peptides, amino acids, anti-inflammatory factors), lipids, metabolites, and relative bioactive substances [25].

Distinguish from liposomes and nanoparticles, exosomes with endogeneity and heterogeneity reveal unique and extensive advantages in the field of pathologic diagnosis and disease treatment [26]. Exosomes are nanoparticles with a diameter ranging from 50 nm to 200 nm, which are adequate to interact with organelles and relative intracellular vesicles [27, 28]. As a unique nanoscale spherical lipid bilayer vesicles, exosomes exhibit a density of 1.13–1.19 g • mL^{-1} according to the sucrose density gradient solution [29]. The conception of "exosomes" is firstly proposed by Trams et al. and referred to the vesicles derived from plasma membrane, which is also regarded as the membrane vesicles with 5′-nucleotide enzyme activity. Currently, exosomes are recognized as nano-particles with multitudinous physiological functions, which can be isolated from the exudation and supernatant of various cells and breezily cross the extracellular matrix and blood vessel wall [7, 30]. For instance, a category of exosomal microRNAs have been involved in the pathogenesis and diagnosis of tumors and immune disorders, which are adequate to mediate exosome-inflammasome crosstalk and epithelial mesenchymal transition (EMT), together with chemoresistance and metastasis of tumor cells [27, 30]. In 2021, Patil et al. reported the novel mechanisms of MSC-exo-mediated phagocytosis and opsonization of dying cardiomyocytes during myocardial ischemic injury both in vitro and in vivo [31].

As reviewed by Zhang et al., the ubiquitous exosomes are advantaged cell-free therapeutic products, which are small in size and thus breezily cross the extracellular matrix and blood vessel wall [7]. For instance, MSC-exo have shown considerable safety and therapeutic effects upon various diseases such as atherosclerosis, and acute and chronic wound model [4, 26]. Govindappa and the colleagues found that diabetic milieu were adequate to stimulate RNA-binding proteins like human antigen R (HuR) expression via increasing pro-fibrogenic and inflammatory responses in fibroblasts and cardiac fibrosis mediated by macrophages-derived exosomes [32]. Meanwhile, the chitosan hydrogel has been proved effective in boosting the stability and retention of exosomes enriched from placenta-derived mesenchymal stem cells (P-MSC-exo) and the contents (e.g., proteins, lipid, microRNAs), together with the resultant enhanced efficacy for hindlimb ischemia treatment and remission [12]. As mentioned above, MSC-derived exosomes (MSC-exo) and the relative sEVs have been reported with diverse application prospects in a variety of refractory and recurrent disease administration, yet the large-scale application for disease management is far from satisfaction, which largely attributes to the inherent disadvantages of exosomes, including the low yield, storage stability, low purity, and weak targeting [27].

3. Biomaterials/MSC-exo composites

Biomaterials with tissue compatibility and inflammatory response mainly function via in contact with biological tissue, which are mainly applied in the medical field for tissue engineering or developing artificial organs for regenerative purposes. Generally, biomaterials can be divided into synthetic polymer biomaterials (silicone rubber, polyurethane, polyester, polyacrylonitrile), natural polymer biomaterials (regenerated fibers, chitin, collagen, hyaluronic acid), medical metal materials (titanium and titanium alloys, stainless steel, titanium-nickel memory alloys), inorganic biomedical materials (bioactive ceramics, carbon materials, glass materials), hybrid biomaterials (e.g., cross-linked hybridization of collagen, polyvinyl alcohol), and composite biomaterials (e.g., bioceramics, glass reinforced with glass fibers).

Current progress in materials and cell biology has extensively indicated the superiority of multiple biomaterials for preclinical and clinical application upon diverse relapse and recurrent diseases, and in particular, the composites of biomaterials and MSC-exo for tissue engineering and regenerative purposes attribute to the unique biocompatibility. In details, biomaterials with biocompatible and biodegradable properties are capable of facilitating the efficacy of MSCs or MSC-exo and enhancing their manifestations during anti-tumor immunity by endowing the therapeutic ability of these encapsulated constituents [33–35]. To date, a variety of biomaterials have been introduced for MSC-exo-based regimens in biomedicine, such as hydrogel acid (HA) (e.g., ε-caprolactone (PCL)/nano-hydroxyapatite (nHA) scaffold, chitosan hydrogel, PCL/nHA + HPCH hybrid scaffolds), gelatin, and nanomaterials [12, 36]. These biomaterials with promising prospective have been proved with the ability to reinforce the biological properties or functions of the encapsulated objectives including

MSC-exo [37]. Of them HA and gelatin are considered as the two major forms of extracellular matrix, which are widely distributed in tissues of the body and benefiting the preparation of the compatible hybrid hydrogels by orchestrating the specific composition, scaffold structure, immune microenvironment, and the concomitant physico-chemical property [38, 39]. For example, as reviewed by Celikkin et al. and Xiao et al., Gelatin methacrylate-based hydrogels exhibit preferable properties over other counterparts in tissue engineering and disease administration on the basis of their biofunctionality as well as unique mechanical tenability (e.g., chemical properties, porosity, physical strength, and conductivity) [40, 41]. Similarly, a number of investigators in the field have also observed the hydrogel encapsulation, exosome-loaded thermosensitive hydorgels, and MSC-exo/hydrogel hybrid patch in controlling the release of paracrine factors, enhancing the maintenance of the biological activity, enhancing corneal epithelium regeneration from MSCs and MSC-exos [42–44].

Longitudinal studies have also suggested the application of multifarious collagens with high biocompatibility is applied as natural scaffolds for tissue engineering, including extracellular matrix (ECM), elastin, proteoglycans, and glycoproteins [45, 46]. For example, the implantation of engineered collagen matrices or resorbable collagen scaffolds has been reported effectively for the remission of meniscus defects by Warth et al. and Patil et al. [47, 48]. Of note, the latest progress has also highlighted the bioprinting of pure collagen or in combination with MSCs and/or MSC-exo for regenerative purposes as well [49]. On the basis of the immunomodulatory properties, MSC-exo have been used as a dermatological nano-therapeutic agent for the administration of oxidative stress-induced skin injury by modulating the NRF2 defense system and H_2O_2-stimulated epidermal keratinocytes [50].

Nanomaterials are defined by their diameters ranging from 1 nm to 100 nm, together with the facilitating effect upon the permeability and retention of the encapsulated cells or cellular components including MSCs and the derivatives (e.g., exosomes, sEVs) [51]. Nanomaterials, together with the nanostructure-mediated physical signals, have been recognized as splendid sources for mimicking ECM and enhancing the therapeutic effect of MSC-exo, which are tightly orchestrated by activating specific signals [52–57]. For example, Luo and the colleagues verified the feasibility of MSC-exo for amelioration of the inflammation-induced astrocyte alterations via the Nrf2-NF-κB signaling pathway [58]. Instead, Zhang et al. verified BM-MSC-derived exosomes (BM-MSC-exo) for promoting remyelination and reducing neuroinflammation via inhibiting the TLR2/IRAK1/NF-κB signaling pathway and increasing polarization of M2 phenotype in the demyelinating central nervous system [59]. Additionally, DiStefano et al. took advantage of Lactic-co-Glycolic Acid and the resultant hydrogel-embedded poly microspheres for the efficient delivery of hMSC-derived exosomes and the promotion of bioactive annulus fibrosus repair [60]. Very recently, Geng et al. reported the generation of the multifunctional antibacterial MSC-Exos@CEC-DCMC HG hydrogel (carboxyethyl chitosan-dialdehyde carboxymethyl cellulose) and BM-MSC-exo composite for accelerating diabetic wound healing [61]. Additionally, with the aid of optimized BM-MSC-exo and unique hierarchical scaffolds, Liu et al. demonstrated the application for bone regeneration by modulating the Smad pathway activated by Bmpr2/Acvr2b competitive receptor [62]. As to the underlying molecular mechanism of various biomaterials in MSC-exo-based regimens, various biomaterials function mainly via orchestrating a series of mode of action, including integrating or incorporating with the encapsulated MSC-exo, benefiting the secretion and maintenance of MSC-exo, serving as substrates or scaffolds, and reinforcing the antioxidant property as well [63–65]. Collectively, biomaterials of different kinds with high biocompatibility have been recognized as momentous components of the formulations for tissue engineering and regenerative medicine [66–70].

4. MSC-exo-based clinical trials

Attributes to the advantaged property, MSC-exo have been extensively explored in clinical trials. According to the ClinicalTrials.gov website (https://www.clinicaltrials.gov/) of National Institute of Health (NIH), a total number of 164 interventional trials have been registered up to February 4th, 2023 (**Figure 2**). Of them, most are in the phase 1 and phase 2 stages, together with the recruiting status (**Table 1**). To date, MSC-exo have been involved in numerous disease administration, including respiratory diseases (e.g., COVID-19, acute respiratory distress syndrome), digestive diseases (e.g., perianal fistula with Crohn's disease, familial hypercholesterolemia, irritable bowel disease, non-alcoholic fatty liver disease), cutaneous diseases (e.g., alopecia, psoriasis, endothelial dysfunction, wounds and injuries, oral mucositis, diabetic foot), vascular diseases (e.g., cerebrovascular disorders, myocardial infarction, myocardial ischemia, myocardial stunning), reproductive diseases (e.g., extreme prematurity, preterm, polycystic ovary syndrome), neurodevelopmental disorders (e.g., neuralgia, refractory depression, anxiety disorders, post-stroke dementia, Alzheimer disease, major depressive disorder, bipolar disorder, mild cognitive impairment, stroke, acute ischemic stroke, Parkinson disease), movement disorders (e.g., knee osteoarthritis, meniscus tear, tibial and knee injuries, arthralgia), endocrine system diseases (e.g., type 1 diabetes mellitus, type 2 diabetes mellitus), immunological disorders (e.g., allergic asthma, severe eosinophilic asthma), and urinary diseases (e.g., chronic kidney failure, bladder cancer, polycystic kidney disease), and even tumors (e.g., metastatic melanoma, colon cancer, non-Hodgkin's

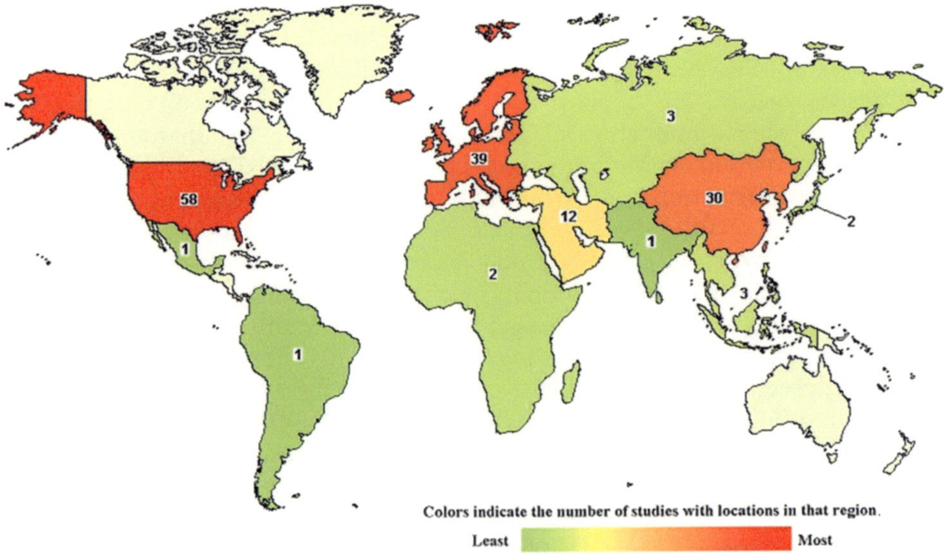

Figure 2.
Illustration of MSC-exo-based clinical trials.

Status	Phases	Cases	Diseases
Recruiting	Not Applicable	20	Hair Loss, Alopecia
Completed	Phase 1	10	Psoriasis
Active	Phase 1, 2	80	Perianal Fistula with Crohn's Disease
Recruiting	Phase 1, 2	80	Fistula Perianal
Unknown	Not Applicable	15	Metastatic Melanoma
Unknown	Phase 1, 2	5	Cerebrovascular Disorders
Completed	Phase 1	24	Coronavirus
Not Recruiting	Not Applicable	10	Extreme Prematurity, Preterm Intraventricular Hemorrhage, Hypoxia-Ischemia, Neurodevelopmental Disorders
Active	Phase 2	155	COVID-19 Disease
Unknown	Early Phase 1	10	Periodontitis
Not recruiting	Phase 1, 2	55	Covid19, Novel Coronavirus Pneumonia, Acute Respiratory Distress Syndrome
Unknown	Early Phase 1	5	Ulcer
Suspended	Not Applicable	100	Neuralgia
Recruiting	Phase 1, 2	20	Myocardial Infarction, Myocardial Ischemia, Myocardial Stunning
Suspended	Not Applicable	300	Refractory Depression, Anxiety Disorders, Neurodegenerative Diseases
Recruiting	Phase 2, 3	60	SARS-CoV-2 Infection
Not recruiting	Phase 1	10	Knee Osteoarthritis
Not recruiting	Not Applicable	60	Multiple Organ Failure
Recruiting	Phase 1, 2	60	Drug-resistant
Recruiting	Phase 1	35	Colon Cancer
Completed	Phase 1	30	Chronic Low Back Pain, Degenerative Disc Disease
Recruiting	Phase 1	35	SARS-CoV-2
Not Recruiting	Phase 1	30	Familial Hypercholesterolemia
Recruiting	Phase 2	30	Knee injury, Meniscus Tear, Tibial and Knee Injuries, Arthralgia
Recruiting	Not Applicable	12	Connective Tissue, Exercise
Recruiting	Phase 2, 3	135	Retinitis Pigmentosa
Recruiting	Not Applicable	90	Non-Hodgkin (B-NHL)
Recruiting	Not Applicable	30	Lung Cancer, Non-Small Cell Lung Cancer
Withdrawn	Not Applicable	0	Polycystic Ovary Syndrome
Unknown	Phase 2, 3	20	Type 1 Diabetes Mellitus
Unknown	Phase 1	60	Corona Virus Infection, Pneumonia
Recruiting	Phase 1, 2	27	Dry Eye
Recruiting	Not Applicable	35	Atrial Fibrillation
Unknown	Not Applicable	100	Endothelial Dysfunction

Status	Phases	Cases	Diseases
Recruiting	Not Applicable	30	Post-stroke Dementia, Acupuncture
Recruiting	Phase 1	28	Metastatic Pancreatic Adenocarcinoma, Pancreatic Ductal Adenocarcinoma, Stage IV Pancreatic Cancer
Recruiting	Not Applicable	40	Insulin Resistance
Not recruiting	Not Applicable	5	Wounds and Injuries
Unknown	Phase 2	90	Covid19, SARS-CoV-2 Pneumonia
Completed	Phase 1, 2	30	Covid19, SARS-CoV-2 Pneumonia
Recruiting	Phase 2	90	Covid19
Completed	Not Applicable	10	Healthy
Completed	Phase 1	24	Healthy
Unknown	Phase 1, 2	169	Acute Respiratory Distress Syndrome
Active	Early Phase 1	44	Macular Holes
Not recruiting	Not Applicable	30	Non-Small Cell Lung Cancer
Completed	Not Applicable	4	Irritable Bowel Disease
Recruiting	Not Applicable	60	HIV Infections
Completed	Not Applicable	18	Blood Coagulation, Platelet Function
Completed	Early Phase 1	9	Larynx, Lip, Oral Cavity, Pharynx
Unknown	Not Applicable	72	Healthy
Completed	Phase 1	60	Head and Neck Cancer, Oral Mucositis
Recruiting	Not Applicable	120	Type 2 Diabetes Mellitus
Terminated	Not Applicable	2	Squamous Cell Carcinoma of the Head and Neck
Unknown	Not Applicable	200	NSCLC Patients
Unknown	Not Applicable	60	NSCLC
Unknown	Not Applicable	60	NSCLC
Recruiting	Phase 1	20	COVID-19 Acute Respiratory Distress Syndrome, Respiratory Distress Syndrome
Recruiting	Not Applicable	80	Metabolism
Completed	Phase 2	41	Non-Small Cell Lung Cancer
Not recruiting	Not Applicable	30	Breast Cancer
Withdrawn	Not Applicable	0	Breast Cancer, Leptomeningeal Metastasis
Completed	Not Applicable	9	Prehypertension
Recruiting	Not Applicable	25	Advanced Breast Cancer
Not recruiting	Not Applicable	30	Diabetic Foot
Unknown	Phase 1, 2	9	Alzheimer Disease
Recruiting	Not Applicable	300	Metastatic Breast Cancer
Recruiting	Not Applicable	1000	Breast Cancer, Digestive Cancer, Gynecologic Cancer, Circulating Tumor DNA
Not recruiting	Phase 1, 2	10	Dystrophic Epidermolysis Bullosa

Status	Phases	Cases	Diseases
Completed	Not Applicable	84	Overweight Children with Type 2 Diabetes Risk
Recruiting	Not Applicable	320	Prostate Cancer
Completed	Not Applicable	71	Cancer
Recruiting	Not Applicable	80	Allergic Asthma, Severe Eosinophilic Asthma
Not recruiting	Not Applicable	1000	Postoperative Delirium, General Anesthesia, Circadian Rhythm Disorders
Active	Not Applicable	48	Sports Drug Abuse
Active	Not Applicable	367	Breast Cancer
Completed	Phase 1	17	Normal Cellular Metabolism
Active	Not Applicable	1000	Cancer of the Prostate
Completed	Phase 1, 2	30	Chronic Kidney Failure, Dialysis-Related Complication
Recruiting	Early Phase 1	9	Recurrent or Metastatic Bladder Cancer
Active	Phase 2, 3	129	Prostatic Neoplasms
Recruiting	Not Applicable	75	Pancreatic Carcinoma, Pancreatic Intraductal Papillary Mucinous Neoplasm
Completed	Not Applicable	19	Port-Wine Stain
Recruiting	Not Applicable	10,000	Major Depressive Disorder, Bipolar Disorder
Not recruiting	Phase 1	20	Alveolar Bone Loss, Alveolar Bone Atrophy, Bone Grafting
Completed	Phase 1	13	Malignant Glioma of Brain
Completed	Phase 1	33	Malignant Glioma, Neoplasms
Completed	Not Applicable	28	Type 1 Diabetes, Diabetes Complications
Recruiting	Phase 1	15	Triple Negative Breast Cancer
Recruiting	Not Applicable	60	Treatment-resistant Depression
Not recruiting	Phase 1	20	Long COVID
Recruiting	Phase 2	20	Mild Cognitive Impairment
Completed	Not Applicable	90	Obesity
Completed	Not Applicable	60	Non-Small Cell Lung Cancer
Recruiting	Phase 1	30	Advanced Hepatocellular Carcinoma, Gastric Cancer Metastatic to Liver, Colorectal Cancer Metastatic to Liver
Not recruiting	Not Applicable	10	Glioma
Recruiting	Not Applicable	72	Acute Myeloid Leukemia
Completed	Phase 1	38	Chronic Ulcer
Terminated	Phase 1, 2	17	T-Cell Lymphoma
Completed	Not Applicable	10	Hypertension
Active	Phase 1, 2	20	COVID-19, Acute Respiratory Distress Syndrome
Completed	Not Applicable	75	Drug Resistant Epilepsy

Status	Phases	Cases	Diseases
Recruiting	Not Applicable	80	Panic Disorder
Completed	Phase 1	19	Polycystic Kidney Disease
Terminated	Not Applicable	28	Carcinoma, Hepatocellular, Colorectal Neoplasms, Melanoma, Kidney Neoplasms
Completed	Phase 2	13	Thyroid
Completed	Not Applicable	13	Insulin Resistance
Terminated	Phase 4	15	Type 2 Diabetes Mellitus, Cardiovascular Diseases
Unknown	Not Applicable	90	Childhood Obesity, Adolescent Obesity
Unknown	Not Applicable	40	Fasting
Not recruiting	Phase 2	78	Esophageal Adenocarcinoma, Esophageal Squamous Cell Carcinoma, Gastroesophageal Junction Carcinoma
Not recruiting	Not Applicable	144	Brugada Syndrome 1
Not recruiting	Phase 1, 2	12	Obstructive Sleep Apnea, Brain Hypoxia, Stroke, Endothelial Dysfunction, Oxidative Stress
Unknown	Not Applicable	102	Pancreas Adenocarcinoma
Recruiting	Phase 3	68	Muscular Dystrophies, Duchenne Muscular Dystrophy, Muscular Disorders, Neuromuscular Diseases, Genetic Diseases, Nervous System Diseases
Completed	Phase 2	63	Covid19
Completed	Phase 2	102	COVID-19, ARDS
Completed	Phase 2	18	Duchenne Muscular Dystrophies, Atrophic Muscular Diseases, Neuromuscular Diseases, Genetic Diseases
Completed	Early Phase 1	14	Heart Failure with Preserved Ejection Fraction
Recruiting	Early Phase 1	6	Recessive Dystrophic Epidermolysis Bullosa
Unknown	Not Applicable	60	Sleep Apnea, Inflammation, Atherosclerosis
Recruiting	Not Applicable	144	Non-alcoholic Fatty Liver Disease, Metabolic Syndrome, Obesity
Recruiting	Not Applicable	300	Obesity, Insulin Resistance
Unknown	Not Applicable	96	Thoracic Surgery, Video-Assisted
Recruiting	Phase 1, 2	30	COVID-19
Terminated	Not Applicable	1	COVID-19
Recruiting	Not Applicable	40	Prostate Cancer
Recruiting	Not Applicable	180	Obesity, Insulin Resistance
Unknown	Not Applicable	260	Body Weight Changes
Not recruiting	Phase 2	203	Locally Advanced Gastric Cancer
Unknown	Not Applicable	180	Rhinitis, Allergic, Perennial
Active	Phase 2	45	Lip, Oral Cavity Squamous Cell Carcinoma, Pharynx, Larynx, Squamous Cell Carcinoma

Status	Phases	Cases	Diseases
Not recruiting	Phase 2	60	Brain Metastases, Non-small Cell Lung Cancer Stage III
Completed	Phase 1	12	Drug–drug Interaction
Recruiting	Not Applicable	120	Heart Failure
Not recruiting	Phase 3	216	Locally Advanced Gastric Cancer
Not recruiting	Phase 1	18	Glioma, Anaplastic Astrocytoma, Anaplastic Oligodendroglioma, Glioblastoma
Unknown	Phase 2	40	Metastatic Colorectal Cancer
Completed	Not Applicable	8	Obesity, Insulin Resistance
Withdrawn	Phase 2	0	Prostate Carcinoma
Not recruiting	Not Applicable	200	Alzheimer Disease
Unknown	Not Applicable	108	Cancer
Completed	Phase 2	25	Non-Small Cell Lung Cancer
Unknown	Phase 2	80	Mild Cognitive Impairment
Recruiting	Phase 2	18	Cutaneous Squamous Cell Carcinoma of the Head and Neck
Terminated	Phase 2	3	Breast Cancer
Unknown	Phase 1	60	Advanced/Metastatic Colorectal Cancer
Completed	Phase 4	40	Non-alcoholic Fatty Liver Disease
Not recruiting	Not Applicable	100	Myocardial Reperfusion Injury, Prognosis, ST Elevation Myocardial Infarction
Active	Phase 2	43	Chordoma
Completed	Not Applicable	45	Stroke, Acute Ischemic Stroke, Cerebrovascular Disorders, Central Nervous System Diseases
Completed	Phase 2	69	Hypothyroidism, Endocrine System Diseases
Completed	Phase 2	26	Prostate Cancer
Recruiting	Not Applicable	124	Multiple System Atrophy
Active	Not Applicable	69	Cardiovascular System, Respiratory System
Recruiting	Phase 2	53	MSS, pMMR, Metastatic Colorectal Adenocarcinoma
Active	Phase 1	46	Resectable Soft Tissue Sarcoma, Soft Tissue Sarcoma
Recruiting	Phase 1, 2	100	Lung Non-Small Cell Carcinoma
Recruiting	Phase 1	30	Lung Non-Small Cell Carcinoma
Completed	Phase 1, 2	4	Minimal Residual Disease, AML
Terminated	Phase 1	10	Neoplasms, Refractory and Recurrent Solid Tumors
Completed	Phase 1, 2	27	Pancreatic Cancer, Pancreatic Ductal Adenocarcinoma
Active	Phase 1	101	Healthy Elderly, Parkinson Disease
Recruiting	Not Applicable	480	Overweight and Obesity, Weight Loss, Pregnancy Related

Table 1.
MSC-exo-based clinical trials.

lymphoma, lung cancer, non-small cell lung cancer, metastatic pancreatic adenocarcinoma, squamous cell carcinoma of the head and neck, advanced breast cancer, triple negative breast cancer, gynecologic cancer, prostate cancer, intraductal papillary mucinous neoplasm, malignant glioma, advanced hepatocellular carcinoma, acute myeloid leukemia, T-cell lymphoma, squamous cell carcinoma, advanced gastric cancer, colorectal cancer).

5. Conclusions

Biomaterials and MSC-exo composites are advantaged sources for tissue engineering and regenerative medicine, which hold superiority over other therapeutic regimens attributes to the unique characteristics. In this chapter, we detailed and introduced the basic conception and latest updates of biomaterials and MSC-exo composites for biomedicine, which will collectively facilitate the further development of MSC-exo-based cell-free regimens in future. Of the multitudinous biomaterials, those with preferable tissue compatibility and minimal inflammatory response would reveal more robust application prospect with MSC-exo in future.

Acknowledgements

The authors would like to thank the members in Key Laboratory of Molecular Diagnostics and Precision Medicine for Surgical Oncology in Gansu Province & NHC Key Laboratory of Diagnosis and Therapy of Gastrointestinal Tumor, Gansu Provincial Hospital, and Chinese Academy of Sciences Hefei Institute of Physical Science for their kind suggestions. This study was supported by grants from, National Natural Science Foundation of China (82260031, 82160534), Gansu Provincial Hospital Intra-Hospital Research Fund Project (22GSSYB-6, 21GSSYB-8, 20GSSY5-2), The 2022 Master/Doctor/Postdoctoral program of NHC Key Laboratory of Diagnosis and Therapy of Gastrointestinal Tumor (NHCDP2022004, NHCDP2022008, NHCDP2022014), the project Youth Fund funded by Shandong Provincial Natural Science Foundation (ZR2020QC097), Science and technology projects of Guizhou Province (QKH-J-ZK[2021]-107), Natural Science Foundation of Jiangxi Province (20224BAB206077, 20212BAB216073), Key project funded by Department of Science and Technology of Shangrao City (2020AB002, 2020 K003, 2021F013, 2022AB003), Jiangxi Provincial Key New Product Incubation Program Funded by Technical Innovation Guidance Program of Shangrao (2020G002), the Non-profit Central Research Institute Fund of Chinese Academy of Medical Sciences (2019PT320005), The 2021 Central-Guided Local Science and Technology Development Fund (ZYYDDFFZZJ-1), Guiding plan for scientific and technological development of Lanzhou (2019-ZD-102), Gansu Key Laboratory of molecular diagnosis and precision treatment of surgical tumors (18JR2RA033), Key talent project of Gansu Province of the Organization Department of Gansu provincial Party committee (2020RCXM076), Young Science and Technology Talent Support Project of Gansu Association for Science and Technology (GXH202220530-17), Natural Science Foundation of Gansu Province (21JR11RA186, 20JR10RA415).

Conflict of interest

The authors declare no conflict of interest.

Notes/thanks/other declarations.

Not applicable.

Appendices and nomenclature

Abbreviation	Nomenclature
MSCs	Mesenchymal stem/stromal cells
OA	Osteoarthritis
MSC-Exo	MSC-derived exosomes
MHC-II	Type II major histocompatibility complex
ACLF	Acute-on-chronic liver failure
P-MSCs	Placental-derived MSCs
ECM	Extracellular matrix
UC-MSCs	Umbilical cord-derived MSCs
PCL	ε-Caprolactone
sEVs	Small extracellular vesicles
PSC-MSCs	Pluripotent stem cell-derived MSCs
ESCs	Embryonic stem cells
iPSCs	Induced pluripotent stem cells
ECM	Extracellular matrix
NCCs	Neural crest cells
PCL	Poly ε-caprolactone
HA	Hyaluronic acid
nHA	Nano-hydroxyapatite
HAP	Hydroxyapatite
P-MSC-exo	Placenta-derived mesenchymal stem cells-derived exosomes
HPCH	Hydroxypropyl chitin hydrogel
MSX2	Msh Homeobox 2
AD	Alzheimer disease
COVID-19	Corona virus disease 2019
NSCLC	Non-small cell lung cancer
ARDS	Acute respiratory distress syndrome
TNBC	Triple negative breast cancer
AML	Acute myeloid leukemia
BM-MSCs	Bone marrow-derived MSCs
NAFLD	Non-alcoholic fatty liver disease
HSCs	Hematopoietic stem cells

Author details

Leisheng Zhang[1,2,3,4*†], Xiaowei Gao[5†], Shixun Ma[1†], Miao Yu[1], Xianghong Xu[1], Yuanguang Zhao[3], Shuang Chen[3], Yonghong Li[1], Xiaonan Yang[6], Tiankang Guo[1] and Hui Cai[1]

1 Laboratory of Molecular Diagnostics and Precision Medicine for Surgical Oncology in Gansu Province and NHC Key Laboratory of Diagnosis and Therapy of Gastrointestinal Tumor, Key Gansu Provincial Hospital, Lanzhou, China

2 CAS Key Laboratory of Radiation Technology and Biophysics in Institute of Biology and Hefei Institute of Physical Science, Chinese Academy of Sciences, Hefei, China

3 Jiangxi Research Center of Stem Cell Engineering, Jiangxi Health-Biotech Stem Cell Technology Co., Ltd., Shangrao, China

4 Department of General Practice, Affiliated Hospital of Xiangnan University, Chenzhou, China

5 Department of Otorhinolaryngology, Second Hospital of Tianjin Medical University, Tianjin, China

6 Department of Plastic and Reconstructive Surgery and Department of Hemangioma and Vascular Malformation, Plastic Surgery Hospital Affiliated to Chinese Academy of Medical Sciences and Peking Union Medical College, Beijing, China

*Address all correspondence to: leisheng_zhang@163.com

† Co-first authors.

References

[1] Whitford W, Guterstam P. Exosome manufacturing status. Future Medicinal Chemistry. 2019;**11**(10):1225-1236

[2] Yang D, Zhang W, Zhang H, Zhang F, Chen L, Ma L, et al. Progress, opportunity, and perspective on exosome isolation - efforts for efficient exosome-based theranostics. Theranostics. 2020;**10**(8):3684-3707

[3] He C, Zheng S, Luo Y, Wang B. Exosome Theranostics: Biology and translational medicine. Theranostics. 2018;**8**(1):237-255

[4] Heo J, Kang H. Exosome-based treatment for atherosclerosis. International Journal of Molecular Sciences. 2022;**23**(2)

[5] Yang B, Chen Y, Shi J. Exosome biochemistry and advanced nanotechnology for next-generation Theranostic platforms. Advanced Materials. 2019;**31**(2):e1802896

[6] Zhang H, Lu J, Liu J, Zhang G, Lu A. Advances in the discovery of exosome inhibitors in cancer. Journal of Enzyme Inhibition and Medicinal Chemistry. 2020;**35**(1):1322-1330

[7] Zhang LS, Yu Y, Yu H, Han ZC. Therapeutic prospects of mesenchymal stem/stromal cells in COVID-19 associated pulmonary diseases: From bench to bedside. World Journal of Stem Cells. 2021;**13**(8):1058-1071

[8] Zhang X, Yang Y, Zhang L, Lu Y, Zhang Q, Fan D, et al. Mesenchymal stromal cells as vehicles of tetravalent bispecific Tandab (CD3/CD19) for the treatment of B cell lymphoma combined with IDO pathway inhibitor D-1-methyl-tryptophan. Journal of Hematology & Oncology. 2017;**10**(1):56

[9] Zhang Y, Li Y, Li W, Cai J, Yue M, Jiang L, et al. Therapeutic effect of human umbilical cord mesenchymal stem cells at various passages on acute liver failure in rats. Stem Cells International. 2018;**2018**:7159465

[10] Zhang L, Wei Y, Chi Y, Liu D, Yang S, Han Z, et al. Two-step generation of mesenchymal stem/stromal cells from human pluripotent stem cells with reinforced efficacy upon osteoarthritis rabbits by HA hydrogel. Cell & Bioscience. 2021;**11**(1):6

[11] Yu H, Feng Y, Du W, Zhao M, Jia H, Wei Z, et al. Off-the-shelf GMP-grade UC-MSCs as therapeutic drugs for the amelioration of CCl4-induced acute-on-chronic liver failure in NOD-SCID mice. International Immunopharmacology. 2022;**113**(Pt A):109408

[12] Zhang K, Zhao X, Chen X, Wei Y, Du W, Wang Y, et al. Enhanced therapeutic effects of mesenchymal stem cell-derived exosomes with an injectable hydrogel for Hindlimb ischemia treatment. ACS Applied Materials & Interfaces. 2018;**10**(36):30081-30091

[13] Zhao Q, Zhang L, Wei Y, Yu H, Zou L, Huo J, et al. Systematic comparison of hUC-MSCs at various passages reveals the variations of signatures and therapeutic effect on acute graft-versus-host disease. Stem Cell Research & Therapy. 2019;**10**(1):354

[14] Zhao M, Li L. Regulation of hematopoietic stem cells in the niche. Science China. Life Sciences. 2015;**58**(12):1209-1215

[15] Friedenstein AJ, Petrakova KV, Kurolesova AI. Frolova GP: Heterotopic of bone marrow. Analysis of

precursor cells for osteogenic and hematopoietic tissues. Transplantation. 1968;**6**(2):230-247

[16] Yao J, Chen N, Wang X, Zhang L, Huo J, Chi Y, et al. Human supernumerary teeth-derived apical papillary stem cells possess preferable characteristics and efficacy on hepatic fibrosis in mice. Stem Cells International. 2020;**2020**:6489396

[17] Du W, Li X, Chi Y, Ma F, Li Z, Yang S, et al. VCAM-1+ placenta chorionic villi-derived mesenchymal stem cells display potent pro-angiogenic activity. Stem Cell Research & Therapy. 2016;**7**:49

[18] Wei Y, Zhang L, Chi Y, Ren X, Gao Y, Song B, et al. High-efficient generation of VCAM-1(+) mesenchymal stem cells with multidimensional superiorities in signatures and efficacy on aplastic anaemia mice. Cell Proliferation. 2020;**53**(8):e12862

[19] Zhang L, Wang H, Liu C, Wu Q, Su P, Wu D, et al. MSX2 initiates and accelerates mesenchymal stem/stromal cell specification of hPSCs by regulating TWIST1 and PRAME. Stem Cell Reports. 2018;**11**(2):497-513

[20] Jiang B, Yan L, Wang X, Li E, Murphy K, Vaccaro K, et al. Concise review: Mesenchymal stem cells derived from human pluripotent cells, an unlimited and quality-controllable source for therapeutic applications. Stem Cells. 2019;**37**(5):572-581

[21] Wei Y, Hou H, Zhang L, Zhao N, Li C, Huo J, et al. JNKi- and DAC-programmed mesenchymal stem/stromal cells from hESCs facilitate hematopoiesis and alleviate hind limb ischemia. Stem Cell Research & Therapy. 2019;**10**(1):186

[22] Fu X, Liu G, Halim A, Ju Y, Luo Q, Song AG. Mesenchymal stem cell migration and tissue repair. Cell. 2019;**8**(8)

[23] Liu H, Li R, Liu T, Yang L, Yin G, Xie Q. Immunomodulatory effects of mesenchymal stem cells and mesenchymal stem cell-derived extracellular vesicles in rheumatoid arthritis. Frontiers in Immunology. 1912;**2020**:11

[24] Lai JJ, Chau ZL, Chen SY, Hill JJ, Korpany KV, Liang NW, et al. Exosome processing and characterization approaches for research and technology development. Advanced Science (Weinh). 2022;**9**(15):e2103222

[25] Kalluri R, LeBleu VS. The biology, function, and biomedical applications of exosomes. Science. 2020;**367**(6478)

[26] Wu P, Zhang B, Shi H, Qian H, Xu W. MSC-exosome: A novel cell-free therapy for cutaneous regeneration. Cytotherapy. 2018;**20**(3):291-301

[27] Zhang Y, Bi J, Huang J, Tang Y, Du S, Li P. Exosome: A review of its classification, isolation techniques, storage, diagnostic and targeted therapy applications. International Journal of Nanomedicine. 2020;**15**:6917-6934

[28] Pegtel DM, Gould SJ. Exosomes. Annual Review of Biochemistry. 2019;**88**:487-514

[29] Miao W, Song B, Shi B, Wan Q, Lv Q, Chen H, et al. Immune thrombocytopenia plasma-derived exosomes impaired megakaryocyte and platelet production through an apoptosis pathway. Thrombosis and Haemostasis. 2021;**121**(4):495-505

[30] Noonin C, Thongboonkerd V. Exosome-inflammasome crosstalk and their roles in inflammatory responses. Theranostics. 2021;**11**(9):4436-4451

[31] Patil M, Saheera S, Dubey PK, Kahn-Krell A, Kumar Govindappa P, Singh S, et al. Novel mechanisms of exosome-mediated phagocytosis of dead cells in injured heart. Circulation Research. 2021;**129**(11):1006-1020

[32] Govindappa PK, Patil M, Garikipati VNS, Verma SK, Saheera S, Narasimhan G, et al. Targeting exosome-associated human antigen R attenuates fibrosis and inflammation in diabetic heart. The FASEB Journal. 2020;**34**(2):2238-2251

[33] Koshy ST, Mooney DJ. Biomaterials for enhancing anti-cancer immunity. Current Opinion in Biotechnology. 2016;**40**:1-8

[34] Lynch RI, Lavelle EC. Immuno-modulatory biomaterials as anti-inflammatory therapeutics. Biochemical Pharmacology. 2022;**197**:114890

[35] Alvarez Echazu MI, Perna O, Olivetti CE, Antezana PE, Municoy S, Tuttolomondo MV, et al. Recent advances in synthetic and natural biomaterials-based therapy for bone defects. Macromolecular Bioscience. 2022;**22**(4):e2100383

[36] Ji X, Yuan X, Ma L, Bi B, Zhu H, Lei Z, et al. Mesenchymal stem cell-loaded thermosensitive hydroxypropyl chitin hydrogel combined with a three-dimensional-printed poly(epsilon-caprolactone) /nano-hydroxyapatite scaffold to repair bone defects via osteogenesis, angiogenesis and immunomodulation. Theranostics. 2020;**10**(2):725-740

[37] Yang J, Zhang YS, Yue K, Khademhosseini A. Cell-laden hydrogels for osteochondral and cartilage tissue engineering. Acta Biomaterialia. 2017;**57**:1-25

[38] Velasco-Rodriguez B, Diaz-Vidal T, Rosales-Rivera LC, Garcia-Gonzalez CA, Alvarez-Lorenzo C, Al-Modlej A, et al. Hybrid Methacrylated Gelatin and hyaluronic acid hydrogel scaffolds. Preparation and systematic characterization for prospective tissue engineering applications. International Journal of Molecular Sciences. 2021;**22**(13)

[39] Madhusudanan P, Raju G, Shankarappa S. Hydrogel systems and their role in neural tissue engineering. Journal of Royal Society Interface. 2020;**17**(162):20190505

[40] Xiao S, Zhao T, Wang J, Wang C, Du J, Ying L, et al. Gelatin methacrylate (GelMA)-based hydrogels for cell transplantation: An effective strategy for tissue engineering. Stem Cell Reviews and Reports. 2019;**15**(5):664-679

[41] Celikkin N, Mastrogiacomo S, Jaroszewicz J, Walboomers XF, Swieszkowski W. Gelatin methacrylate scaffold for bone tissue engineering: The influence of polymer concentration. Journal of Biomedical Materials Research. Part A. 2018;**106**(1):201-209

[42] Khayambashi P, Iyer J, Pillai S, Upadhyay A, Zhang Y, Tran SD. Hydrogel encapsulation of mesenchymal stem cells and their derived exosomes for tissue engineering. International Journal of Molecular Sciences. 2021;**22**(2)

[43] Tang Q, Lu B, He J, Chen X, Fu Q, Han H, et al. Exosomes-loaded thermosensitive hydrogels for corneal epithelium and stroma regeneration. Biomaterials. 2022;**280**:121320

[44] Han M, Yang H, Lu X, Li Y, Liu Z, Li F, et al. Three-dimensional-cultured MSC-derived exosome-hydrogel hybrid microneedle Array patch for spinal cord repair. Nano Letters. 2022;**22**(15):6391-6401

[45] Blackstone BN, Gallentine SC, Powell HM. Collagen-based electrospun

materials for tissue engineering: A systematic review. Bioengineering (Basel). 2021;**8**(3)

[46] Rezvani Ghomi E, Nourbakhsh N, Akbari Kenari M, Zare M, Ramakrishna S. Collagen-based biomaterials for biomedical applications. Journal of Biomedical Materials Research. Part B, Applied Biomaterials. 2021;**109**(12):1986-1999

[47] Warth RJ, Rodkey WG. Resorbable collagen scaffolds for the treatment of meniscus defects: A systematic review. Arthroscopy. 2015;**31**(5):927-941

[48] Patil VA, Masters KS. Engineered collagen matrices. Bioengineering (Basel). 2020;**7**:4

[49] Lee JM, Suen SKQ, Ng WL, Ma WC, Yeong WY. Bioprinting of collagen: Considerations, potentials, and applications. Macromolecular Bioscience. 2021;**21**(1):e2000280

[50] Wang T, Jian Z, Baskys A, Yang J, Li J, Guo H, et al. MSC-derived exosomes protect against oxidative stress-induced skin injury via adaptive regulation of the NRF2 defense system. Biomaterials. 2020;**257**:120264

[51] Stater EP, Sonay AY, Hart C, Grimm J. The ancillary effects of nanoparticles and their implications for nanomedicine. Nature Nanotechnology. 2021;**16**(11):1180-1194

[52] Zhao C, Tan A, Pastorin G, Ho HK. Nanomaterial scaffolds for stem cell proliferation and differentiation in tissue engineering. Biotechnology Advances. 2013;**31**(5):654-668

[53] Hu B, Cheng Z, Liang S. Advantages and prospects of stem cells in nanotoxicology. Chemosphere. 2022;**291**(Pt 2):132861

[54] Mahapatra C, Lee R, Paul MK. Emerging role and promise of nanomaterials in organoid research. Drug Discovery Today. 2022;**27**(3):890-899

[55] Liu G, Zhou Y, Zhang X, Guo S. Advances in hydrogels for stem cell therapy: Regulation mechanisms and tissue engineering applications. Journal of Materials Chemistry B. 2022;**10**(29):5520-5536

[56] Hofmann MC. Stem cells and nanomaterials. Advances in Experimental Medicine and Biology. 2014;**811**:255-275

[57] Kong Y, Duan J, Liu F, Han L, Li G, Sun C, et al. Regulation of stem cell fate using nanostructure-mediated physical signals. Chemical Society Reviews. 2021;**50**(22):12828-12872

[58] Xian P, Hei Y, Wang R, Wang T, Yang J, Li J, et al. Mesenchymal stem cell-derived exosomes as a nanotherapeutic agent for amelioration of inflammation-induced astrocyte alterations in mice. Theranostics. 2019;**9**(20):5956-5975

[59] Zhang J, Buller BA, Zhang ZG, Zhang Y, Lu M, Rosene DL, et al. Exosomes derived from bone marrow mesenchymal stromal cells promote remyelination and reduce neuroinflammation in the demyelinating central nervous system. Experimental Neurology. 2022;**347**:113895

[60] DiStefano TJ, Vaso K, Panebianco CJ, Danias G, Chionuma HN, Kunnath K, et al. Hydrogel-embedded poly(lactic-co-glycolic acid) microspheres for the delivery of hMSC-derived exosomes to promote bioactive annulus Fibrosus repair. Cartilage. 2022;**13**(3):1947

[61] Geng X, Qi Y, Liu X, Shi Y, Li H, Zhao L. A multifunctional antibacterial

and self-healing hydrogel laden with bone marrow mesenchymal stem cell-derived exosomes for accelerating diabetic wound healing. Biomaterial Advance. 2022;**133**:112613

[62] Liu A, Lin D, Zhao H, Chen L, Cai B, Lin K, et al. Optimized BMSC-derived osteoinductive exosomes immobilized in hierarchical scaffold via lyophilization for bone repair through Bmpr2/Acvr2b competitive receptor-activated Smad pathway. Biomaterials. 2021;**272**:120718

[63] Tian H, Yuan L, Song Y, Deng J, Qi XW. A review of recent advances in nanomaterial-based stem cell therapy and the corresponding risks. Current Stem Cell Research & Therapy. 2022;**17**(3):195-206

[64] Pinho S, Macedo MH, Rebelo C, Sarmento B, Ferreira L. Stem cells as vehicles and targets of nanoparticles. Drug Discovery Today. 2018;**23**(5):1071-1078

[65] Shi M, Xu Q, Ding L, Xia Y, Zhang C, Lai H, et al. Cell infiltrative inner connected porous hydrogel improves neural stem cell migration and differentiation for functional repair of spinal cord injury. ACS Biomaterials Science & Engineering. 2022;**8**(12):5307-5318

[66] Rochlin DH, Inchauste S, Zelones J, Nguyen DH. The role of adjunct nanofibrillar collagen scaffold implantation in the surgical management of secondary lymphedema: Review of the literature and summary of initial pilot studies. Journal of Surgical Oncology. 2020;**121**(1):121-128

[67] Sharma S, Rai VK, Narang RK, Markandeywar TS. Collagen-based formulations for wound healing: A literature review. Life Sciences. 2022;**290**:120096

[68] Murshed M. Mechanism of bone mineralization. Cold Spring Harbour Perspective Medicine. 3 Dec 2018;**8**(12):a031229

[69] Huang J, Heng S, Zhang W, Liu Y, Xia T, Ji C, et al. Dermal extracellular matrix molecules in skin development, homeostasis, wound regeneration and diseases. Seminars in Cell & Developmental Biology. 2022;**128**:137-144

[70] Brett D. A review of collagen and collagen-based wound dressings. Wounds. 2008;**20**(12):347-356

Section 2

Exosomes and Infectious Diseases

Chapter 3

Effectiveness of Exosomes in the Immune Cascade

Gözde Atila Uslu and Hamit Uslu

Abstract

In order to treat and/or control a disease or prevent its occurrence, first of all, physiological pathways must be understood very well. In the previous 10 years, there has been a lot of interest in the function of exosomes in intercellular communication, particularly in studies on cancer and neurodegenerative disorders. This has led to plenty of research in this area. Exosomes are tiny transmembrane vesicles that are produced by endocytosis and are found in a variety of bodily fluids, including blood, saliva, cerebrospinal fluid, and breast milk. They are also released by a variety of tissues. Exosomes have a varied composition depending on where they come from, but they are often rich in cytosolic and cell surface proteins, lipids, DNA, and RNA. In recent years, the interactions between exosomes and the immune system have been frequently studied. However, despite all the researches, the physiological purposes of exosomes are still largely unclear.

Keywords: exosomes, immune system, T cells, NK cells, mast cells

1. Introduction

Exosomes; although it was first defined as microparticles released from neoplastic cell lines, it was later determined that these structures were secreted by almost all cells in the body, and it was concluded that it would be more accurate to call them membrane-bound extracellular vesicles produced with endosomal division [1, 2]. It is stated that these microvesicles have an average diameter range of 40–160 nm and are formed by endocytic cellular pathways consisting of three different stages that have been identified so far. First stage; It is stated that is the invagination of the cell membrane from endocytic vesicles and leads to the formation of an early-shorting endosome (ESE), after which either novo formation occurs or can directly fuse with a pre-existing ESE, moreover golgi apparatus and the endoplasmic reticulum participate in this process. In the second stage, it is stated that ESEs can mature into late-shorting endosomes (LSEs) and multivesicular bodies are formed by accumulation of intraluminal vesicles in these bodies. In the third stage, it has been determined that multivesicular bodies can undergo proteosomal degradation, function as a temporary storage area (for major histocompatibility complex (MHC) class II), or combine with the plasma membrane to release exosomes (**Figure 1**) [3–7]. Exosomes can enter cells directly by different mechanisms or can be produced by cells by the process of endocytosis as mentioned above. It has been determined that exosome production, release,

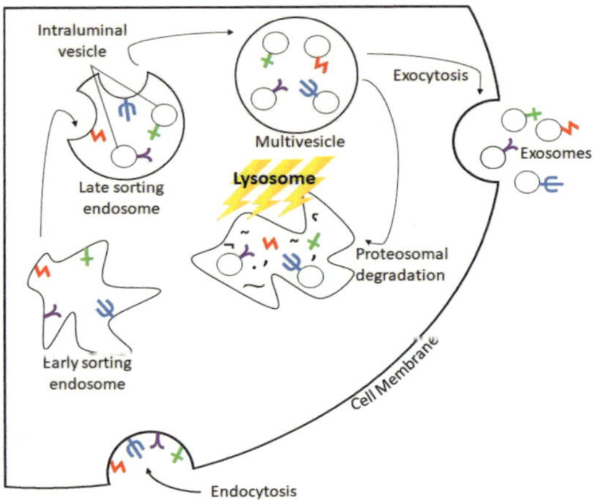

Figure 1.
Exosome biogenesis.

and uptake may change with oxidative stress, radiation, inhibiting a proton pump, altering cellular pH decrease in membrane cholesterol and increase in intracellular calcium level [8–11]. Numerous proteins, including the tetraspanins CD63, CD81, and CD9, TSG101, Alix, and HSP70, have been discovered to be present in exosomes. In addition, cell type-specific proteins may vary due to their endosomal origin, but they also have conserved proteins identified in almost all exosomes (hsc70, tetraspanin, CD63) [3]. It has been reported that exosomes also have lipid bilayer, which is mostly composed of phosphatidylcholine (PC), ganglioside GM3, phosphatidyl ethanolamine (PE), sphingomyelin (SM), and cholesterol [12]. Exosomes contain a wide variety of RNAs; some of these have been shown to be mRNA, miRNA, rRNA, tRNA, lncRNA, piRNA, snRNA, and small nucleolar RNA [13].

Although the functions of exosomes are not entirely understood and are still the subject of debate, they are involved in remodeling the extracellular matrix, homeostasis and adaptation of plasma membranous glycoprotein models, signal transduction between cells, immunity, tissue homeostasis, and many aspects of human health and disease which including cancer and neurodegenerative diseases have stated that have important functions [14–17]. They may have a role in the spread of prions throughout the body and the exchange of membranes between cells in infectious neurodegenerative illnesses, also known as prion diseases [18]. In their study on the synaptic physiology of neurons, Chivet et al. [19] found that the lipids, proteins, and RNAs in the exosomes released by neurons in response to synaptic activity can directly alter signal transmission and protein expression in recipient cells and play a crucial role in information transfer between synapses. It has been emphasized that intercellular communication has a very important role in vascular remodeling, and although direct intercellular contact or paracrine effects are focused on in this process, recently, it may be effective in this process in extracellular vesicles. When the effectiveness of exosomes in the neovascularization process was investigated, it was shown that they can act with the Notch signaling pathway, which is one of the cell interaction mechanisms, and an increase in blood vessel frequency and bifurcation number [20]. In order to treat and/or control a disease or prevent its occurrence, the physiological pathways must first be understood very well. Exosomes can also have an impact on the immune system by directly contacting the cell's plasma membrane during this process and then inducing intracellular signal cascades. The immune system plays a significant role in the emergence and development of disease pathophysiology as well as the emergence of acute and chronic complications.

2. Exosomes and T cells

In the case of contact with foreign antigens, such as in the case of infection, several days are needed for the formation of the immune responses, which we call cell-mediated or cellular immunity, by the effector T cells. For this reason, this type of immunity is also called delayed-type immune response. Antigen presenting cells (APC) such as macrophages, dendritic cells, and B cells are needed in this process. These constructs process antigenic constructs and antigen processing and presentation is performed with MHC class I or MHC class II. The term human leukocyte antigen (HLA) can also be used instead of MHC proteins in humans. AHS binary signaling is triggered by the binding of the intracellular adhesion molecule (ICAM) on the ASH surface and the lymphocyte function-associated antigen 1 (LFA-1) on T cells. This process can be opened as follows: (1) Recognition of the antigen by the T cell receptor and its co-receptor (CD8 molecules on cytotoxic T cells and CD4 molecules on helper T cells are called co-receptors). (2) The binding of the B7 protein in ASH and the CD28 protein on the T cells leads to rapid proliferation, clonal expansion, and differentiation in T cells [21]. In addition, suppression mediated by regulatory T (Treg) cells had found to be effective in making the immune system tolerant to most autoantigens and preventing host damage [22]. As mentioned above, a large number of extracellular and intracellular signals are needed to initiate the rapid proliferation, differentiation, and migration of T cells to peripheral infection sites (**Figure 2**).

Exosomes, which have been determined to be secreted by almost all cells in the body, are also secreted from various hematopoietic cell types such as reticulocytes, B lymphocytes, platelets, T lymphocytes, and dendritic cells. It is known that exosomes secreted from dendritic cells contain proteins such as MHC class I and II and CD86 (provide necessary signals for T cell activation and survival) and these structures

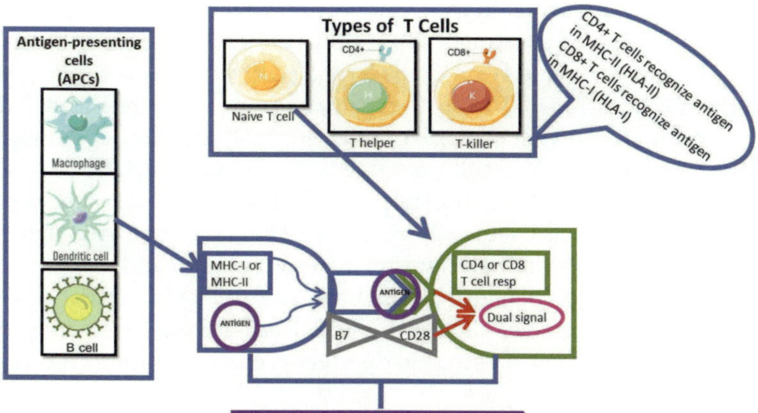

Figure 2.
T cell activation.

are effective in T cell stimulation. Exosome production may occur in peripheral tissues, after dendritic cells have traveled to lymph nodes, or in both cases, according to reports, but there is currently insufficient evidence to make a firm determination [23]. Exosomes that are loaded with specific peptides or antigens serve as vehicles for antigen presentation and can activate T cells (CD4+ and CD8+) also in the lack of dendridic cell. It has been established that exosomes have a positive impact on the immune system through various activities such as antigen presentation, stimulation, suppression, and tolerance of immunity [24]. It is also mentioned that some exosomes can express chemokine sequences like CCL2-5, CCL7, CCL20, CCL28, CXCL1-2, and CXCL16 because they can start other leukocytes like T cells from migrating to the infection sites [25, 26]. It is known that dendritic cell-T cell interactions cause an increase in calcium mobilization and Interleukin-2 and Interferon-gamma levels, resulting in T-cell activation. In addition, it is emphasized that co-stimulatory molecules such as CD86 strengthen intercellular interactions and T-cell functional activation in this process [27]. Zitvogel et al. [28] found that tumor peptide-pulsed dendritic cells-derived exosomes could eradicate or suppress the growth of tumors in a T-cell-dependent manner.

While it has been reported that synoviocyte-produced microparticles in inflammatory conditions like rheumatoid arthritis may exacerbate cartilage damage by increasing the synthesis of inflammatory mediators and cartilage-degrading enzymes [29, 30], other studies have suggested that T cell-stimulated TRAIL- and FasL-containing microvesicules produced in the synovium may also be helpful in preventing autoimmune damage in rheumatoid diseases [31]. In fact, exosomes originating from immunosuppressive dendritic cells have been shown to be more efficient and safe than modified dendritic cells in the therapies of autoimmune disorders like rheumatoid arthritis [32]. However, there are studies showing that exosomes produced from cancer cells could disturb the functions of T and B cells, monocytes/macrophages, NK cells and dendritic cells [33–35]. Exosomes synthesized from other cells could affect T cell functions, and the T-cells themselves too synthesize exosomes. It has been shown that these exosomes have a lipid bilayer and contain structures such as CD2, CD3/TCR, CD4, CD8, CD11c, CD25, CD69, LFA-1, CXCR4, FasL [36]. Tregs are subtypes of T cells, and it has been determined that the expression of CD73 by these cells shows a suppressive effect by converting extracellular adenosine 5-monophosphate to adenosine, in the same way that exosomes secreted from these cells also contain CD73 and exerting a suppressive effect with same pathway [37]. It is stated that exosomes derived from Tregs have a suppressive role in acute rejection and inhibit the proliferation of T cells, therefore exosomes released from Tregs may be a good alternative to prevent transplant rejection [38]. In another study, it is stated that the antigen-specific CD41 T-cell exosome (expressing CD4, TCR, LFA-1, CD25, and Fas ligand) may act as an immunosuppressant in the transplant rejection and treatment of autoimmune diseases [39]. Scientists have demonstrated that exosomes isolated from CD3+ T cells stimulated with IL-2 interact with and promote proliferation in resting autologous T cells [40]. It has been emphasized that high-level regulation of the miR-765/PLP2 axis of CD45RO-CD8+ T cell-derived exosomes can limit the cancer-supporting effects of estrogen on uterine corpus endometrial cancer [41].

3. Exosomes and natural killer (NK) cells

While NK cells were at first idea to be large granular lymphocytes with built-in cytotoxicity against tumor cells, they have since been identified as a distinct class of lymphocytes with effector capabilities that enable them to produce cytokines in addition to their natural cytotoxicity [42]. Since it was not known at the time what strategies NK cells use to differentiate between normal and abnormal cells and thus participate in the defense mechanism, the missing self hypothesis was suggested. According to this theory, NK cells recognize and eliminate cells that do not express their MHC Class-1 (MHC) molecules [43]. However, it is now known that NK cells have a large number of activating and inhibitory receptors that can combine MHC class-1 molecules, MHC class-1-like molecules and non-MHC related molecules [44]. Although not previously known, it is now well established that NK cells, in addition to their cytotoxic effector functions, can secrete cytokines and serve to control the immune system as regulatory lymphocytes that can interact with both innate and adaptive immune cells such as monocytes and macrophages, dendritic cells and T lymphocytes [45, 46]. Detailed studies have shown that conventional NK cells (cNK) are distributed in circulation in the blood, spleen, and bone marrow [47–49]. However, it has also been shown that NK cells can infiltrate tissues. They also have resident NK cells, defined as resident NK cells (trNK), in the lungs, skin, kidneys, lymph nodes, liver, intestines, and virgin uterus [47, 49, 50]. In addition to the peritoneal region and placenta, NK cells are also present in peripheral circulation, where they account for 10–15% of all lymphocytes [51].

Defined as a subgroup of extracellular vesicles of endocytic origin [52–55], 30–150 nm sized exosomes [53–57] are secreted by various cell types and are involved in complex physiological and pathological processes [58]. Exosomes can move far within the body and have been found in a variety of bodily secretions, including blood, saliva, cerebrospinal fluid, breast milk, urine, gastric juice, and semen [55]. Exosomes are produced by a wide variety of cell types, but it is known that exosomes released by cancer cells are specifically taken up by different immune cells, including Treg, dendritic cells, and NK cells, and are therefore successful in controlling their functions [59, 60]. Exosomes excreted by cancer cells are thought to help tumor cells escape immune surveillance in their microenvironment by stimulating angiogenesis and metastasis, as well as inhibiting the function of immune cells (**Figure 3**) [61]. Despite all this information, how exosomes secreted from tumor cells affect the health of individuals with cancer has not been fully elucidated [60, 61]. Exosomes can carry many different molecules with the ability to stimulate the immune system depending on the cell of origin from which they are secreted.

In particular, exosomes secreted from dendritic cells have been shown to carry ligands that can activate NK cells and can also be loaded with antigen to activate invariant NKT (a subset of T cells with characteristics of NK cells and conventional T cells) cells and induce T and B cell responses that are specific to the antigen [62]. Several studies in the last decade have provided evidence supporting the important role of cancer-originate exosomes in regulating the cancer microenvironment [63, 64]. Exosomes released by human tumors like myeloid leukemia, cervical cancer, breast cancer, hepatoblastoma, T cell cancer, pancreatic cancer, and multiple myeloma that are dyed with PKH67 membrane have been shown to associate with, infiltrate, and be engulfed by NK cells [65–67]. Li et al. [60] showed that exosomes derived from genetically modified K562 cells secreting IL-15, IL-18, and 4-1BBL on their surface carry the proteins of these three molecules similar to the source cell, and that these exosomes can increase the activity of NK cells after 4 h of treatment and even strengthen their cytotoxicity on some tumor types. In contrast, they reported that prolonged treatment (48 h) may suppress the cytotoxicity of NK cells by inhibiting the expression of activated receptors on NK cells. In mouse B16 melanoma, MC38 colon adenocarcinoma, and KLN205 squamous cell carcinoma cell lines, both

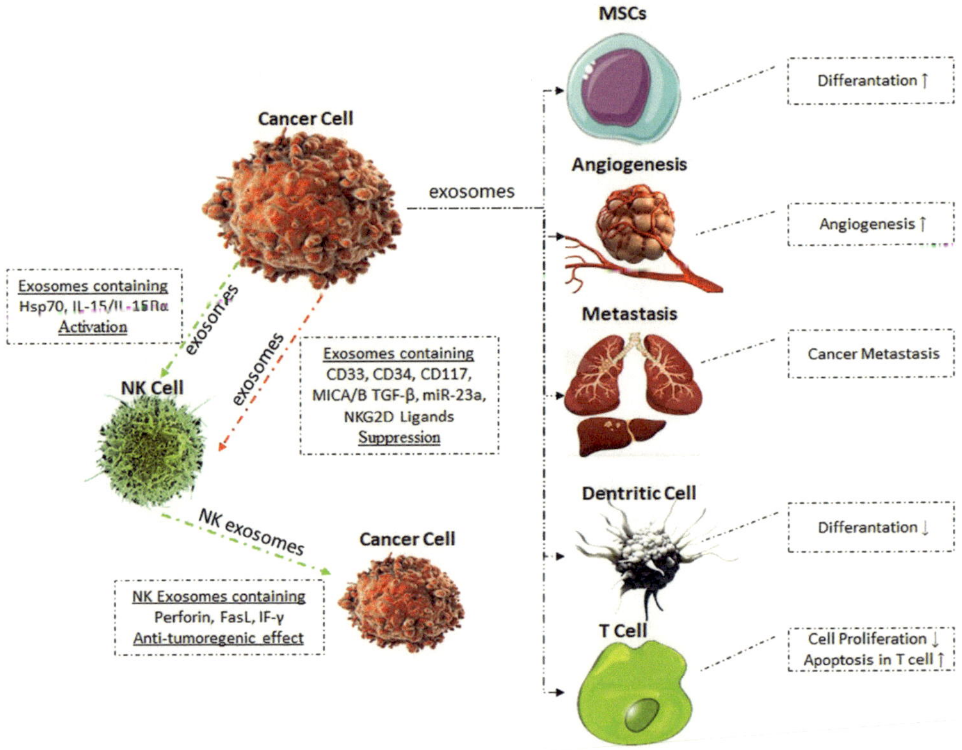

Figure 3.
Some roles of cancer cell-derived exosomes.

dendritic cells and exosomes secreted from dendritic cells can cause caspase activation and apoptosis, and exosomes released from dendritic cells can activate NK cells, according to research by Munich et al. [68]. In addition, TNF generated by exosomes of dendritic cells stimulates interferon gamma secretion by binding with NK cell TNF receptors. Jiang et al. [69] in NK92 and NK92-hIL-15 cell lines exposed to hypoxia for 48 h, they demonstrated that cytotoxicity was significantly increased and that hypoxia increased FasL, perforin, and granzyme B secretion. They revealed that exosomes produced from these NK cell lines under hypoxic conditions were effective in inhibiting both cell proliferation and migration while promoting apoptosis of breast cancer (MCF-7) and ovarian cancer (A2780) cells. However, this strategy, which encourages the overproduction of exosomes from NK cells as a consequence of NK cell hypoxia induction, might be a hopeful one for treating malignancy.

As a result, it is widely believed that exosomes produced by immune cells can strengthen immunity against cancer. In contrast, exosomes derived from cancer cells may decrease immunity and even alter the tumor microenvironment to promote self-enhancement and metastasis [70].

4. Exosomes and mast cells

Paul Ehrlich discovered mast cells 145 years ago and named them "mastzellen," meaning "nourishing cells," because of their appearance [71]. CD34+ progenitor cells, which are mast cell precursors of hematopoietic stem cells (CD34−), are produced in the bone marrow during hematopoiesis and are introduced into the bloodstream [72]. These hematopoietic progenitor cells are thought to stay undifferentiated in the circulation but mature into mast cells in the presence of different growth factors secreted from the microenvironment of the tissues where they must settle. C-kit ligand and stem cell proteins are a few of these [73]. Mature mast cells are not detected in circulation under normal circumstances. However, under the control of stem cell factor (SCF) and a number of mediators, CD34+ progenitor cells move to regions where they finish differentiating into mast cells [73, 74]. Mast cells are distributed in the skin and mucosal tissues such as the stomach, intestines, and respiratory tract, which are the entry points of antigens, as well as in the peritoneum and chest cavities, smooth muscle tissue, connective tissue surrounding hair follicles, the central nervous system, and all tissues with blood vessels except the retina [73, 75–77]. Mast cells are mainly recognized for their role in allergy. They are also known to mediate vital symptoms such as skin blistering and flare reactions, bronchospasms in asthma, congestion and excessive mucus secretion in allergy-induced rhinitis and even systemic anaphylaxis [77, 78].

On the membrane of every mast cell, there is a high affinity IgE receptor called FcεRI. Due to its high affinity, IgE molecules can no longer detach after binding to the receptor and consequently mast cells are coated with IgE. This stimulation leads to the secretion of exosomes containing a large number of proinflammatory mediators (proteases, chemokines, amines, and cytokines) that are stored and newly synthesized in mast cells [79, 80]. Of course, this extra vesicular composition varies according to the stimulation received by mast cells, but they frequently cause the secretion of numerous cytokines, growth factors, and mitogens such as TNF-α, IL-1β, IL-2, IL-3, IL-4, IL-5, IL-6, IL-9, IL-10, IL-11, IL-11, IL-12, IL-13, IL-16, IL-33, EGF, FG2, GM-CSF, IF-γ, NGF, PDGF, SCF, FGF-β1, and VEGF (**Figure 4**) [80].

Mast cells contribute to the promotion of angiogenesis. Mast cells promote angiogenesis, or the bud-like growth of new blood vessels from old ones, by secreting angiogenic factors like bFGF, VEGF, TGF-β, IL-8, and TNF-α. Mast cells also exude proteases that exude pro-angiogenic factors that bind to heparin and promote their release. However, there is also a proof that mast cells promote angiogenesis in the development of cancerous cells [73, 81]. Exosomes released by human mast cells have been shown by Ekström et al. [82] to be capable of RNA cell-to-cell transmission. They also showed that these exosomes have enough mRNA to equal 15% of the content of the source cell. Xiao et al. [83] also reported that exosomes containing KIT (labeled with PKH67), a cytokine receptor expressed mainly on the surface of hematopoietic stem cells, were secreted from a human mast cell line (HMC-1) and that these exosomes could be taken up by the lung epithelial cell line A549, and could also cause increased proliferation in recipient cancer cells by activation of the PI3K signaling pathway. Exosomes from human adipose-derived mesenchymal stem cells have been shown to effectively suppress atopic dermatitis in mice with the condition by lowering blood eosinophil counts, serum IgE levels, and the expression of the cytokines IL-4, IL-23, IL-31, and TNF- at the mRNA level [84]. However, in a model of cerebral malaria in C57BL/6 mice infected with Plasmodium berghei ANKA strain, it has been shown that intravenous administration of exosomes derived from mast cells to infected animals increases the incidence of the disease, exacerbates both liver and brain damage, contributes to disruption of the brain vascular endothelial structure, and increases the corruption of the blood-brain barrier (**Figure 5**) [85].

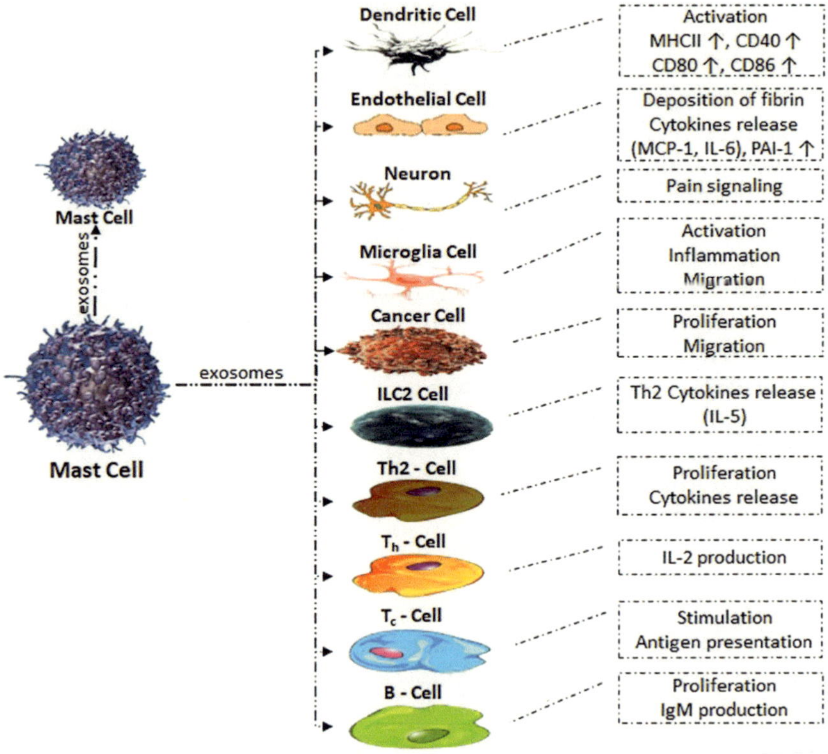

Figure 4.
Interactions of exosomes produced from mast cells with some other cells.

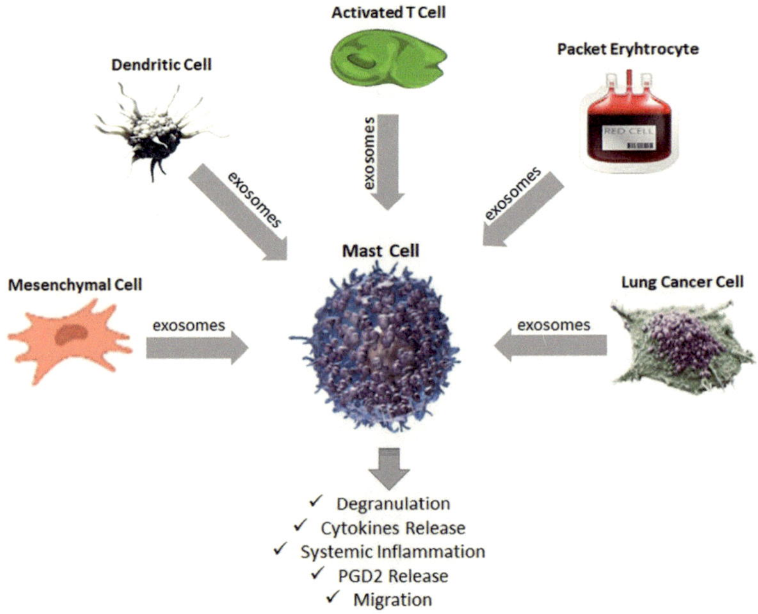

Figure 5.
Various cells' released exosomes' effects on the activation of mast cells.

5. Conclusion

In the literature reviews, it was observed that the activity of exosomes on the immune system has not been fully elucidated. Exosomes formed by other cells under normal physiological conditions and affecting cells in the immune system and exosomes expressed by cells that are effective in the immune system may have different activities. In addition, it has been determined that exosomes secreted under normal physiological conditions and exosomes secreted under pathological conditions have different routes of action (one of the main reasons for this difference is surface proteins), therefore, exosomes can exhibit immunomodulatory effects by showing both immunosuppressive and immunostimulatory effects depending on the current conditions.

Funding

There is no organization that financed this study.

Conflict of interest

The authors declare that there are no conflicts of interest.

Author details

Gözde Atila Uslu* and Hamit Uslu
Faculty of Medicine, Department of Physiology, Erzincan Binali Yıldırım University, Erzincan, Turkey

*Address all correspondence to: gzd.gozde@hotmail.com

References

[1] Johnstone RM, Adam M, Hammond JR, Orr L, Turbide C. Vesicle formation during reticulocyte maturation. Association of plasma-membrane activities with released vesicles (exosomes). The Journal of Biological Chemistry. 1987;**262**:9412-9420

[2] Théry C, Zitvogel L, Amigorena S. Exosomes: Composition, biogenesis and function. Nature Reviews Immunology. 2002;**2**(8):569-579

[3] Mathivanan S, Ji H, Simpson RJ. Exosomes: extracellular organelles important in intercellular communication. Journal of Proteomics. 2010;**73**(10):1907-1920

[4] Batista BS, Eng WS, Pilobello KT, Hendricks-Muñoz KD, Mahal LK. Identification of a conserved glycan signature for microvesicles. Journal of Proteome Research. 2011;**10**(10):4624-4633

[5] Qin J, Xu Q. Functions and application of exosomes. Acta Poloniae Pharmaceutica. 2014;**71**(4):537-543

[6] Kalluri R, LeBleu VS. The biology, function, and biomedical applications of exosomes. Science. 2020;**367**(6478):eaau6977

[7] Kleijmeer M, Ramm G, Schuurhuis D, Griffith J, Rescigno M, Ricciardi-Castagnoli P, et al. Reorganization of multivesicular bodies regulates MHC class II antigen presentation by dendritic cells. The Journal of Cell Biology. 2001;**155**(1):53-64

[8] Zhang W, Liu R, Chen Y, Wang M, Du J. Crosstalk between oxidative stress and exosomes. Oxidative Medicine and Cellular Longevity. 2022;**2022**:3553617

[9] Hazawa M, Tomiyama K, Saotome-Nakamura A, Obara C, Yasuda T, Gotoh T, et al. Radiation increases the cellular uptake of exosomes through CD29/CD81 complex formation. Biochemical and Biophysical Research Communications. 2014;**446**(4):1165-1171

[10] Pant S, Hilton H, Burczynski ME. The multifaceted exosome: biogenesis, role in normal and aberrant cellular function, and frontiers for pharmacological and biomarker opportunities. Biochemical Pharmacology. 2012;**83**(11):1484-1494

[11] Parolini I, Federici C, Raggi C, Lugini L, Palleschi S, De Milito A, et al. Microenvironmental pH is a key factor for exosome traffic in tumor cells. Journal of Biological Chemistry. 2009;**284**(49):34211-34222

[12] de Gassart A, Géminard C, Février B, Raposo G, Vidal M. Lipid raft-associated protein sorting in exosomes. Blood. 2003;**102**(13):4336-4344

[13] Huang X, Yuan T, Tschannen M, Sun Z, Jacob H, Du M, et al. Characterization of human plasma-derived exosomal RNAs by deep sequencing. BMC Genomics. 2013;**14**:319

[14] Wang L, Hu L, Zhou X, Xiong Z, Zhang C, Shehada HM, et al. Exosomes secreted by human adipose mesenchymal stem cells promote scarless cutaneous repair by regulating extracellular matrix remodelling. Scientific Reports. 2017;**7**(1):13321

[15] Staubach S, Razawi H, Hanisch FG. Proteomics of MUC1-containing lipid

rafts from plasma membranes and exosomes of human breast carcinoma cells MCF-7. Proteomics. 2009;**9**(10):2820-2835

[16] Van Niel G, Mallegol J, Bevilacqua C, Candalh C, Brugiere S, Tomaskovic-Crook E, et al. Intestinal epithelial exosomes carry MHC class II/peptides able to inform the immune system in mice. Gut. 2003;**52**(12):1690-1697

[17] De Toro J, Herschlik L, Waldner C, Mongini C. Emerging roles of exosomes in normal and pathological conditions: new insights for diagnosis and therapeutic applications. Frontiers in Immunology. 2015;**6**:203

[18] Fevrier B, Vilette D, Archer F, Loew D, Faigle W, Vidal M, et al. Cells release prions in association with exosomes. Proceedings of the National Academy of Sciences. 2004;**101**(26):9683-9688

[19] Chivet M, Javalet C, Hemming F, Pernet-Gallay K, Laulagnier K, Fraboulet S, et al. Exosomes as a novel way of interneuronal communication. Biochemical Society Transactions. 2013;**41**(1):241-244

[20] Sheldon H, Heikamp E, Turley H, Dragovic R, Thomas P, Oon CE, et al. New mechanism for Notch signaling to endothelium at a distance by Delta-like 4 incorporation into exosomes. Blood. 2010;**116**:2385-2394

[21] Silbernagl S, Despopoulos A. Color Atlas of Physiology. 6th ed. New York: Thieme; 2009. 978-3-13-545006-3

[22] O'garra A, Vieira P. Regulatory T cells and mechanisms of immune system control. Nature Medicine. 2004;**10**(8):801-805

[23] Théry C, Duban L, Segura E, Véron P, Lantz O, Amigorena S. Indirect activation of naïve CD4+ T cells by dendritic cell–derived exosomes. Nature Immunology. 2002;**3**(12):1156-1162

[24] Admyre C, Johansson SM, Paulie S, Gabrielsson S. Direct exosome stimulation of peripheral humanT cells detected by ELISPOT. European Journal of Immunology. 2006;**36**(7):1772-1781

[25] Chen T, Guo J, Yang M, Zhu X, Cao X. Chemokine-containing exosomes are released from heat-stressed tumor cells via lipid raft-dependent pathway and act as efficient tumor vaccine. Journal of Immunology. 2011;**186**:2219-2228

[26] McKelvey KJ, Powell KL, Ashton AW, Morris JM, McCracken SA. Exosomes: mechanisms of uptake. Journal of Circulating Biomarkers. 2015;**4**:7

[27] Lim TS, Goh JKH, Mortellaro A, Lim CT, Hämmerling GJ, Ricciardi CP. CD80 and CD86 differentially regulate mechanical interactions of T cells with antigen-presenting dendritic cells and B-cells. PLoS One. 2012;7(9):e45185

[28] Zitvogel L, Regnault A, Lozier A, Wolfers J, Flament C, Tenza D, et al. Eradication of established murine tumors using a novel cell-free vaccine: dendritic cell derived exosomes. Nature Medicine. 1998;**4**(5):594-600

[29] Berckmans RJ, Nieuwland R, Kraan MC, Schaap MC, Pots D, Smeets TJ, et al. Synovial microparticles from arthritic patients modulate chemokine and cytokine release by synoviocytes. Arthritis Research & Therapy. 2005;7:1-9

[30] Cicero AL, Majkowska I, Nagase H, Di Liegro I, Troeberg L. Microvesicles shed by oligodendroglioma cells and

rheumatoid synovial fibroblasts contain aggrecanase activity. Matrix Biology. 2012;**31**(4):229-233

[31] Martínez-Lorenzo MJ, Anel A, Saez-Gutierrez B, Royo-Cañas M, Bosque A, Alava MA, et al. Rheumatoid synovial fluid T cells are sensitive to APO2L/TRAIL. Clinical Immunology. 2007;**122**(1):28-40

[32] Kim SH, Bianco NR, Shufesky WJ, Morelli AE, Robbins PD. Effective treatment of inflammatory disease models with exosomes derived from dendritic cells genetically modified to express IL-4. The Journal of Immunology. 2007;**179**(4):2242-2249

[33] Wen SW, Sceneay J, Lima LG, Wong CS, Becker M, Krumeich S, et al. The biodistribution and immune suppressive effects of breast cancer-derived exosomes. Cancer Research. 2016;**76**(23):6

[34] Schuler PJ, Saze Z, Hong CS, Muller L, Gillespie DG, Cheng D, et al. Human CD4+ CD39+ regulatory T cells produce adenosine upon co-expression of surface CD73 or contact with CD73+ exosomes or CD73+ cells. Clinical and Experimental Immunology. 2014;**177**(2):531-543

[35] Liu Y, Xiang X, Zhuang X, Zhang S, Liu C, Cheng Z, et al. Contribution of MyD88 to the tumor exosome-mediated induction of myeloid derived suppressor cells. The American Journal of Pathology. 2010;**176**(5):2490-2499

[36] Lu J, Wu J, Tian J, Wang S. Role of T cell-derived exosomes in immunoregulation. Immunologic Research. 2018;**66**:313-322

[37] Smyth LA, Ratnasothy K, Tsang JY, Boardman D, Warley A, Lechler R, et al. CD73 expression on extracellular vesicles derived from CD4+ CD25+ Foxp3+ T cells contributes to their regulatory function. European Journal of Immunology. 2013;**43**(9):2430-2440

[38] Yu X, Huang C, Song B, Xiao Y, Fang M, Feng J, et al. CD4+ CD25+ regulatory T cells-derived exosomes prolonged kidney allograft survival in a rat model. Cellular Immunology. 2013;**285**(1-2):62-68

[39] Zhang H, Xie Y, Li W, Chibbar R, Xiong S, Xiang J. CD4+ T cell-released exosomes inhibit CD8+ cytotoxic T-lymphocyte responses and antitumor immunity. Cellular & Molecular Immunology. 2011;**8**(1):23-30

[40] Wahlgren J, Karlson TDL, Glader P, Telemo E, Valadi H. Activated human T cells secrete exosomes that participate in IL-2 mediated immune response signaling. PLoS One. 2012;**7**(11):e49723

[41] Zhou WJ, Zhang J, Xie F, Wu JN, Ye JF, Wang J, et al. CD45RO-CD8+ T cell-derived exosomes restrict estrogen-driven endometrial cancer development via the ERβ/miR-765/PLP2/Notch axis. Theranostics. 2021;**11**(11):5330

[42] Vivier E, Tomasello E, Baratin M, Walzer T, Ugolini S. Functions of natural killer cells. Nature Immunology. 2008;**9**(5):503-510

[43] Ljunggren HG, Kärre K. In search of the 'missing self': MHC molecules and NK cell recognition. Immunology Today. 1990;**11**:237-244

[44] Caligiuri MA. Human natural killer cells. Blood, The Journal of the American Society of Hematology. 2008;**112**(3):461-469

[45] Mattiola I, Pesant M, Tentorio PF, Molgora M, Marcenaro E, Lugli E, et al. Priming of human resting NK cells by

autologous M1 macrophages via the engagement of IL-1β, IFN-β, and IL-15 pathways. Journal of Immunology. 2015;**195**:2818-2828

[46] Di Vito C, Mikulak J, Mavilio D. On the way to become a natural killer cell. Frontiers in Immunology. 2019;**10**:1812

[47] Habif G, Crinier A, André P, Vivier E, Narni-Mancinelli E. Targeting natural killer cells in solid tumors. Cellular & Molecular Immunology. 2019;**16**(5):415-422

[48] Diefenbach A, Colonna M, Koyasu S. Development, differentiation, and diversity of innate lymphoid cells. Immunity. 2014;**41**:354-365

[49] Sojka DK, Yang L, Yokoyama WM. Uterine natural killer cells. Frontiers in Immunology. 2019;**10**:960

[50] Victorino F, Sojka DK, Brodsky KS, McNamee EN, Masterson JC, Homann D, et al. Tissue-resident NK cells mediate ischemic kidney injury and are not depleted by anti-asialo-GM1 antibody. Journal of Immunology. 2015;**195**:4973-4985

[51] Cooper MA, Fehniger TA, Caligiuri MA. The biology of human natural killer-cell subsets. Trends in Immunology. 2001;**22**(11):633-640

[52] Guo W, Gao Y, Li N, Shao F, Wang C, Wang P, et al. Exosomes: New players in cancer (Review). Oncology Reports. 2017;**38**:665-675

[53] Zhang X, Yuan X, Shi H, Wu L, Qian H, Xu W. Exosomes in cancer: Small particle, big player. Journal of Hematology & Oncology. 2015;**8**:83

[54] Rajagopal C, Harikumar KB. The origin and functions of exosomes in cancer. Frontiers in Oncology. 2018;**8**:66

[55] Batista IA, Quintas ST, Melo SA. The interplay of exosomes and NK cells in cancer biology. Cancers. 2021;**13**(3):473

[56] Ruivo CF, Adem B, Silva M, Melo SA. The biology of cancer exosomes: Insights and new perspectives. Cancer Research. 2017;**77**:6480-6488

[57] Thakur BK, Zhang H, Becker A, Matei I, Huang Y, Costa-Silva B, et al. Double-stranded DNA in exosomes: A novel biomarker in cancer detection. Cell Research. 2014;**24**:766-769

[58] Yáñez-Mó M, Siljander P, Andreu Z, Zavec A, Borràs F, Buzas E, et al. Biological properties of extracellular vesicles and their physiological functions. Journal of Extracellular Vesicles. 2015;**4**:27066

[59] Whiteside TL. Immune modulation of T-cell and NK (natural killer) cell activities by TEXs (tumour-derived exosomes). Biochemical Society Transactions. 2013;**41**(1):245-251

[60] Li Q, Huang Q, Huyan T, Wang Y, Huang Q, et al. Bifacial effects of engineering tumour cell-derived exosomes on human natural killer cells. Experimental Cell Research. 2018;**363**(2):141-150

[61] Taylor DD, Gercel-Taylor C. Exosomes/microvesicles: Mediators of cancer-associated immunosuppressive microenvironments. Seminars in Immunopathology. 2011;**33**:441-454

[62] Gehrmann U, Näslund TI, Hiltbrunner S, Larssen P, Gabrielsson S. Harnessing the exosome-induced immune response for cancer immunotherapy. Seminars in Cancer Biology. 2014;**28**:58-67

[63] Kahlert C, Kalluri R. Exosomes in tumor microenvironment influence

cancer progression and metastasis. Journal of Molecular Medicine. 2013;**91**:431-437

[64] Wang Z, Chen JQ, Liu J, Tian L. Exosomes in tumor microenvironment: Novel transporters and biomarkers. Journal of Translational Medicine. 2016;**14**:297

[65] Huyan T, Du Y, Huang Q, Huang Q, Li Q. Uptake characterization of tumor cell-derived exosomes by natural killer cells. Iranian Journal of Public Health. 2018;**47**:803-813

[66] Zhao J, Schlößer H, Wang Z, Qin J, Li J, Popp F, et al. Tumor-derived extracellular vesicles inhibit natural killer cell function in pancreatic cancer. Cancers. 2019;**11**:874

[67] Vulpis E, Cecere F, Molfetta R, Soriani A, Fionda C, Peruzzi G, et al. Genotoxic stress modulates the release of exosomes from multiple myeloma cells capable of activating NK cell cytokine production: Role of HSP70/TLR2/NF-kB axis. Oncoimmunology. 2017;**6**:e1279372

[68] Munich S, Sobo-Vujanovic A, Buchser WJ, Beer-Stolz D, Vujanovic NL. Dendritic cell exosomes directly kill tumor cells and activate natural killer cells via TNF superfamily ligands. Oncoimmunology. 2012;**1**(7):1074-1083

[69] Jiang Y, Jiang H, Wang K, Liu C, Man X, Fu Q. Hypoxia enhances the production and antitumor effect of exosomes derived from natural killer cells. Annals of Translational Medicine. 2021;**9**(6):473

[70] Shoae-Hassani A, Hamidieh AA, Behfar M, Mohseni R, Mortazavi-Tabatabaei SA, Asgharzadeh S. NK cell-derived exosomes from NK cells previously exposed to neuroblastoma cells augment the antitumor activity of cytokine-activated NK cells. Journal of Immunotherapy (Hagerstown, Md.: 1997). 2017;**40**(7):265

[71] Ehrlich P. Beiträge zur theorie und praxis der histologischen Färbung. In: The Collected Papers of Paul Ehrlich. Pergamon, Turkey: Elsevier; 2013. pp. 29-64

[72] Shea-Donohue T, Stiltz J, Zhao A, Notari L. Mast cells. Current Gastroenterology Reports. 2010;**12**:349-357

[73] Krystel-Whittemore M, Dileepan KN, Wood JG. Mast cell: A multi-functional master cell. Frontiers in Immunology. 2016;**6**:620

[74] Zhang T, Finn DF, Barlow JW, Walsh JJ. Mast cell stabilisers. European Journal of Pharmacology. 2016;**778**:158-168

[75] da Silva EZ, Jamur MC, Oliver C. Mast cell function: A new vision of an old cell. The Journal of Histochemistry and Cytochemistry. 2014;**62**(10):698-738

[76] Galli SJ, Tsai M. Mast cells in allergy and infection: Versatile effector and regulatory cells in innate and adaptive immunity. European Journal of Immunology. 2010;**40**(7):1843-1851

[77] Weller CL, Collington SJ, Williams T, Lamb JR. Mast cells in health and disease. Clinical Science. 2011;**120**(11):473-484

[78] Collington SJ, Williams TJ, Weller CL. Mechanisms underlying the localisation of mast cells in tissues. Trends in Immunology. 2011;**32**(10):478-485

[79] Lecce M, Molfetta R, Milito ND, Santoni A, Paolini R. FcεRI signaling in the modulation of allergic response:

Role of mast cell-derived exosomes. International Journal of Molecular Sciences. 2020;**21**(15):5464

[80] Mukai K, Tsai M, Saito H, Galli SJ. Mast cells as sources of cytokines, chemokines, and growth factors. Immunological Reviews. 2018;**282**(1):121-150

[81] Norrby K. Mast cells and angiogenesis. APMIS. 2002;**110**(5):355-371

[82] Ekström K, Valadi H, Sjöstrand M, Malmhäll C, Bossios A, Eldh M, et al. Characterization of mRNA and microRNA in human mast cell-derived exosomes and their transfer to other mast cells and blood CD34 progenitor cells. Journal of Extracellular Vesicles. 2012;**1**(1):18389

[83] Xiao H, Lässer C, Shelke GV, Wang J, Rådinger M, Lunavat TR, et al. Mast cell exosomes promote lung adenocarcinoma cell proliferation—role of KIT-stem cell factor signaling. Cell Communication and Signaling. 2014;**12**:1-10

[84] Cho BS, Kim JO, Ha DH, Yi YW. Exosomes derived from human adipose tissue-derived mesenchymal stem cells alleviate atopic dermatitis. Stem cell Research & Therapy. 2018;**9**(1):1-5

[85] Huang K, Huang L, Zhang X, Zhang M, Wang Q, Lin H, et al. Mast cells-derived exosomes worsen the development of experimental cerebral malaria. Acta Tropica. 2021;**224**:106145

Chapter 4

Perspective Chapter: Exosome-Mediated Pathogen Transmission

Kundave Rajendran Venkataswamy

Abstract

Exosomes are membrane-bound vesicles. They are considered as waste-management system of cells, crucial for intercellular communication of information and have emerged to be mediators of pathogen transmission. Pathogen derived exosomes advance infections by suppression of host immune response, transmission of pathogen-related molecules and immune evasion. The ability of exosomes derived from the virus infected cells to modulate the host immune response and/or further viral replication in the host has been reported in several viruses infecting human and animals. Apart from the virus infected cells, parasites have also known to release exosomes, parasite derived exosomes help in the attachment of parasite to the host and facilitate evasion of host immune responses. Tick-derived exosomes aid transmission of vector-borne pathogens. Similar to certain viral and parasitic infections, exosomes derived from bacteria infected cells could also play a key role in dissemination of the infection. An understanding of the exosome mediated pathogen transmission, its pathway and host-pathogen interactions could pave way to discovery of novel therapeutic targets.

Keywords: exosomes, intercellular communication, pathogen transmission, immune response, viral replication, attachment of parasite, bacteria, therapeutic targets

1. Introduction

Exosomes are small extracellular vesicles ranging from 50 to 100 nm, that were first described in the late 1980s as "garbage bags" for cells to dispose the unwanted material and cellular waste from the cytosol. However, it has ever since become clear that they play a much broader role in intercellular communication by transferring bioactive molecules between cells [1]. Exosomes are composed of diverse bioactive molecules, such as proteins, lipids, and nucleic acids, such as DNA and RNA. These molecules can be taken up by other cells and influence cellular behavior, making exosomes a potentially important mode of intercellular communication. The two mechanisms of exosome biogenesis are the ESCRT-dependent and ESCRT-independent pathways [2]. The ESCRT-dependent pathway utilizes the endosomal sorting complexes required for transport (ESCRT) machinery which consists of several protein complexes (ESCRT-0, -I, -II, and -III) that recognize and cluster cargo molecules on the endosomal membrane and facilitate the

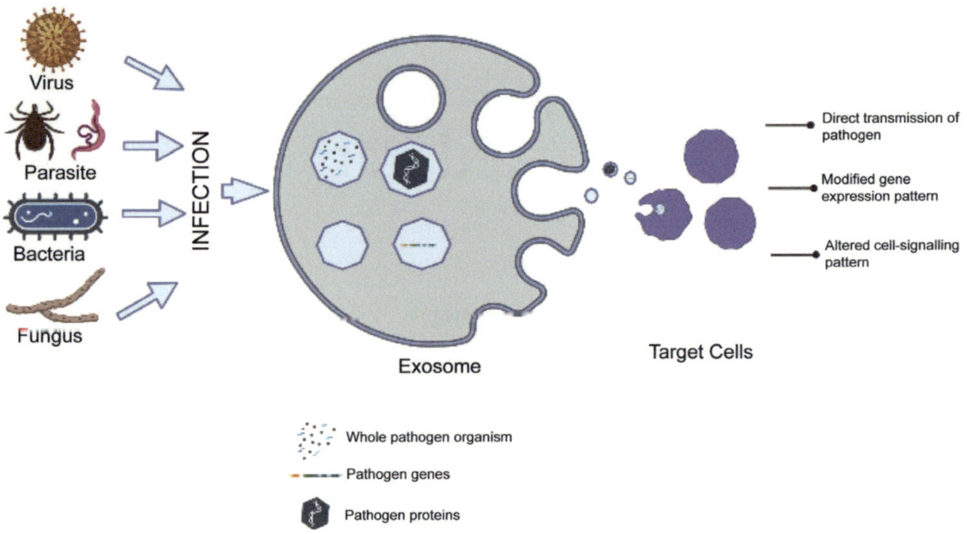

Figure 1.
Exosomes mediate further infection. Exosomes mediate further infection through transferring pathogen-related molecules (pathogenic genes and proteins) or even the entire pathogens. Therefore, exosomes can be either directly infectious, alter nuclear gene expression, or mediate toxic reactions.

budding of intraluminal vesicles (ILVs) within the lumen of late endosomes or multivesicular bodies (MVBs). After the formation of MVBs containing (ILVs), the MVBs either fuse with lysosomes for degradation or fuse with the plasma membrane for exosome release. The ESCRT-independent pathway, on the other hand, does not require the ESCRT machinery for cargo sorting and ILV formation. Instead, it involves the direct budding of the plasma membrane to form exosomes. This process is thought to be mediated by lipid rafts and tetraspanin-enriched microdomains on the plasma membrane, which recruit specific cargo molecules and drive the formation of small membrane vesicles [3, 4]. The resulting vesicles are then released into the extracellular space as exosomes. Exosomes are known to play a crucial role in infections as carriers of pathogen-related molecules. Microorganisms such as bacteria, Protozoa, and fungi have been found to secrete various types of microvesicles, including exosomes, which are used by pathogens to spread infection and evade the host immune system. In addition to these microorganisms, viruses, have been shown to stimulate the production of exosomes in host cells, which in turn can regulate the host immune response [5]. Exosomes can directly transmit substances of pathogen origin and also indirectly influence the progression of infection by modulating processes such as immune evasion and apoptosis (**Figure 1**). Thus, the study of microvesicles and their role in host-pathogen interactions is an important area of research that could lead to the development of new therapeutics for infectious diseases.

2. Exosome-mediated parasite transmission

Exosome research in parasite infections is particularly intriguing because it suggests that the communication between the host and the parasite via exosomes may play a key role in pathogenesis. Exosomal vesicles are an important component of microbial communication and can facilitate the exchange of genetic material, which can have significant implications for microbial evolution and adaptation [6].

2.1 Haemoprotozoan parasites

Studies have shown that promastigote and amastigote forms of *Leishmania donovani* and *Leishmania major* can release exosomes, which are detected in host cells and selectively induce IL-8 secretion from macrophages [7, 8]. The chemokinetic recruitment of neutrophils helps *Leishmania* invade cells and gain access to macrophages upon phagocytosis of the infected neutrophils. This process is thought to occur through the release of chemoattractants by the infected macrophages, which then recruit neutrophils to the site of infection [9, 10]. This suggests that exosomes released by *Leishmania* species may play a role in modulating the host immune response and contributing to the pathogenesis of leishmaniasis. Research has demonstrated that *Leishmania* exosomes can induce the release of the immunosuppressive cytokine IL-10 while inhibiting the inflammatory cytokine tumor necrosis factor (TNF) in human monocyte-derived dendritic cells (DCs) in response to interferon gamma (IFNg). Dendritic cells are a type of immune cell that play a crucial role in initiating and regulating immune responses. The inhibition of TNF and induction of IL-10 by *Leishmania* exosomes can have important implications for the ability of the immune system to effectively respond to and clear *Leishmania* infections. TNF is a pro-inflammatory cytokine that helps to recruit immune cells to sites of infection and activate their antimicrobial functions, while IL-10 is an immunosuppressive cytokine that can dampen immune responses and promote the persistence of pathogens [9]. Several protozoan parasites, including *Leishmania* species and *T. cruzi*, have been shown to release exosomes and/or microvesicles [11–13]. *Leishmania* species are the parasites that cause human leishmaniasis, while *T. cruzi* causes Chagas disease. Similarly, studies have shown that *T. cruzi* can release exosomes that contain parasite-derived molecules, such as proteins and nucleic acids, which can modulate the host immune response and aid in parasite survival and proliferation. *T. cruzi*-derived exosomes have also been shown to induce pro-inflammatory cytokine production and apoptosis in host cells [14]. *T. cruzi*-derived exosomes have also been shown to contain immunomodulatory molecules, including miRNAs, which can regulate theexpression of host immune genes and contribute to the pathogenesis of Chagas disease. *T. cruzi* induces the release of exosomes from infected host cells, which expresses TGF-β, which has proven to facilitate parasite invasion and maturation in host cells [15]. The exosomes are known to protect extracellular life cycle stages of *T. cruzi*, such as epimastigotes from the vector and trypomastigotes from ruptured cells, from complement-mediated attack, facilitating parasite invasion of host cells [16]. The secretion of exosomes by *Leishmania* spp. and *T. cruzi* induce the release of exosomes from the cells that they infect [7]. Extracellular vesicles (EVs) have been shown to play a role in intercellular communication between parasites. Recent studies have shown that microvesicles play a crucial role in the transmission of malaria caused by the *Plasmodium falciparum* parasite (DEBS). These microvesicles are small membrane-bound particles that are released by infected red blood cells and can interact with uninfected cells in the vicinity. It has been found that these microvesicles contain specific molecules that can influence the behavior of the parasite. In particular, they can increase the commitment of asexual parasites to differentiate into sexual stages, known as gametocytes. This is important for the transmission of the parasite, as only the sexual stages can be transmitted to mosquitoes and therefore continue the life cycle of the parasite. By increasing the production of gametocytes, the microvesicles can effectively enhance the transmission potential of the parasite, making it more likely to be passed on to mosquitoes and therefore increase the spread of malaria [17, 18].

2.1.1 *Plasmodium falciparum*

Malaria parasite *Plasmodium falciparum* has been found to use exosomes for communication between infected red blood cells. This communication between infected and uninfected red blood cells via exosomes is thought to play a key role in the pathogenesis of malaria [7]. Exosomal vesicles released from *P. falciparum* infected erythrocytes have been shown to help in parasite survival, transmission, density sensing and differentiation of gametocytes [19–21]. *Plasmodium falciparum*-infected RBCs (iRBCs) can communicate with each other via different mechanisms, including the exchange of genetic material through a process called cell cell transfer or tunneling nanotubes (TNTs). This communication can result in the increased production of gametocytes, which are the parasite's sexual forms that can be transmitted to mosquito vectors and infect other hosts. In addition to TNTs, iRBCs can also release exosome-like vesicles that contain different types of cargo, including proteins, lipids, and nucleic acids. These vesicles can be taken up by other iRBCs or host cells, modulating their functions and promoting parasite survival in different environments, such as drug pressure or immune attack. One of the proteins that play a critical role in exosome-like vesicle production in *P. falciparum* is PfPTP2. This protein is a phosphatase that regulates different signaling pathways in the parasite, including those involved in vesicle biogenesis and secretion. Disrupting PfPTP2 function can reduce exosome-like vesicle production and affect parasite survival and virulence.

2.2 Protozoan parasites

2.2.1 *Trichomonas vaginalis*

Trichomonas vaginalis, a parasitic protozoan that is responsible for the common sexually transmitted infection trichomoniasis, has been shown to release functional exosomes that play a role in both parasite-to-parasite and parasite-to-host communication. One study published in 2013 showed that *T. vaginalis* exosomes contained virulence products that could specifically downregulate the secretion of the pro-inflammatory cytokine IL-8 by ectocervical cells [22]. This downregulation of IL-8 secretion could potentially limit neutrophil migration, which in turn could prevent pathogen clearance and facilitate the establishment of infection. Furthermore, *T. vaginalis* exosomes have been shown to contain a range of other bioactive molecules, including proteins, lipids, and nucleic acids, that are capable of modulating host cell behavior. They are known to induce cell death in host immune cells, impair host cell signaling pathways, and modulate host cell gene expression. The detection of exosomes secreted by *T. vaginalis* suggests a potential role for these extracellular vesicles in the pathogenesis of trichomoniasis. Furthermore, the detection of specific parasite proteins in T. vaginalis exosomes suggests that these vesicles may also play a role in the parasite's adherence to host epithelial cells, which is a critical step in the infection process.

2.2.2 *Toxoplasma gondii*

Toxoplasmosis is known to be caused by *Toxoplasma gondii*. The human foreskin fibroblasts infected with *T. gondii* release a type of exosome-like vesicle that contains abundant miRNAs and shows a significant increase in mRNAs compared to uninfected fibroblasts. The mRNAs that are most enriched in these vesicles include thymosin beta 4, eukaryotic elongation factor-1α (EF-1α), Rab-13, and LLP homolog.

These mRNAs have been previously associated with neurologic activitysuggesting that *T. gondii* exosomes may play a role in mediating neurologic effects in toxoplasmosis, a parasitic disease caused by *T. gondii* [23].

2.3 Helminths

Various helminths, including trematodes like *Fasciola hepatica* and *Echinostoma caproni*, secrete exosomes and other extracellular vesicles (EVs) that can be internalized by host cells. Electron microscopy images have been used to study the morphology and distribution of EVs released by these helminths, including those that can be detected on the tegumental surface. The tegument is the outermost layer of the parasite, and it plays a critical role in the host-parasite interaction. By releasing EVs that can interact with the tegument, these helminths may be able to modulate the host immune response and evade host defenses [24]. Exosomes released by *Heligmosomoides polygyrus* (*H. polygyrus*), a parasitic helminth, can block the activation of type 2 innate lymphoid cells (ILC2s), which are immune cells that play a critical role in the host response to helminth infections. This blockade of ILC2 activation is thought to contribute to the ability of *H. polygyrus* to establish chronic infections in its host [25]. Furthermore, *H. polygyrus*-derived exosomes have downstream effects on eosinophilic recruitment. Eosinophils are immune cells that play a role in the host response to helminth infections, and studies have shown that *H. polygyrus*-derived exosomes can induce the recruitment of eosinophils to sites of infection. This recruitment is thought to be mediated by the activation of IL-5, a cytokine that plays a role in the production and recruitment of eosinophils. Analyses of the secretion products of the tapeworm *E. granulosus* have revealed the presence of exosome-associated proteins, including CD63-like tetraspanins. CD63 is a transmembrane protein that is commonly used as a marker of exosomes, and tetraspanins are a family of proteins that are associated with the membrane of exosomes and play a role in their biogenesis and function. The presence of CD63-like tetraspanins in the secretion products of *E. granulosus* suggests that the parasite is capable of releasing exosomes, which could play a role in the pathogenesis of echinococcosis [26]. Exosomes released by parasites such as *Heligmosomoides polygyrus*, *Schistosoma mansoni*, and *Schistosoma japonicum* have been shown to contain immunomodulatory molecules, including proteins and miRNAs, which can modulate the host immune response and aid in parasite survival and proliferation. Exosome-like extracellular vesicles (EVs) was isolated from excretory-secretory (ES) products of fourth stage larvae (Tci-L4ES) of *Telodorsagia circumcincta*, a parasitic nematode that affects sheep. Proteomic characterization of these EVs and identified several proteins involved in various functions such as structure and metabolism of the parasite. Importantly, it was found that some of these proteins can be bound by two types of antibodies, IgA and IgG, in *T. circumcincta*-infected sheep suggesting that these proteins may have potential as vaccine targets for the development and production of a vaccine against *T. circumcincta* infection [27]. Proteomic analysis could identify proteins carried by extracellular vesicles (EVs) released by tapeworms. Parasite-derived proteins such as antigen-5, severin/gelsolin/villin lipid transport protein, alpha-mannosidase, and malate-dehydrogenase, as well as host-origin proteins such as carbonic anhydrase, fructose-bisphosphate aldolase, peroxiredoxin, hemoglobin alpha and beta, pyruvate kinase, serum albumin, and triose phosphate isomerase were identified in the EVs. The study also revealed that the EVs carried virulence factors, including highly immunogenic and tolerogenic antigens and peptidases, that were associated with cyst survival. This finding suggests that EVs may play a crucial role in tapeworm infection [28].

2.3.1 Filarial parasites

Lymphatic filariasis is a parasitic disease caused by filarial worms, including *Brugia malayi*, *Wuchereria bancrofti*, and *Brugia timori*, which are transmitted through the bites of infected mosquitoes. Studies have suggested that extracellular vesicles (EVs), including exosomes, released by these worms may play a role in the pathogenesis of the disease [29]. Exosome-like vesicles secreted by the infective L3 stage of *B. malayi* are designated a set of proteins, including actin, EF-1α, EF-2, Rab-1, and HSP70, as exosome markers based on their presence in the vesicles. These proteins are known to be involved in various cellular processes, such as cytoskeletal organization, protein synthesis, and vesicle trafficking, suggesting that the EVs may play a role in modulating the host immune response and promoting parasite survival.

3. Exosome-mediated pathogen transmission by arthropods

Arthropods, such as ticks and mosquitoes, have been shown to release extracellular vesicles (EVs) in their saliva during feeding. EVs are double-layer vesicles that are secreted by all cells and play a critical role in cell-to-cell communication. These vesicles contain various molecules, including proteins, lipids, and nucleic acids, that can be transferred to other cells to influence their behavior. In the context of pathogen transmission, infected cells can secrete EVs that carry infectious cargo, such as viral RNA, which can enhance pathogen transmission and replication. This has been demonstrated in the case of Zika virus, where infected mosquito saliva was found to contain EVs that carry viral RNA and can promote infection in recipient cells. Ticks are ectoparasites that feed on the blood of their hosts, and their saliva contains a complex mixture of proteins, lipids, and other molecules that help them to obtain a blood meal and evade the host immune response. It is likely that EVs are also present in tick saliva and play a role in modulating the host immune response. The argasid tick *Ornithodoros moubata* secretes immunomodulatory proteins in the saliva. Proteomic analysis of tick saliva has revealed several exosome-associated proteins, such as aldolase and enolase, as well as lipocalins that have anti-inflammatory properties. These lipocalins can scavenge leukotrienes, which are inflammatory mediators, and adenosine nucleotides, which can modulate the immune response. It is reported that exosomes are critical for the transmission life cycle of Langat virus (LGTV), a tick-borne virus closely related to tick-borne encephalitis virus (TBEV), which is a causative agent of a neurological tick-borne disease [30]. A study demonstrated that LGTV can infect tick cells and replicate within them. The virus is then secreted into the extracellular space via. Exosomes, which are taken up by neighboring cells, including both tick and mammalian cells. The exosomes containing LGTV were found to be infectious and could transfer the virus from infected to uninfected cells, indicating that exosomes play a crucial role in LGTV transmission. Furthermore, research shows that the exosomal cargo of LGTV-infected tick cells contained viral RNA and proteins, which could induce an antiviral response in uninfected cells, potentially limiting viral spread. It is also suggested that exosomes derived from neuronal cells are likely able to mediate transmission of tick-borne flavivirus RNA and proteins from one neuronal cell to the other in the CNS. These findings suggest that exosomes play a complex role in the transmission and pathogenesis of LGTV, and potentially other related tick-borne viruses such as TBEV. RNAi-mediated silencing of synaptobrevin expression in *A. americanum* adult ticks resulted in a significant decrease in feeding success. Specifically, the silenced ticks exhibited increased mortality, premature detachment from the host, and lower engorgement weights compared to control ticks. These findings suggest that synaptobrevin is critical for successful tick feeding and survival [31]. Arthropods such as mosquitoes are known to be important vectors for the transmission of flaviviruses, including DENV. Recent studies have shown that arthropod-derived EVs can contain viral RNA, including full-length viral genomes, and can transfer this RNA to neighboring cells or even to other hosts, potentially leading to the spread of infection. In addition to DENV, other flaviviruses such as Zika virus, Japanese encephalitis virus, and West Nile virus have also been shown to be transmitted by arthropod vectors and may potentially be contained within EVs. The mechanisms by which flaviviruses are packaged into arthropod-derived EVs and how they are transmitted to new hosts are not yet fully understood, and further research is needed to elucidate these processes. However, the discovery of viral RNA in arthropod EVs suggests that these structures may play an important role in the transmission and dissemination of flaviviruses.

4. Exosome mediated fungal transmission

In addition to the parasites, other eukaryotes such as pathogenic fungi also release extracellular vesicles (EVs) that play important role in mediating the pathogenesis. Exosomes can play a role in the proliferation of fungal infections by several mechanisms. Firstly, fungal exosomes can carry virulence factors and antigens that can directly contribute to the pathogenesis of the infection. For example, fungal exosomes have been shown to contain proteins and lipids that promote the adhesion and invasion of host cells, as well as molecules that suppress the immune response and promote the survival of the pathogen within the host. Secondly, exosomes secreted by infected host cells can also indirectly promote the proliferation of fungal infections by modulating immune responses. For instance, exosomes released by infected immune cells can contain cytokines and other immune modulators that suppress the activity of immune cells, such as macrophages and neutrophils, which are crucial for controlling fungal infections. This, in turn, can facilitate the proliferation of the fungus within the host. Moreover, recent studies suggest that exosomes may play a role in the horizontal transfer of antifungal resistance among fungal populations. Fungal exosomes can carry genetic material, such as RNA and DNA, which can be transferred to other fungi, leading to the acquisition of antifungal resistance. Exosomes can proliferate fungal infections by carrying virulence factors, modulating immune responses. For example, the pathogenic fungus *Paracoccidioides brasiliensis* releases highly immunogenic EVs that contain the carbohydrate galactose-/-1,3-galactose (/-Gal), which is not found in human cells. These/-Gal-enriched EVs may generate a robust immune response in the host, but they may also be beneficial to the pathogen by binding to host lectins and potentially stimulating a suppressive type 2 response. Other opportunistic fungi, including *Cryptococcus neoformans*, *Candida albicans*, and *Histoplasma capsulatum*, also release EVs that contain virulence-associated factors such as polysaccharides and lipids [32]. For example, *C. neoformans* EVs are enriched in virulent capsular components such as glucosylceramide and glucuronoxylomannan (GXM), and a recent study has shown that phospholipid translocases (flippases) are important for *C. neoformans* exosome packaging and transport [33]. Interestingly, fungus-released EVs can also induce antimicrobial activity by host cells. *C. neoformans* EVs are taken up by macrophages and stimulate the production of TNF, IL-10, TGF-b, and nitric oxide [34]. EVs released by *Malassezia sympodialis*, a component of human flora, can generate IL-4 and TNF secretion from peripheral blood mononuclear cells, enhancing an inflammatory response in cases of atopic dermatitis [35].

5. Exosome mediated bacteria transmission

Extracellular vesicles (EVs) have been identified as a mechanism for dissemination of bacterial components. Gram-negative bacteria such as *Escherichia coli* and *Salmonella* have been shown to produce outer membrane vesicles (OMVs) that contain lipopolysaccharide (LPS), a potent endotoxin that can trigger an inflammatory response in host cells. OMVs have also been shown to carry other virulence factors, such as adhesins and toxins, and can promote bacterial survival and dissemination within the host. Similarly, Gram-positive bacteria such as *Staphylococcus aureus* and *Streptococcus pyogenes* have been shown to release membrane vesicles that carry lipoteichoic acid (LTA), another pathogen-associated molecular pattern (PAMP) that can activate host immune responses. In addition to OMVs and membrane vesicles, bacteria can also release exosomes, which are thought to originate from the bacterial cytoplasmic membrane and can carry a range of bacterial components, including nucleic acids, proteins, and lipids. Extracellular vesicles (EVs) are a newly described mechanism for bacterial dissemination and can contribute to the pathogenesis of bacterial infections.

5.1 *Mycobacterium* spp.

In the case of bacterial infections, much of our understanding of exosome production and function comes from studies on *Mycobacteria*. Additionally, there is increasing evidence that other bacterial species also produce exosomes that contribute to disease pathogenesis. Mycobacterial exosomes have been shown to carry bacterial components that modulate host immune responses and promote bacterial survival, as well as contributing to the dissemination of mycobacteria to other cells and tissues in the host. *Mycobacterium avium*-infected macrophages release vesicles that can stimulate a pro-inflammatory response in neighboring macrophages that are not infected [36]. *Mycobacterium tuberculosis* PAMPs can be transported from the phagosome to the MVB during macrophage infection, and these PAMPs are also found in extracellular vesicles released by infected macrophages [37]. These vesicles have been shown to have markers of a late endosomal/lysosomal compartment and are released through calcium-dependent exocytosis, suggesting that they are exosomes [38]. The content of these exosomes can be detected inside neighboring uninfected cells, suggesting a potential role in intercellular communication during infection. The release of pro-inflammatory exosomes has also been observed in macrophages infected with *Mycobacterium tuberculosis* or *Mycobacterium bovis* BCG. These exosomes carry mycobacterial components that can stimulate an immune response and contribute to disease pathogenesis. The pro-inflammatory response is thought to be mediated by the activation of pattern recognition receptors (PRRs) on the surface of the macrophages, which recognize the mycobacterial components carried by the exosomes. This activation leads to the production of pro-inflammatory cytokines and chemokines that recruit and activate other immune cells to the site of infection. While mycobacterial exosomes have been shown to stimulate pro-inflammatory responses in macrophages, it is also possible that the mycobacterial components present on or in the exosomes could function to suppress the immune response. Mycobacterial exosomes can carry immunosuppressive components, such as mycobacterial lipids, that can downregulate the immune response and promote bacterial survival within host cells. In addition to carrying immunosuppressive components, mycobacterial exosomes may also promote bacterial persistence by facilitating intercellular communication and promoting the formation of bacterial aggregates within host cells. This can protect the bacteria from immune surveillance and promote their survival within the host. Exosomes have been shown to play a role in anthrax infection by serving as carriers of anthrax toxin components [39]. Tissue factor, is a blood coagulation protein that is also involved in a variety of cellular processes such as cell proliferation, migration, and apoptosis. It has been found on the surface of various cell types, including endothelial cells and macrophages.

5.2 *Helicobacter pylori*

miRNA expression in exosomes plays a role in the regulation of inflammation in macrophages and can affect the infectivity and pathogenicity of *Helicobacter pylori*. Specifically, miR-155 expression in exosomes derived from *H. pylori*-infected macrophages was found to increase significantly and could be delivered to surrounding macrophages to induce a stronger inflammatory response. Moreover, miR-155 loaded in exosomes derived from *H. pylori*-infected macrophages was found to promote the production of cytokines such as TNF-α, IL-6, and IL-23 to regulate inflammatory responses, thereby enhancing the expressions of cellular signal transduction proteins such as CD40, CD63, CD81, and MHC-I for immune-regulation responses. However, overactive macrophages can produce a multitude of proinflammatory cytokines and chemokines, leading to inflammation-related diseases or autoimmune diseases. During *H. pylori* infection, exosomes may act as vectors to carry virulence factors or proteins of *H. pylori* to host cells and target organs, thus playing a role in the pathogenicity of *H. pylori* [18].

5.3 *Bacteroides fragilis*

Bacteroides fragilis, a representative strain of *Bacteroides* spp., has been found to enhance immune function. This is achieved through the transfer of bacterial lipopolysaccharide to intestinal dendritic cells via exosomes. This process promotes the secretion of IL-10 and IL-6 by dendritic cells and the differentiation of T lymphocytes, which in turn intensifies the immune reactions of the host. Exosomes, which are closely associated with bacterial infection, are believed to act as signal transduction messengers [40].

5.4 Other bacteria

It is shown that "microparticles" released from *Chlamydia pneumoniae*-infected cells contain tissue factor, and that these microparticles can activate NF-κB, a transcription factor involved in the regulation of TF expression in endothelial cells suggesting that *Chlamydia pneumoniae* may use exosomes or exosome-like vesicles as a mechanism for spreading the infection and modulating host cell responses [37]. Other bacterial species, such as *Pseudomonas aeruginosa*, *Burkholderia cenocepacia*, and *Staphylococcus aureus*, also produce exosomes that carry virulence factors and other bacterial components, which can modulate host immune responses and promote bacterial survival and dissemination. *Chlamydia trachomatis* is an intracellular bacterial pathogen that causes a variety of diseases in humans, including sexually transmitted infections and ocular infections. To establish and maintain infection, *C. trachomatis* has evolved several mechanisms to interact with host cells and manipulate host cellular processes.

One such mechanism is the release of host cell vesicles that contain bacterial effector proteins. These vesicles can be internalized by neighboring cells, allowing *C. trachomatis* to spread and establish new infection foci. Several cytotoxic and secreted proteins have been identified in these host vesicles, and they are believed to play a role in the delivery of virulence factors. One such protein is CT166, a cytotoxic protein that has been shown to induce cell death in host cells. Another is CT694, a secreted protein that has been shown to interact with host proteins involved in cell signaling pathways. These proteins, along with others found in host vesicles, likely play a critical role in *C. trachomatis* pathogenesis by facilitating the delivery of virulence factors and manipulating host cellular processes to the bacterium's advantage. Exosomes have been found to play a role in the pathogenicity of *Staphylococcus aureus*, specifically through the actions of the pore-forming α-toxin [41]. This toxin targets human non-virally transformed keratinocytes (HaCaT cells) and can be endocytosed by the cells to prevent cell lysis. The toxin-containing vesicles are then transported to late endosomes and incorporated into exosomes, which are secreted by the cells [42]. Interestingly, these exosomes contain both mono- and multi-meric toxins, which can be activated after being taken up by naive cells. This mechanism allows the bacteria to spread its virulence factors and evade the immune system, ultimately leading to the development of infections.

6. Exosome-mediated viral transmission

Exosomes have been shown to play a role in a range of viral infections, including HIV, Hepatitis B and C, Influenza, and Zika virus, among others. Exosomes can contribute to viral pathogenesis by promoting viral replication and spread, inducing apoptosis in infected cells, and modulating the immune response to favor viral persistence. Additionally, exosomes can serve as vehicles for the transfer of viral components, including nucleic acids and proteins, between cells, facilitating viral spread and potentially contributing to the development of chronic infections. Viruses can hijack the host cell's exosomal pathway to promote the transfer of viral components, including nucleic acids such as viral RNA or DNA, between cells. Exosomes containing viral genomes can be taken up by susceptible cells, potentially leading to the establishment of a productive viral infection. When a cell is infected with a virus, it may secrete exosomes that contain viral components. These exosomes can then be taken up by other cells, potentially leading to the spread of the virus. Exosomes derived from viral-infected cells can contain a range of viral components, including viral proteins, nucleic acids (such as RNA or DNA), and even intact viruses themselves. These exosomes can therefore serve as a means of exporting viral components from the infected cell, potentially contributing to viral pathogenesis [43, 44]. The viral components contained within exosomes derived from viral-infected cells can contribute to the pathophysiological effects on recipient cells. These effects can be mediated by a variety of mechanisms, including the activation of cellular signaling pathways, the induction of inflammation, and the suppression of antiviral responses.

6.1 Human immunodeficiency virus (HIV)

Exosomes derived from HIV-infected cells have been shown to contain viral proteins that can induce apoptosis (programmed cell death) in recipient cells. Similarly, exosomes derived from cells infected with the Respiratory Syncytial Virus (RSV) have been shown to contain viral proteins that can trigger an inflammatory response in recipient cells. HIV-1 is known to exploit exosomes to facilitate viral spread and evade host immune responses. The transfer of HIV-1 coreceptors CCR5 and CXCR4 within exosomes from infected to uninfected cells is one mechanism by which the virus can enhance its infectivity and spread to new cells. Exosomes from HIV-1-infected cells can transfer viral proteins and RNA to uninfected cells, leading to the activation of host immune responses and the promotion of viral replication and dissemination [45, 46]. In addition to promoting viral spread, exosomes can also serve as a mechanism for the virus to evade host immune surveillance. HIV-1 has been shown to use exosomes to downregulate host immune responses by transferring viral proteins such as Nef and Vpu to immune cells, leading to the degradation of host immune factors such as CD4 and MHC class I molecules [47].

6.2 Hepatitis A virus (HAV)

Exosomes can acquire Hepatitis A Virus (HAV) components after HAV-infected plasmacytoid dendritic cells. These exosomes can protect HAV from neutralization by HAV antibodies and assist in the transmission of HAV among liver cells. Additionally, these HAV-carrying exosomes can also directly invade and infect uninfected cells with modest pathogenicity. In the case of HAV, infected plasmacytoid dendritic cells can release exosomes containing HAV components, which can then be taken up by uninfected liver cells. These exosomes can protect HAV from neutralization by HAV antibodies, allowing the virus to more easily infect liver cells and spread throughout the liver [48].

6.3 Hepatitis C virus (HCV)

In the case of HCV, studies have shown that the virus can incorporate into exosomes either as whole virions or as nucleocapsids, envelope proteins, and replication-competent viral RNA. The mechanism by which HCV incorporates into exosomes and how this process is regulated is not yet fully understood. However, it is believed that the incorporation of HCV into exosomes may help the virus to evade the immune system and spread throughout the body and play a role in the pathogenesis of HCV infection [49]. Hepatitis C virus (HCV) is a small enveloped virus with a positive-sense single-stranded RNA genome, belonging to the Flaviviridae family. Recent research has shown that the assembly and release of HCV virions in hepatocytes are closely correlated with the exosome secretory pathway. This pathway can incorporate either the whole virions or only nucleocapsids, envelope proteins, and replication-competent viral RNA into exosomes. In addition to classical transmission by free viral particles, HCV can also be transferred by exosomes to naive human hepatoma Huh7.5.1 cells, resulting in productive infection with efficiency like that of free infectious particles. Exosomes derived from HCV-infected Huh7.5 cells or individuals both contain miR-122, which promotes HCV replication and transfer. Exosomes can transmit HCV to naive cells and modestly protect antibodies from being neutralized by HCV. This suggests that HCV may use transmission via exosomes as an immune evasion mechanism, allowing it to resist neutralization by anti-HCV antibodies.

6.4 Epstein-Barr virus (EBV)

Epstein-Barr virus (EBV), exosomes are known to play a role in the maintenance of latent infection. EBV is a virus that can cause infectious mononucleosis and is associated with several types of cancer. When EBV infects a cell, it can enter a latent phase in which it remains in the host cell without causing any symptoms. During this phase, the virus can be reactivated and start replicating, leading to the production of new viral particles and the spread of infection. EBV can exploit exosomes to deliver its genetic material, including proteins, RNA, and miRNA, to target cells. This allows the virus to maintain its latent infection in the host by regulating the expression of viral and host genes [50]. Apart from Burkitt lymphoma and nasopharyngeal carcinoma, EBV has also been linked to other malignancies, including Hodgkin's lymphoma, gastric cancer, and certain types of lymphomas and leukemias. Exosomes released by EBV-infected cells can play a role in the pathogenesis of these diseases by transferring viral proteins, RNA, and miRNA to surrounding cells and tissues. This can lead to the activation of signaling pathways that promote tumor growth and metastasis, as well as the suppression of host immune responses against the virus and cancer cells. Therefore, understanding the role of exosomes in EBV-associated malignancies may provide new insights into the mechanisms of tumor progression and immune evasion, as well as potential targets for therapeutic intervention [51].

6.5 Herpes simplex virus (HSV)

Exosomes derived from Herpes Simplex Virus (HSV) infected cells have been shown to contain viral proteins, RNA, and miRNAs that can be transmitted to uninfected cells and modulate their gene expression to promote viral replication and transmission [52]. The presence of these viral components in exosomes suggests that they may play a role in HPV-mediated immune evasion and tumor progression. Furthermore, the ability of exosomes to transfer their contents to neighboring cells may contribute to the spread of HPV infection. Dias et al. [53]. found that the prion protein (PRNP) plays a role in directing multivesicular bodies (MVBs) containing intraluminal vesicles (ILVs) toward the plasma membrane for the release of exosomes. Specifically, PRNP was shown to interact with components of the endosomal sorting complex required for transport (ESCRT) machinery, which is involved in the formation of ILVs within MVBs. This interaction was found to promote the association of MVBs with the plasma membrane and the subsequent release of exosomes. These findings suggest that PRNP may play a key role in regulating the secretion of exosomes in various physiological and pathological contexts.

6.6 Porcine reproductive and respiratory syndrome virus (PRRSV)

Exosomes derived from Porcine Reproductive and Respiratory Syndrome Virus (PRRSV)-infected cells can contain viral RNAs and transfer productive infections to naive cells, even in the presence of PRRSV-specific neutralizing antibodies (NAbs). PRRSV is a highly contagious virus that causes significant economic losses to the swine industry worldwide. The virus is known to replicate in the respiratory tract and can cause respiratory distress in infected pigs, as well as reproductive failure in pregnant sows. Recent studies have shown that exosomes derived from PRRSV-infected cells can contain viral RNAs, proteins, and even infectious virions. These exosomes can then be taken up by naive cells, which can lead to the establishment of a productive infection. It has been shown that PRRSV-specific NAbs are not effective in neutralizing the virus when it is packaged within exosomes. This suggests that exosomes may provide a mechanism for PRRSV to evade the host immune response and spread the infection to other cells [54].

6.7 West Nile virus (WNV)

It has been demonstrated that exosomes containing mosquito-borne West Nile Virus (WNV) can facilitate the transmission of viral RNA and proteins from one neuronal cell to others, suggesting a potential role for exosomes in WNV neuropathogenesis. West Nile Virus is a neurotropic virus that can cause severe neurological disease in humans and animals. The virus is thought to replicate in neurons and can spread from cell to cell within the nervous system. Recent studies have shown that exosomes derived from WNV-infected cells can contain viral RNA and proteins, which can be transferred to neighboring neuronal cells. This suggests that exosomes may play a role in the spread of WNV within the nervous system [44]. Furthermore, it has been suggested that exosomes may also be involved in the development of WNV neuropathogenesis, as the transfer of viral RNA and proteins to neighboring cells may alter the function of the recipient cells and contribute to disease progression.

7. Conclusion

In conclusion, exosomes play a significant role in mediating pathogen transmission between cells. Through their ability to transfer various types of bioactive molecules, including nucleic acids, proteins, and lipids, exosomes can facilitate the transfer of infectious agents, including bacteria, viruses, and parasites. Exosomes have been shown to act as vectors for the spread of several human pathogens, including HIV, HCV, and prion proteins. In addition, exosomes released from infected cells can promote the spread of infection by suppressing the host immune response and facilitating pathogen replication. However, the mechanisms by which exosomes mediate pathogen transmission are still not fully understood, and further research is needed to better characterize the specific roles of exosomes in the pathogenesis of different infectious diseases. Additionally, the potential use of exosomes as diagnostic markers or therapeutic targets for infectious diseases warrants further investigation. Despite the remaining uncertainties, the emerging evidence suggests that exosome-mediated pathogen transmission is a crucial aspect of infectious disease biology and has significant implications for the development of new diagnostic and therapeutic approaches.

Author details

Kundave Rajendran Venkataswamy
Tanuvas Veterinary College and Research Institute, Orathanadu, Tamil Nadu, India

*Address all correspondence to: kun.vet@gmail.com

References

[1] Jaiswal R, Sedger LM. Intercellular vesicular transfer by exosomes, microparticles and oncosomes-implications for cancer biology and treatments. Frontiers in Oncology. 2019;**9**:125

[2] Yousef MH, Abdelnaser A. Exosomes: Biological couriers with transformative messages. Journal of Biomedicine. 2019;**4**:14-34

[3] Platta HW, Stenmark H. Endocytosis and signaling. Current Opinion in Cell Biology. 2011;**23**(4):393-403

[4] Beach A, Zhang HG, Ratajczak MZ, Kakar SS. Exosomes: An overview of biogenesis, composition and role in ovarian cancer. Journal of Ovarian Research. 2014;**7**:1-11

[5] Schwab A, Meyering SS, Lepene B, Iordanskiy S, Van Hoek ML, Hakami RM, et al. Extracellular vesicles from infected cells: Potential for direct pathogenesis. Frontiers in Microbiology. 2015;**6**:1132

[6] Silverman JM, Chan SK, Robinson DP, Dwyer DM, Nandan D, Foster LJ, et al. Proteomic analysis of the secretome of *Leishmania donovani*. Genome Biology. 2008;**9**:1-21

[7] Coakley G, Maizels RM, Buck AH. Exosomes and other extracellular vesicles: The new communicators in parasite infections. Trends in Parasitology. 2015;**31**(10):477-489

[8] Levings MK, Reiner NE, Lynn MA, McMaster WR, Foster LJ, Wang AY, et al. Leishmania exosomes modulate. Journal of Immunology. 2010;**185**:5011-5022

[9] Silverman JM, Clos J, Horakova E, Wang AY, Wiesgigl M, Kelly I, et al. Leishmania exosomes modulate innate and adaptive immune responses through effects on monocytes and dendritic cells. The Journal of Immunology. 2010;**185**(9):5011-5022

[10] van Zandbergen G, Klinger M, Mueller A, Dannenberg S, Gebert A, Solbach W, et al. Cutting edge: Neutrophil granulocyte serves as a vector for Leishmania entry into macrophages. The Journal of Immunology. 2004;**173**(11):6521-6525

[11] Bayer-Santos E, Aguilar-Bonavides C, Rodrigues SP, Cordero EM, Marques AF, Varela-Ramirez A, et al. Proteomic analysis of Trypanosoma cruzisecretome: Characterization of two populations of extracellular vesicles and soluble proteins. Journal of Proteome Research. 2013;**12**(2):883-897

[12] Garcia-Silva MR, Cura das NevesRF, Cabrera-CabreraF, SanguinettiJ, MedeirosLC, RobelloC, et al. Extracellular vesicles shed by Trypanosoma cruzi are linked to small RNA pathways, life cycle regulation, and susceptibility to infection of mammalian cells. Parasitology Research. 2014;**113**:285-304

[13] Torrecilhas ACT, Tonelli RR, Pavanelli WR, da Silva JS, Schumacher RI, de Souza W, et al. Trypanosoma cruzi: Parasite shed vesicles increase heart parasitism and generate an intense inflammatory response. Microbes and Infection. 2009;**11**(1):29-39

[14] Lovo-Martins MI, Malvezi AD, Zanluqui NG, Lucchetti BFC, Tatakihara VLH, Mörking PA, et al. Extracellular vesicles shed by Trypanosoma cruzi potentiate infection and elicit lipid body formation and PGE2

production in murine macrophages. Frontiers in Immunology. 2018;**9**:896

[15] Cestari I, Ansa-Addo E, Deolindo P, Inal JM, Ramirez MI. Trypanosoma cruzi immune evasion mediated by host cell-derived microvesicles. The Journal of Immunology. 2012;**188**(4):1942-1952

[16] Cestari I, Ramirez MI. Inefficient complement system clearance of Trypanosoma cruzi metacyclic trypomastigotes enables resistant strains to invade eukaryotic cells. PLoS One. 2010;**5**(3):e9721

[17] Mantel PY, Hoang AN, Goldowitz I, Potashnikova D, Hamza B, Vorobjev I, et al. Malaria-infected erythrocyte-derived microvesicles mediate cellular communication within the parasite population and with the host immune system. Cell Host & Microbe. 2013;**13**(5):521-534

[18] Regev-Rudzki N, Wilson DW, Carvalho TG, Sisquella X, Coleman BM, Rug M, et al. Cell-cell communication between malaria-infected red blood cells via exosome-like vesicles. Cell. 2013;**153**(5):1120-1133

[19] Vimonpatranon S, Roytrakul S, Phaonakrop N, Lekmanee K, Atipimonpat A, Srimark N, et al. Extracellular vesicles derived from early and late stage plasmodium falciparum-infected red blood cells contain invasion-associated proteins. Journal of Clinical Medicine. 2022;**11**(14):4250

[20] Nilsson SK, Childs LM, Buckee C, Marti M. Targeting human transmission biology for malaria elimination. PLoS Pathogens. 2015;**11**(6):e1004871

[21] Mwangi JS. The Impact of Plasmodium falciparum Small-Sized Extracellular Vesicles (PfsEVs) and Plasmodium falciparum-Infected Red Blood Cells (PfiRBCs) on Host Immune Cells in Vitro (Doctoral dissertation. JKUAT-COHES; 2022

[22] Twu O, de Miguel N, Lustig G, Stevens GC, Vashisht AA, Wohlschlegel JA, et al. Trichomonas vaginalis exosomes deliver cargo to host cells and mediate host: parasite interactions. PLoS Pathogens. 2013;**9**(7):e1003482

[23] Dlugonska H, Gatkowska J. Exosomes in the context of toxoplasma gondii-host communication. Annals of Parasitology. 2016;**62**(3)

[24] Marcilla A, Trelis M, Cortés A, Sotillo J, Cantalapiedra F, Minguez MT, et al. Extracellular vesicles from parasitic helminths contain specific excretory/secretory proteins and are internalized in intestinal host cells; PLoS ONE. 2012;**7**(9):e45974

[25] Humphreys NE, Xu D, Hepworth MR, Liew FY, Grencis RK. IL-33, a potent inducer of adaptive immunity to intestinal nematodes. The Journal of Immunology. 2008;**180**(4):2443-2449

[26] Parkinson J, Wasmuth JD, Salinas G, Bizarro CV, Sanford CA, et al. Transcriptomic Analysis of Echinococcus Granulosus Larval Stages: Implications for Parasite Biology and Host Adaptation. PLoS Negl Trop Dis. 2012;**6**(11):e1897

[27] Machín C, Corripio-Miyar Y, Hernández JN, Pérez-Hernández T, Hayward AD, Wright HW, et al. Cellular and humoral immune responses associated with protection in sheep vaccinated against Teladorsagia circumcincta. Veterinary Research. 2021;**52**(1):89

[28] Siles-Lucas M, Sánchez-Ovejero C, González-Sánchez M, González E, Falcón-Pérez JM, Boufana B, et al. Isolation and characterization of

exosomes derived from fertile sheep hydatid cysts. Veterinary Parasitology. 2017;**236**:22-33

[29] Zamanian M, Fraser LM, Agbedanu PN, Harischandra H, Moorhead AR, Day TA, et al. Release of small RNA-containing exosome-like vesicles from the human filarial parasite Brugia malayi. PLoS Neglected Tropical Diseases. 2015;**9**(9):e0004069

[30] Zhou W, Woodson M, Neupane B, Bai F, Sherman MB, Choi KH, et al. Exosomes serve as novel modes of tick-borne flavivirus transmission from arthropod to human cells and facilitates dissemination of viral RNA and proteins to the vertebrate neuronal cells. PLoS Pathogens. 2018;**14**(1):e1006764

[31] Karim S, Miller NJ, Valenzuela J, Sauer JR, Mather TN. RNAi-mediated gene silencing to assess the role of synaptobrevin and cystatin in tick blood feeding. Biochemical and Biophysical Research Communications. 2005;**334**(4):1336-1342

[32] Rodrigues ML, Nimrichter L, Oliveira DL, Nosanchuk JD, Casadevall A. Vesicular trans-cell wall transport in fungi: A mechanism for the delivery of virulence-associated macromolecules? Lipid Insights. 2008;**2**:LPI-S1000

[33] Rodrigues ML, Nakayasu ES, Oliveira DL, Nimrichter L, Nosanchuk JD, Almeida IC, et al. Extracellular vesicles produced by Cryptococcus neoformans contain protein components associated with virulence. Eukaryotic Cell. 2008;**7**(1):58-67

[34] Rizzo J, Oliveira DL, Joffe LS, Hu G, Gazos-Lopes F, Fonseca FL, et al. Role of the Apt1 protein in polysaccharide secretion by Cryptococcus neoformans. Eukaryotic Cell. 2014;**13**(6):715-726

[35] Gehrmann U, Qazi KR, Johansson C, Hultenby K, Karlsson M, Lundeberg L, et al. Nanovesicles from Malassezia sympodialis and host exosomes induce cytokine responses–novel mechanisms for host-microbe interactions in atopic eczema. PLoS One. 2011;**6**(7):e21480

[36] Bhatnagar S, Schorey JS. Exosomes released from infected macrophages contain Mycobacterium avium glycopeptidolipids and are proinflammatory. Journal of Biological Chemistry. 2007;**282**(35):25779-25789

[37] Schorey JS, Cheng Y, Singh PP, Smith VL. Exosomes and other extracellular vesicles in host–pathogen interactions. EMBO Reports. 2015;**16**(1):24-43

[38] Mohammadzadeh R, Ghazvini K, Farsiani H, Soleimanpour S. Mycobacterium tuberculosis extracellular vesicles: Exploitation for vaccine technology and diagnostic methods. Critical Reviews in Microbiology. 2021;**47**(1):13-33

[39] Abrami L, Brandi L, Moayeri M, Brown MJ, Krantz BA, Leppla SH, et al. Hijacking multivesicular bodies enables long-term and exosome-mediated long-distance action of anthrax toxin. Cell Reports. 2013;**5**(4):986-996

[40] Wang J, Deng Z, Wang Z, Wu J, Gu T, Jiang Y, et al. MicroRNA-155 in exosomes secreted from helicobacter pylori infection macrophages immunomodulates inflammatory response. American Journal of Translational Research. 2016;**8**(9):3700

[41] Samuelson JC, Caulfield JP. The cercarial glycocalyx of Schistosoma mansoni. The Journal of Cell Biology. 1985;**100**(5):1423-1434

[42] Husmann M, Beckmann E, Boller K, Kloft N, Tenzer S, Bobkiewicz W, et al.

Elimination of a bacterial pore-forming toxin by sequential endocytosis and exocytosis. FEBS Letters. 2009;**583**(2):337-344

[43] Tamai K, Shiina M, Tanaka N, Nakano T, Yamamoto A, Kondo Y, et al. Regulation of hepatitis C virus secretion by the Hrs-dependent exosomal pathway. Virology. 2012;**422**(2):377-385

[44] Zhang W, Jiang X, Bao J, Wang Y, Liu H, Tang L. Exosomes in pathogen infections: A bridge to deliver molecules and link functions. Frontiers in Immunology. 2018;**9**:90.Z

[45] Mack M, Kleinschmidt A, Brühl H, Klier C, Nelson PJ, Cihak J, et al. Transfer of the chemokine receptor CCR5 between cells by membrane-derived microparticles: A mechanism for cellular human immunodeficiency virus 1 infection. Nature Medicine. 2000;**6**(7):769-775

[46] Rozmyslowicz T, Majka M, Kijowski J, Murphy SL, Conover DO, Poncz M, et al. Platelet-and megakaryocyte-derived microparticles transfer CXCR4 receptor to CXCR4-null cells and make them susceptible to infection by X4-HIV. AIDS. 2003;**17**(1):33-42

[47] Kadiu I, Narayanasamy P, Dash PK, Zhang W, Gendelman HE. Biochemical and biologic characterization of exosomes and microvesicles as facilitators of HIV-1 infection in macrophages. The Journal of Immunology. 2012;**189**(2):744-754

[48] Arakawa M, Morita E. Flavivirus replication organelle biogenesis in the endoplasmic reticulum: Comparison with other single-stranded positive-sense RNA viruses. International Journal of Molecular Sciences. 2019;**20**(9):2336

[49] Ramakrishnaiah V, Thumann C, Fofana I, Habersetzer F, Pan Q, de Ruiter PE, et al. Exosome-mediated transmission of hepatitis C virus between human hepatoma Huh7. 5 cells. Proceedings of the National Academy of Sciences. 2013;**110**(32):13109-13113

[50] Sato Y, Yaguchi M, Okuno Y, Ishimaru H, Sagou K, Ozaki S, et al. Epstein–Barr virus tegument protein BGLF2 in exosomes released from virus-producing cells facilitates de novo infection. Cell Communication and Signaling. 2022;**20**(1):1-12

[51] Zhao M, Nanbo A, Sun L, Lin Z. Extracellular vesicles in Epstein-Barr virus' life cycle and pathogenesis. Microorganisms. 2019;7(2):48

[52] Zhou X, Wang L, Zou W, Chen X, Roizman B, Zhou GG. hnRNPA2B1 associated with recruitment of RNA into exosomes plays a key role in herpes simplex virus 1 release from infected cells. Journal of Virology. 2020;**94**(13):e00367-e00320

[53] Dias MV, Teixeira BL, Rodrigues BR, Sinigaglia-Coimbra R, Porto-Carreiro I, Roffé M, et al. PRNP/prion protein regulates the secretion of exosomes modulating CAV1/caveolin-1-suppressed autophagy. Autophagy. 2016;**12**(11):2113-2128

[54] Wang T, Fang L, Zhao F, Wang D, Xiao S. Exosomes mediate intercellular transmission of porcine reproductive and respiratory syndrome virus. Journal of Virology. 2018;**92**(4):e01734-e01717

Chapter 5

Role of Exosomes in Tuberculosis: Looking towards a Future Road Map

Sushanta Kumar Barik and Jyotirmayee Turuk

Abstract

Exosomes are generated by the multivesicular degradation of plasma membrane fusion, lysosomal, and extracellular release of intracellular vesicles. The exosome ranges from 30 to 150 nm in size. Exosomes are "bioactive vesicles" that promote intercellular communication. Exosomes contain a variety of biologically active substances packaged with proteins, lipids, and nucleic acids. After any microbe infection into the exosomes, the content of the exosomes changes and is released into the bloodstream. Such type of exosome content could be useful for basic research on exosome biology. Tuberculosis (TB) is a serious infectious disease caused by *Mycobacterium tuberculosis* (*Mtb*). During the *Mtb* infection, the exosomes played an important role in the body's infection and immune response by releasing several exosome components providing new ideas for diagnosis, prevention, and therapeutic treatment of *Mtb* infection. The detection of the low abundance of the *Mtb* numbers or secreted peptides in the serum of TB patients is not possible. The best way of findings for diagnosis and treatment of TB could be possible by the exploration of exosome content analysis through various useful technologies. The study and analysis of exosome content would produce a road map for the future early diagnosis, prognosis estimation, efficacy monitoring, research, and application for TB.

Keywords: exosome, TB, *Mtb*, content, roadmap, serum

1. Introduction

Tuberculosis (TB) is an infectious disease caused by *Mycobacterium tuberculosis* (*Mtb*). *Mtb* is an intracellular bacteria engulfed by the macrophages through the process of phagocytosis. After invades into the host body, some of them eliminates and survives by immune escape mechanism as well but cause TB or latent tuberculosis infection (LTI). The exosomes size ranges 30–100 nm and is secreted by all living cells. Exosomes are circulating in the human body fluids rich in proteins, nucleic acids, lipids, etc. The components of the exosomes released by the body after *Mtb* infection play an important role in body's immune response and infection by providing new ideas on the diagnosis, treatment, and prevention of TB infection [1]. The vesicles were isolated through centrifugation at 10,000 *g* for

IntechOpen

90 minutes from in vitro culture of sheep reticulocytes during the maturation of reticulocytes. These vesicles were called "exosomes" coined by Johnstone in the year 1987 [2]. Those vesicular exosomes were released during the maturation of the sheep reticulocyte and contained a few numbers of plasma membrane functions. These vesicles contained the transferrin receptor and also contain other plasma membrane activities such as nucleoside transporter and acetylcholinesterase. The formation of exosomes is a natural phenomenon with the release of the transferrin receptor [3]. Exosomes were observed in both nucleated and non-nucleated reticulocytes. The protein content of exosomes is equal to the protein content of plasma membrane. The protein content of the exosomes may vary on the origin of the species. Exosomes contain a non-transmembrane protein HSP70, a major cellular chaperone protein. The externalized proteins are the intact proteins retaining the catalytic activity and native ligand binding activity. The small exosome structures relatively contain many proteins play an important role in controlling serious human pathological problems by various pathogens. Revisiting the functions of exosomes in human pathological problems since the discovery could possibly to making a roadmap [4].

Exosomes were involved in intercellular information transmission and potential medical applications. The special insight on the biological significance of the exosome is very essential for various applications in the human biological field [4]. The characterization of exosomes is very essential during immune response for a better announcement of host-pathogen interactions. Based on exosome characterization, development of various approaches would be possible to fight infections through various pathogens. When macrophages infected with the *Mtb* release from cells small vesicles known as exosomes that contain pathogen-associated molecular patterns (PAMPs). When exosomes were exposed to the uninfected macrophages, they were stimulated with a proinflammatory response in a toll-like receptor and myeloid differentiation factor 88-dependent manner. The cell culture media along with fetal calf serum (FCS) at a centrifugal speed of 100,000 *g* for 15 h had been used to isolate contaminating exosomes [5]. The exosomes are controlling *Mtb* infection through exosome biogenesis. During *Mtb* infection, exosomes played an important role in recruiting and regulating host cells. *Mtb*-infected RAW264.7 cells secreted chemokines from C57BL/6 mouse-derived bone marrow macrophages treated with exosomes and also induced the migration of CFSE-labeled macrophages and splenocytes. Exosomes were purified using Exo Quick purification system (System Biosciences, CA) on an average of 20 μg purified exosomes from 10 million cells [6].

Mtb peptides were detected in serum extracellular vesicles with latent tuberculosis-infected (LTBI) individuals. The identification of biomarkers from a serum source of latent *Mtb*-infected patients could be a better target for preventive therapy. Multiple reaction monitoring mass spectrometry (MRM-MS) assays detected 40 *Mtb* peptides from 19 LTBI patients. Mtb peptide detection in serum extracellular vesicles is a useful technique in diagnosis of LTBI [7]. Exosomes containing highly antigenic proteins could be an alternative approach for the development of a TB vaccine [8]. Extracellular vesicles (EVs) delivered Mycobacterium RNA into the host to promote host immunity by killing the bacteria. This technology is a novel approach to treat drug-resistant TB [9]. Exosomes were used as a tool for rapid diagnosis of TB. The detection of *Mtb* lipoarabinomannan and CFP-10 from the urinary EVs of pulmonary tuberculosis (PTB) and extrapulmonary tuberculosis (EPTB) patients would be helpful in the rapid diagnosis of TB [10].

Mtb-infected exosome contains a lot of proteins, nucleic acids for the rapid or slow manner detection and diagnosis of TB whether PTB or LTBI or drug-resistant (DR-TB). The collection of various *Mtb*-infected exosome materials from various research papers could give a better road map on the diagnosis of TB in a better way and plan out the future for rapid diagnosis on the development, detection, and cure of TB in the world.

2. Exosomes response to the *Mtb*

The host interactions with the pathogens are always a challenge in chronic diseases and to understand the mechanism, complexities, and sequential events. TB is a major worldwide disease and the understanding of TB immunology become a major refined since the identification of *Mtb*. Understanding the mechanism of how the immune cells are recognizing *Mtb* can be an important issue for development of therapeutic strategies and vaccine development. Several classes of pattern recognition receptors (PRRS) including toll-like receptors (TLRs), C-type lectin receptors (CLRs), and nod-like receptors (NLRs) were involved in the recognition of *Mtb*. TLRs family such as TLR1, TLR2, TLR4, TLR9, IL-1β, and IL-18 played an important role in the pathogenesis of TB [11].

Exosomes are the potential mediator of T cell activation. The released exosomes from mouse *Mtb* infection contribute significantly to T cell response. Rab27a played an important role in exosome biogenesis. The Rab27a deficiency mice showed diminishing of the protein components to exosomes and *Mtb* strains. Exosomes function to promote T cell immunity during *Mtb* infection and an important source of extracellular antigen [12]. Exfoliated vesicles with 5′-nucleotidase activity was reflected from the culture of various normal and neoplastic cell lines. Exfoliated membrane vesicles were served in physiologic function and referred to as exosomes. It was observed by electron microscopy that the shredded vesicles were a constituted part of plasma membrane [13].

EVs were packed with proteins, nucleic acids, and lipids released from the mammalian and bacterial cells. EVs played an important role through the intercellular transduction acts like a messenger. The *Mtb*-infected EVs released cells played an important regulatory role in the anti-*Mtb* immune response. EVs regulate innate and acquired immune responses of the body against *Mtb* and for this key immune response, EVs were considered an important factor in the development of *Mtb* vaccine [14]. The microbial and host interaction components were spread through exosomes either activate or suppress the immune system of the host. Exosomes were involved in multiple infection processes including formation or modification of the infection, T or B cells activation, and interaction with nonimmune cells such as fibroblasts and endothelial cells (**Figures 1–3**). When the bacteria exposure to the exosome, the release of cellular components begins with the activation/submersion of the immune response of the host [15].

Proteins secreted from the Mycobacterium species were identified those were contributed to the protective immunity. Mycobacterial surface proteins were analyzed from infected macrophages. The fibronectin and 85 kDa protein complexes were identified among the mycobacterial proteins released by the infected macrophages [16].

The exosomes promoted the macrophages for the release of chemotactic factors by activating immune cells in vivo and in vitro [6]. The microvesicles and exosomes

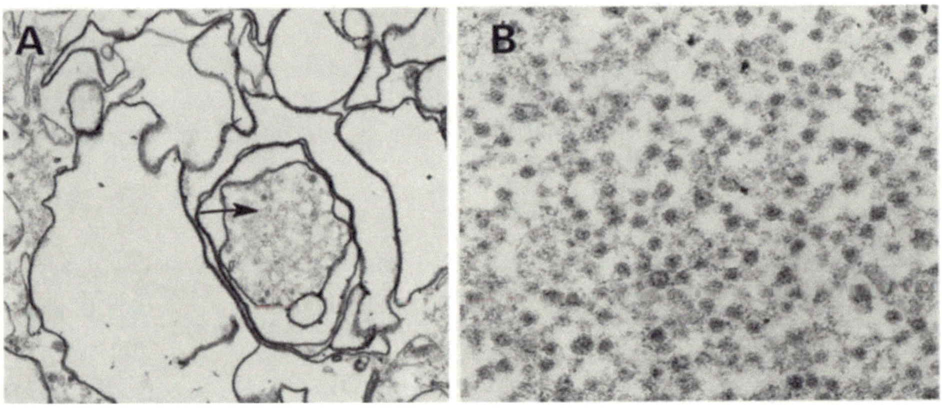

Figure 1.
(A) Electron photomicrograph of vesicular particles sedimented from superfusate of C-6 rat glioma monolayer cultures. Particles in conditioned medium. (magnification X 33 600). Note smaller vesicles contained within the larger vesicles (arrow). (B) Small vesicle population at greater magnification (glutaraldehyde fixed, magnification X 78 400) [13].

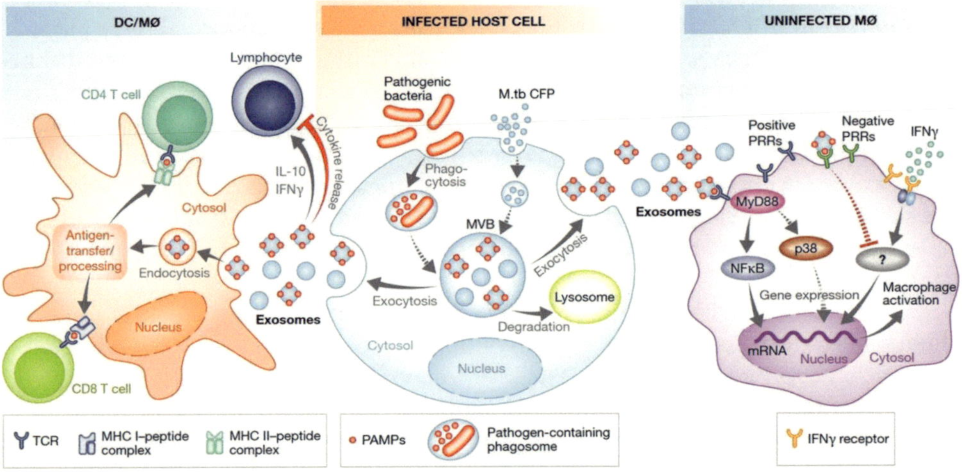

Figure 2.
Exosomes from bacteria-infected macrophages release exosomes containing antigens that induce cross-priming to activate antigen-specific $CD4^+$ and $CD8^+$ T cells. Some exosomes released from infected cells inhibit cytokine production by T cells. Exosomes from infected cells also contain PAMPs that stimulate macrophage production of proinflammatory mediators like TNF-α or limit the macrophage response to IFN-Y. Dashed line indicates unknown mechanism [15].

from the *Mtb* macrophages could activate T cells in response to antigen presentation. Adenosine triphosphate (ATP) induced exosomes were generated very rapidly and yielded much higher allowing significant time and cost advantages. *Mtb* interacted with ATP to induce the release of exosomes. These induced exosomes contained the major histocompatibility complex class-II (MHC-II) molecules for antigen presentation. ATP-induced exosomes could be used for a therapeutic purpose as an alternative to conventional exosomes [17].

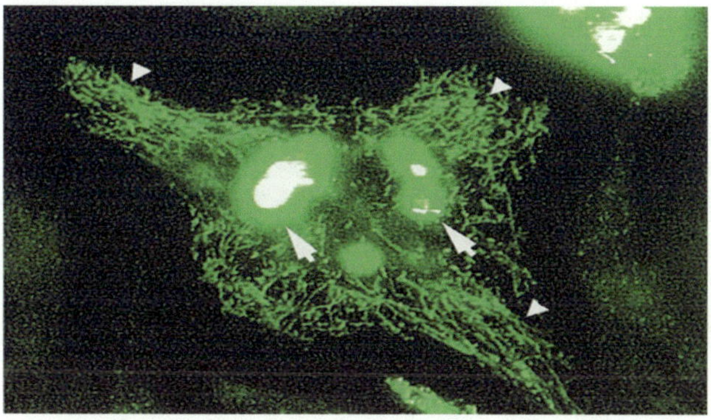

Figure 3.
The release of mycobacterial proteins from the phagosome in infected macrophages. Release of labeled mycobacterial proteins from the phagosome in infected macrophages. Live BMMf infected for 24 h with fluorescein succinimidyl ester-labeled BCG were analyzed by fluorescence microscopy. Labeled bacterial proteins were released from the mycobacterial phagosome into subcellular compartments of the infected macrophage (small arrowheads). The labeled bacteria are intensely fluorescent and are indicated by the large arrows [16].

3. Exosome contents and proteomic profiles of exosome proteins with TB

Exosomes are nanovesicles secreted by most but not all cells and specifically mediate intercellular communication through the transfer of genetic information of coding and noncoding RNA to recipient cells. The exosomes played an important biological role in the regulation of normal physiological and pathological processes through altered gene regulatory networks. Exosomes were targeted for the delivery of human genetic therapies through exogenous genetic cargoes such as siRNA [18]. *Mtb* is always in a dormant state for many years in the host system which is the cause of latent tuberculosis (LTB). Exosome contains a lot of *Mtb* antigens may be used as an alternative approach to develop the TB vaccine. A study was reported through the LC–MS/MS technique identified 41 *Mtb* proteins such as antigen 85-C, PckA, GabD1, β-1,3-Glucanase precursor, DnaK, LpdC, LprA, EST-6, etc. These were presented in exosomes released from *Mtb*-infected J774 cells and 29 *Mtb* proteins such as antigen 85-C, PckA, Fba, PepN, SahH, GroES, etc. Many of the released exosome proteins were highly immunogenic [8]. Flow cytometry analysis is a suitable method to characterize the surface markers of the extracellular vesicle's subpopulations in cells. The surface marker proteins were detected those were unique to exosomes naïve and *Mtb* infected THP-1 macrophages. The most similar findings of the surface protein markers such as CD63, CD9, CD81, and CD29 were detected in the exosomes of THP-1 cell culture supernatants by flow cytometry method. The purpose of characterization of the exosome surface proteins from the cell culture supernatants. Thus, the establishment of more sensitive methods enables the researcher to characterize the *Mtb* proteins in exosomes [19]. The main function of exosomes is interaction between cells through contact and exchange of soluble materials.

In TB patients, the exosomes were released from the *Mtb*-infected cells. The plasma of active TB patients generally contains the lipids and proteins derived from the exosome. Exosomes of all TB patients contains a lot of proteins such as sphingomyelins (SM), phosphatidylcholines, phosphatidylcholine inositol, free fatty acids, triglycerols, cholesteryl esters, etc. *Mtb* infections to the host proteins changed the host protein composition of a total of 37 proteins. Proteomic study indicates the expression of low levels of proteins such as apolipoproteins, antibacterial proteins cathelicidin, scavenger receptor cystine rich family member, ficolin3, etc. were observed in TB patients but the adhesion proteins (integrins, intercellular adhesion molecule2 (ICAM2), CD151, proteoglycan4 were highly prevalent in PTB patients. Analysis of these exosome proteins in TB patients is a new achievement in the host-pathogen interaction and helps the development of new vaccines and therapies in TB research [20].

Exosomes were loaded with the microbial proteins after *Mtb* infection. After *Mtb* infection into the exosome, there must be changes in the composition of exosomal proteins and the study of the exosomal proteins could contribute to the understanding of the progression of TB after *Mtb* infection and open the way to understand the development of a specific biomarker for diagnosis of the TB. An experimental analysis of the *Mtb*-infected cells by the tandem mass spectrometry analysis specifically showed that the 41 proteins were significantly more abundant in exosomes. Some of the proteins were identified through the novel biotinylation strategy to confirm the protein localization in the exosomal membrane. The *Mtb* influenced the changes in the protein composition of exosomes released from the *Mtb*-infected cells [21]. These proteins are given in **Tables 1–3**.

A study investigated the regulation of protein N-glycosylation in human macrophages and their secreted microparticles (MPs) after *Mtb* infection. Upon *Mtb* infection, the protein N-glycosylation of macrophages rapidly and significantly occurred following *Mtb* infection [22]. Always searching for a rapid and sensitive biomarker is useful for the diagnosis of TB. Exosome markers were stable within the double membrane of the exosome. Heat shock protein HSP16.3 was an important capsule protein produced by *Mtb*. The HSP16.3 protein was secreted in excess amount in exosomes from the U937 cells infected with *Mtb* and an amount of HSP16.3 proteins was detected in blood exosomes of ATB patients. Thus, the HSP16.3 protein act as an exosome-based TB biomarker for *Mtb* diagnosis [23]. Blood-secreted exosome-based "biosignature" through the multiple reactions monitoring mass spectrometry assay (MRM-MS) could be used as a diagnostic biomarker for active TB [24]. The details of the peptides are given in **Tables 4** and **5**.

Exosome RNA sequencing analysis were derived from the clinical samples of ATB, LTB revealed the gene expression profiles. The selective packaging of RNA cargoes into exosomes in different stages of *Mtb* infection would facilitate the potential targets for prevention, treatment, and diagnosis of TB. The gene enrichment analysis of the *Mtb* RNA in exosomes identified a lot of functions in active and LTB patients [25]. The details of total function of *Mtb* exosome are given in **Figure 4**.

These gene-enrichment analysis of the *Mtb*-infected exosome gives an idea of the future roadmap of the TB diagnosis in active population level. Generally, TB diagnosis was performed through microscopy, PCR amplification, or culture of *Mtb* DNA from sputum or the biopsy of infected tissue from human beings. The current improvement of detection methods for diagnosis of TB in serum samples could possible by advanced methods. Sometimes the detection of Mycobacterial products in serum is not possible due to the low abundance number of *Mtb.* The exploration of the exosome enrichment advance assay would require to improve the sensitivity of the assay.

No. of proteins	Identified proteins
1.	60S acidic ribosomal protein P0
2.	Coronin-1 C
3.	Lupus La Protein
4.	Heterogenous nuclear ribonucleoprotein K
5.	Heat shock 70KDa protein 4
6.	Alanine -tRNA ligase, cytoplasmic
7.	Calreticulin
8.	Protein disulphide isomerase A3
9.	L-amino acid oxidase
10.	Moesin
11.	Nucleolin
12.	Vimentin
13.	Protein disulfide-isomerase A6
14.	Spliceosome RNA helicase DDX39B
15.	Fermitin family homolog 3
16.	Programmed cell death -6 interacting protein
17.	S-adenosylmethionine synthase isoform type -2
18.	Glyceral dehyde -3 phosphate dehydrogenase
19.	ATP dependent RNA helicase A
20.	60 kDa heatshock protein, mitochondrial
21.	Cytosol aminopeptidase
22.	Ubiquitin like modifier activating enzyme-1
23.	ITIH4 protein
24.	Serine/threonine protein phosphatase 2A 65kDa regulatory subunit A alpha isoform
25.	Tryptophan t-RNA ligase cytoplasmic
26.	Transketolase
27.	Zyxin (fragment)
28.	Heat shock protein HSP90-beta
29.	Tyrosine-tRNA ligase, cytoplasmic
30.	6-Phosphogluconate dehydronase, decarboxylating
31.	X-ray repair cross complementing protein-6
32.	78kDa glucose regulated protein
33.	Eukaryotic initiation factor 4A-I
34.	Thrombospondin -4
35.	Bifunctional purine biosynthesis protein PURH
36.	Staphylococcal nuclease domain containing protein-1
37.	Heat shock cognate 71kDa protein
38.	Integrin beta-1

No. of proteins	Identified proteins
39.	UDP glucose 6-dehydronase
40.	Purine nucleoside phosphorylase
41.	Lamin B-1
42.	Transforming growth factor beta induced protein ig-h3
43.	Palmitoyl protein thioesterase -1
44.	Complement C4- A

Table 1.
Proteins significantly different between exosomes from Mtb-infected and control macrophages.

No. of proteins	Membrane associated proteins
1.	60S acidic ribosomal protein P0
2.	Coronin-1 C
3.	Heterogenous nuclear ribonucleoprotein K
4.	Alanine -tRNA ligase, cytoplasmic
5.	Calreticulin
6.	Protein disulphide isomerase A3
7.	Moesin
8.	Nucleolin
9.	Vimentin
10.	Protein disulfide-isomerase A6
11.	Fermitin family homolog 3
12.	Programmed cell death -6 interacting protein
13.	Glyceral dehyde -3 phosphate dehydrogenase
14.	ATP dependent RNA helicase A
15.	60 kDa heatshock protein, mitochondrial
16.	Cytosol aminopeptidase
17.	Serine/threonine protein phosphatase 2A 65kDa regulatory subunit A alpha isoform
18.	Transketolase
19.	Heat shock protein HSP90-beta
20.	78kDa glucose regulated protein
21.	Eukaryotic initiation factor 4A-I
22.	Bifunctional purine biosynthesis protein PURH
23.	Staphylococcal nuclease domain containing protein-1
24.	Heat shock cognate 71 kDa protein
25.	Integrin beta-1
26.	Lamin-B1

Table 2.
Membrane-associated proteins significantly more abundant in exosomes from Mtb infected cells and their biotinylation pattern.

No. of proteins	Protein name and sequences
1.	Eukaryotic initiation factor 4AI and EVQkLQMEAPHIIVGTPGRVF
2.	Glyceral dehyde 3 phosphate dehydrogenase and DNFGIVEGLMTTVHAITATQkTV
3.	Heat shock cognate 71 kDa protein and DPVEkALR
4.	Heat shock protein HSP90-beta and ERIMkAQALR
5.	Moesin and EFAkEALLQASR
6.	Nucleoside diphosphate kinase and ERTFIAIkP
7.	Vimentin and DVRQQYESVAAkNLQEA

Table 3.
List of proteins and specific peptides labeled with LC-LC biotin.

An enhanced MRM-MS is a method to detect ultra-low abundance of ultra-*Mtb* peptides in human serum exosomes. This MRM-MS technology could be useful for the detection and diagnosis of low-abundance *Mtb* peptides in the circulating serum exosome for the search of biomarkers [26]. As TB is a chronic infectious disease, attention to be paid to the non-coding RNA of exosome content of *Mtb* patients. Research on progress reported by Shu-hui et al. [27] on exosome non-coding RNA of *Mtb* patients could be useful as a potential biomarker on TB. A comprehensive proteomic analysis of the serum exosome proteins was analyzed in active TB (ATB) patients. A total of 123 differential proteins were identified in the serum exosome of ATB patient's. The characterization and identification of proteins in exosome of serum-active patients could consider a potential biomarker for TB [28]. The details of upregulated and downregulated proteins are given in **Tables 6** and 7.

The study and analysis of exosome contents are suitable for the development of a suitable biomarker for the diagnosis and treatment of TB. The exosome protein components were identified.

Sequence	Protein
a. PTB patient	
FALNAANAR	GlcB
VYQNAGGTHPTTTYK	Mpt64
AFDWDQAYR	Mpt64
EAPYELNITSATYQSAIPPR	Mpt64
b. EPTB patient	
PGLPVEYLQVPSPSMGR	Ag85
FLEGLTLR	Ag85c
LYASAEATDSK	Mpt32
ATIEQLLTIPLAK	GlcB
DGQLTIK	HspX
SEFAYGSFVR	HspX

Table 4.
Peptides that distinguish (a) pulmonary tuberculosis (PTB) or (b) extra-PTB patients from non-Tb patients.

Sequence	Protein
FALNAANAR	GlcB
DGQLTIK	HspX
SEFAYGSFVR	HspX
WHDPWVHASLLAQNNTR	Mpt51
GSVTPAVSQFNAR	Mpt63
VYQNAGGTHPTTTYK	Mpt64
EAPYELNITSATYQSAIPPR	Mpt64
IPDEDLAGLR	AcpM
ATIEQLLTIPLAK	GlcB

Table 5.
Peptides specifically detected in active Tb patients.

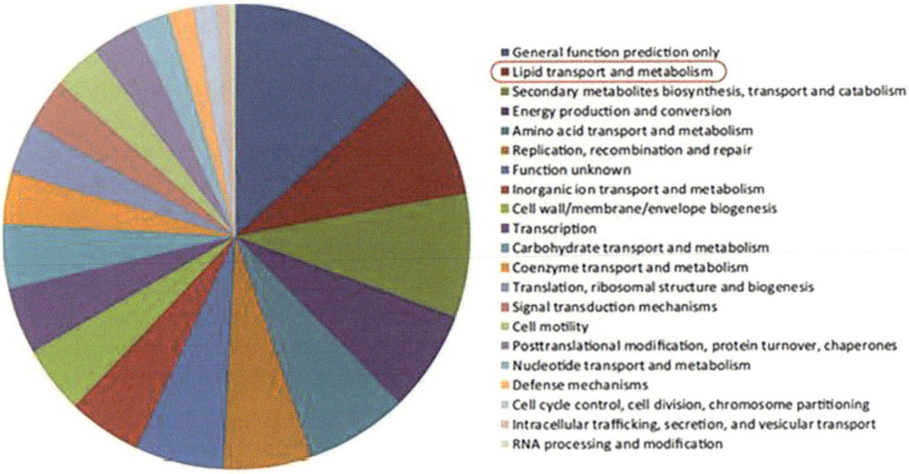

Figure 4.
Total function of Mtb exosome.

4. Exosome miRNA as a biomarker source for diagnosis and treatment of TB

Serum exosomes expressed CD81, the exosome marker protein. When these exosomes were infected with the *Mtb,* contains the increased level of miRNA such as miR484, miR 425, and miR96 in TB patients compared with the healthy control. As these markers were associated with active PTB, the expression of these miR could possibly increase the diagnostic power for diagnosis of TB patients as a biomarker [29]. Selection of biomarkers for diagnosis and treatment of TB is the most important issue. Analysis of blood samples from TB patients showed that the upregulation of miR-106b-5p was increased in exosomes. miR106b-5p promoted lipid droplet accumulation through the regulation of Creb5-SOAT1-CIDEC and suppressed macrophage apoptosis via Creb5-CASP9-CASP3 pathway leads to survival of *Mtb* in the host. The miR-106b-5p could be used as a biomarker for diagnosis of TB patients [30].

Now a days, TB is a threat to human health problem has an accuracy to the current TB diagnosis. Circulating exosome could be used as a diagnostic biomarker in TB. The study was examined the expression of the biomarkers for the diagnosis of TB infection. The miR-484, miR425, and miR96 were significantly increased in TB patients as compared with the healthy control and was examined the expression of miRNA as biomarker candidates for diagnosis of TB infection [31]. miRNA and electronic health records (EHRs) could be used to develop diagnostic models for

Number	Protein	Protein name	Gene
1	P02671	Fibrinogen alpha chain	FGA
2	G3V1N2	HCG1745306, isoform CRA_a	HBA2
3	A0N071	Delta globin	HBD
4	A0A024R035	Complement component C9	C9
5	V9HWE3	Carbonic anhydrase	HEL-S-11
6	Q9Y6C2	EMILIN-1	EMILIN-1
7	A0A024RC61	Aminopeptidase	ANPEP
8	Q8TCF0 L	Lipopolysaccharide-binding protein	LBP
9	P02786	Transferrin receptor protein 1	TFRC
10	P01023	Alpha-2-macroglobulin;α-2	A2M
11	C9JB55	Serotransferrin	TF
12	P19652	Alpha-1-acid glycoprotein 2	ORM2
13	Q1L857	Ceruloplasmin	N/A

Table 6.
Upregulated proteins with significant interesting in exosomes from ATB patients.

Number	Protein	Protein name	Gene
1	A3KPE2	Apolipoprotein C-III	APOC3
2	V9HVZ4	Glyceraldehyde-3-phosphate dehydrogenase	HEL-S-162eP
3	B0UXD8	HLA-DRA	HLA-DRA
4	P04899	Guanine nucleotide-binding protein G(i) subunit alpha-2	GNAI2
5	E7EU05	Glycoprotein IIIb	CD36
6	P23229	Integrin alpha-6	ITGA6
7	A0A024R4F1	2-phospho-D-glycerate hydro-lyase	HEL-S-17
8	G8GBV0	MHC class I antigen	HLA-A
9	P07737	Profilin-1	PFN1
10	L7UUZ7	Integrin beta	ITGB3
11	Q5JP53	Tubulin beta chain	TUBB
12	V9HWF0	Integrin-linked protein kinase	HEL-S-28

Number	Protein	Protein name	Gene
13	A0A024R611	Coronin	CORO1A
14	V9HWN7	Fructose-bisphosphate aldolase	HEL-S-87p
15	G9FP35	Guanine nucleotide binding protein	GNAQ
16	D3DVF0	Junctional adhesion molecule 1	F11R
17	Q9NZN3	EH domain-containing protein 3	EHD3
18	A0A024R3Q0	ADP-ribosylation factor 1, isoform CRA_a	ARF1
19	V9HWF5	Peptidyl-prolyl cis-trans isomerase	HEL-S-69p
20	B0V023	C6orf25	C6orf25
21	X6RJP6	Transgelin-2	TAGLN2
22	Q12913	Receptor-type tyrosine-protein phosphatase eta	PTPRJ
23	P08567	Pleckstrin	PLEK
24	P48059	LIM and senescent cell antigen-like-containing domain protein 1	LIMS1
25	Q86UX7	Fermitin family homolog 3	FERMT3
26	Q9Y490	Talin-1	TLN1
27	P21333	Filamin-A	FLNA
28	V9HWI5	Cofilin, non-muscle isoform	HEL-S-15
29	P61160	Actin-related protein 2	ACTR2
30	A8K0T9	F-actin-capping protein subunit alpha	N/A

Table 7.
Down-expressed proteins with significant interesting in exosomes from ATB patients.

PTB and tuberculosis meningitis (TBM) in a selective cohort study with the support vector machine (SVM) algorithm. Exosomal miRNAs (miR 20b, miR191 and miR486) along with EHR data through a machine learning algorithm could suggest for the diagnosis of the PTB and TBM [32]. The development of potential molecular targets for the detection and diagnosis of latent and active TB is possible by the miRNAs and repetitive region-derived small RNAs in exosomes. The most possible specifically expressed miRNA in LTBI patients were (hsa-let-7e-5p, hsa-let-7d-5p, hsa-miR-450a-5p, and hsa-miR-140-5p) and in TB patients were (hsa-miR-1246, hsa-miR-2110, hsa-miR-370-3P, hsa-miR-28-3P, and hsa-miR-193b-5p). Over all findings on miRNA, indicates the presence of biomarkers on the detection and diagnosis of the LTBI and TB patients [33].

The emerging role of functional and diagnostic potential of the several exosomal miRNA was studied by the several investigators and could explore as a possible diagnostic and therapeutic biomarker in *Mtb* infection [34]. TB biomarkers are generally predicting the treatment efficacy, cure of active tuberculosis, induction of protein immune responses by vaccination and reactivation of LTI. The suitable efforts are needed for development of suitable biomarker to meet the future challenges to cure the TB.

5. Exosomal DNA as a novel diagnostic biomarker for TB

Exosome is suitable for the detection of pathogen-derived nucleic acids. A novel approach was adopted for diagnosis of TB using exosomal DNA (exoDNA) through the droplet digital PCR (ddPCR). The ddPCR platform was used for detection of *Mtb* DNA in suspected PTB cases. The exosomal DNA was the primary method for the detection of the *Mtb* DNA in the ddPCR. The ddPCR is more sensitive than the real-time PCR. Therefore, the detection of exoDNA would be a sensitive and accurate method for diagnosis of *Mtb* infection [35].

6. Basic needs of exosomes as a biomarker content in the diagnosis and treatment of TB

Mtb causes the high morbidity and mortality for human TB. The pathogenesis of *Mtb* is very complex and is difficult to explained the mechanism of infection into human beings. The current TB diagnosis tools is inadequate and had several shortcomings on *Mtb* pathobiology. The study of the genetic diversity, pathogenesis of the *Mtb* through multi-omics approach leads to development of host biomarker in early diagnosis of TB. The discovery of new biomarkers has a great challenge on TB prevention and treatment. The search of a suitable biomarker for early diagnosis of TB is a great achievement in clinical context. TB remains a worldwide problem of human health. In order to prevent the TB infection, we must need the accurate vaccine development and reliable diagnostic tools.

Exosomes were isolated from human body fluids and considered for early detection of *Mtb* for diagnosis. From the above descriptive research papers, the research on the *Mtb*-derived exosomes (Mtbexo) is still at the preliminary stage and miRNA, protein, or DNA content of the *Mtb*-derived exosome from TB patients could possible for making a road map for biomarker discovery for the early diagnosis, treatment, and prevention of TB.

7. Conclusion

Exosome emerged as a potent genetic information for therapeutic potential through transfer agents corroborating a range of biological processes. Exosomes were used as a research tool for diagnosis and treatment of TB because the exosomes were released from cells packaged with biochemical materials. The characterization and detection of various packaged biochemical materials in exosome could make a future roadmap for the diagnosis and treatment of TB in human population level.

Acknowledgements

Indian Council of Medical Research, Govt. of India is acknowledged. N S Manisha, Odisha University of Agriculture and Technology, Odisha, India is highly praised for assisting making tables and pictures in the book chapter. Thanks to Mrs. Usha Padhee, Indian Administrative Service, Principal Secretary for a supportive stand on the road map for Tuberculosis.

Author details

Sushanta Kumar Barik* and Jyotirmayee Turuk*
Tuberculosis Division, ICMR-Regional Medical Research Centre, Chandrasekharpur, Bhubaneswar, Odisha, India

*Address all correspondence to: sushantakumarbarik82@gmail.com and drjyotirmayeetruk@gmail.com

References

[1] Jia L, Sha Y, Zhou H. The role of exosomes in Mycobacterium tuberculosis infection and their application value. International Journal of Pediatrics. 2021;**6**:538-542

[2] Johnstone RM et al. Vesicle formation during reticulocyte maturation. Association of plasma membrane activities with released vesicles (exosomes). Journal of Biological Chemistry. 1987;**262**(19):9412-9420

[3] Johnstone RM, Bianchini A, Teng K. Reticulocyte maturation and exosome release: Transferrin receptor containing exosomes shows multiple plasma membrane functions. Blood. 1989;**74**(5):1844-1851

[4] Johnstone RM. Revisiting the road to the discovery of exosomes. Blood Cells, Molecules, and Diseases. 2005;**34**(3):214-219

[5] Bhatnagar S et al. Exosomes released from macrophages infected with intracellular pathogens stimulate a proinflammatory response in vitro and in vivo. Blood, The Journal of the American Society of Hematology. 2007;**110**(9):3234-3244

[6] Singh PP et al. Exosomes isolated from mycobacteria-infected mice or cultured macrophages can recruit and activate immune cells in vitro and in vivo. The Journal of Immunology. 2012;**189**(2):777-785

[7] Mehaffy C et al. Identification of *Mycobacterium tuberculosis* peptides in serum extracellular vesicles from persons with latent tuberculosis infection. Journal of Clinical Microbiology. 2020;**58**(6):e00393-20

[8] Giri PK et al. Proteomic analysis identifies highly antigenic proteins in exosomes from M. tuberculosis-infected and culture filtrate protein-treated macrophages. Proteomics. 2010;**10**(17):3190-3202

[9] Cheng Y, Schorey JS. Extracellular vesicles deliver Mycobacterium RNA to promote host immunity and bacterial killing. EMBO Reports. 2019;**20**(3):e46613

[10] Dahiya B et al. Detection of *Mycobacterium tuberculosis* lipoarabinomannan and CFP-10 (Rv3874) from urinary extracellular vesicles of tuberculosis patients by immuno-PCR. Pathogens and disease. 2019;**77**(5):ftz049

[11] Mortaz E et al. Interaction of pattern recognition receptors with *Mycobacterium tuberculosis*. Journal of Clinical Immunology. 2015;**35**:1-10

[12] Smith VL et al. Exosomes function in antigen presentation during an in vivo *Mycobacterium tuberculosis* infection. Scientific Reports. 2017;**7**:1, 1-12

[13] Trams EG et al. Exfoliation of membrane ecto-enzymes in the form of micro-vesicles. Biochimica et Biophysica Acta (BBA) - Biomembranes. 1981;**645**(1):63-70

[14] Yan Z et al. Regulatory roles of extracellular vesicles in immune responses against *Mycobacterium tuberculosis* infection. World Journal of Clinical Cases. 2021;**9**(25):7311

[15] Schorey JS et al. Exosomes and other extracellular vesicles in host–pathogen interactions. EMBO Reports. 2015;**16**(1):24-43

[16] Beatty WL, Russell DG. Identification of mycobacterial surface proteins released into subcellular compartments of infected macrophages. Infection and Immunity. 2000;**68**(12):6997-7002

[17] Ramachandra L et al. *Mycobacterium tuberculosis* synergizes with ATP to induce release of microvesicles and exosomes containing major histocompatibility complex class II molecules capable of antigen presentation. Infection and Immunity. 2010;**78**(12):5116-5125

[18] Lee Y, El Andaloussi S, Wood MJA. Exosomes and microvesicles: Extracellular vesicles for genetic information transfer and gene therapy. Human Molecular Genetics. 2012;**21**(R1):R125-R134

[19] Biadglegne F et al. Exosomes in serum-free cultures of THP-1 macrophages infected with *Mycobacterium tuberculosis*. Molecular Medicine Reports. 2021;**24**(5):1-9

[20] Biadglegne F et al. *Mycobacterium tuberculosis* affects protein and lipid content of circulating exosomes in infected patients depending on tuberculosis disease state. Biomedicine. 2022;**10**(4):783

[21] Diaz G et al. Changes in the membrane-associated proteins of exosomes released from human macrophages after *Mycobacterium tuberculosis* infection. Scientific Reports. 2016;**6**(1):37975

[22] Hare NJ et al. *Mycobacterium tuberculosis* infection manipulates the glycosylation machinery and the N-glycoproteome of human macrophages and their microparticles. Journal of Proteome Research. 2017;**16**(1):247-263

[23] Huang C et al. Hsp16.3 of *mycobacterium tuberculosis* in exosomes as a biomarker of tuberculosis. European Journal of Clinical Microbiology & Infectious Diseases. 2021;**40**(11):2427-2430

[24] Kruh-Garcia NA et al. Detection of *Mycobacterium tuberculosis* peptides in the exosomes of patients with active and latent *M. tuberculosis* infection using MRM-MS. PLoS One. 2014;**9**(7):e103811

[25] Lv L et al. RNA profiling analysis of the serum exosomes derived from patients with active and latent *Mycobacterium tuberculosis* infection. Frontiers in Microbiology. 2017;**8**:1051

[26] Mehaffy C et al. Second generation multiple reaction monitoring assays for enhanced detection of ultra-low abundance *Mycobacterium tuberculosis* peptides in human serum. Clinical Proteomics. 2017;**14**:1, 1-10

[27] Shuhui GAO, Junwei ZHAO. Research progress of exosomal non-coding RNA as potential biomarkers of tuberculosis. Chinese Journal of Antituberculosis. 2020;**42**(3):282-285

[28] Zhang M et al. Proteomics analysis of exosomes from patients with active tuberculosis reveals infection profiles and potential biomarkers. Frontiers in Microbiology. 2022;**12**:800807

[29] Alipoor SD et al. Serum exosomal miRNAs are associated with active pulmonary tuberculosis. Disease Markers. 2019;**2019**:1907426

[30] Chen H et al. Exosomal miR-106b-5p promotes Mtb survival via targeting CREB5 followed by SOAT1-CIDEC and CASP9-CASP3 pathway. bioRxiv. 11 Aug 2021:1-29

[31] Mortaz E et al. Exosomal miRNAs and association with pulmonary

tuberculosis. European Respiratory Journal. 2019;**54**(63):PA5444

[32] Hu X et al. Integrating exosomal microRNAs and electronic health data improved tuberculosis diagnosis. eBioMedicine. 2019;**40**:564-573

[33] Lyu L et al. Small RNA profiles of serum exosomes derived from individuals with latent and active tuberculosis. Frontiers in Microbiology. 2019;**10**:1174

[34] Mirzaei R et al. The emerging role of exosomal miRNAs as a diagnostic and therapeutic biomarker in *Mycobacterium tuberculosis* infection. Molecular Medicine. 2021;**27**:1-31

[35] Cho SM et al. A novel approach for tuberculosis diagnosis using exosomal DNA and droplet digital PCR. Clinical Microbiology and Infection. 2020;**26**(7):942-e1

Section 3

Applications of Exosomes

Chapter 6

Perspective Chapter: Tissue Specificity of Exosomes and Their Prospects as a Drug Delivery System

Alisa Petkevich, Aleksandr Abramov and Vadim Pospelov

Abstract

This chapter reviewed the various sources of exosomes and their characteristics. Exosomes, which in the context of the proposed chapter are the synonym for extracellular vesicles up to 200 nm, play a pivotal role in cell to cell communication thus leading to the involvement of exosomes in inflammation and cancer development. This brings exosomes to the forefront of promising markers of a sub-clinical stage of the disease, which makes identifying exosome's source and destination one of the main goals in exosome research. However, due to some biogenesis features and technological difficulties, which are discussed further, identification of a certain exosome's address, or its specificity for a certain tissue or cell type, becomes a non-trivial task. The chapter covers the following questions: some of the main barriers on the way of testing tissue specificity hypothesis of exosomes, exosomes from synovial fluid and CSF and their features, exosomes from mesenchymal stem cells (MSCs) of different origins, and some membrane and cargo exosomal markers for tissue specificity and the prospect of exosomes as a drug delivery approach.

Keywords: exosomes, tissue specificity, synovial fluid, cerebrospinal fluid, mesenchymal stem cells of different origins, drug delivery

1. Introduction

The term "exosome" has been known since the beginning of 1970s, when it was first used in papers published in "The Proceedings of the National Academy of Sciences (PNAS)" and dedicated to the transfer of DNA fragments between Drosophila or Neurospora cells. The term in that context had little in common with lipid bilayer vesicles, which may contain a wide variety of nucleic acids and proteins and was mainly related to DNA fragments that are not integrated into the exome and eliminated during meiosis [1]. The first use of the term "exosomes" in the extracellular vesicles context happened in 1980s, when Trams et al. in 1981 described vesicles that are produced directly by outward budding at the plasma membrane [2]. Nowadays, the ISEV (International Society for Extracellular Vesicles) consensus recommendation on nomenclature is to use "extracellular vesicle" as the "generic term for particles naturally released from the cell that is delimited by a lipid bilayer and cannot replicate" and to modify "EV" based on clear, measurable characteristics such as the cell of origin, molecular markers, size, density, function, etc [1]. In this paper we assume exosomes and extracellular vesicles (EV) as synonym terms. They are assumed to be a tool for intracellular communication and are promising biomarkers in different pathologies, including tumor growth. Another perspective trend for exosome' application is the use of the latter as a delivery system for various therapeutic targets. These microvesicles have some of the features of an ideal drug delivery system such as high biocompatibility, minimal toxicity, and tissue specificity. The latter feature may seem difficult to be objectively determined as far as the experimental design for confirmation or refutation of exosomes` tissue specificity is troublesome. This chapter proposes to discuss various aspects of the tissue specificity of exosomes, including some of the main barriers on the way of testing the tissue specificity hypothesis of exosomes, exosomes from synovial fluid and CSF and their features, exosomes from mesenchymal stem cells (MSCs) of different origin and some of membrane and cargo exosomal markers for tissue specificity the prospect of exosomes as a drug delivery approach.

2. Some of the main barriers on the way of testing the tissue specificity hypothesis of exosomes

First of all, culturing difficulties should be admitted. The difference between cell lines and even the corresponding primary cell cultures is obvious and does not allow to extrapolation of data obtained on cell lines to corresponding cells of an organism without limitations. Barriers in experiments with exosomes on the primary cell cultures lie on the surface: during obtaining the ex vivo culture of human cells successive steps should be performed, including dissection and/or disaggregation of the tissue, which may be accompanied by the formation of vesicles as the result of mechanical destruction of cells, especially in working with dense tissues, requiring preliminary mechanical grinding [3]. Another barrier, and perhaps more serious, is time limits. It is well known, that the longer primary cell cultures exist the less they reflect the ex vivo state of the corresponding tissue. Anyway, the latter reason along with others such as changes in morphology and signaling under the influence of antibiotics, culture flask, absence of tissue architectonics, etc., is not unique to exosome experiments.

Secondly, in terms of biogenesis exosomes are secreted intraluminal vesicles (ILVs), which sequester specific proteins, lipids, and cytosolic components, whilst multivesicular bodies (MVBs), and late endosomes are a subset of specialized endosomal compartments rich in intraluminal vesicles. ILVs are generated by the inward budding of endosomal membranes and MVBs get transported to plasma membrane *via* cytoskeletal and microtubule network, after that they undergo exocytosis post-fusion with the cell surface whereby the ILVs get secreted as exosomes [4]. The biology of this process does not allow us to make a firm assumption, that exosomes, even secreted by different cell types, have distinct superficial/membrane markers, identifying their specificity. Nevertheless, there is a probability of determining exosome's cell or tissue origin or tissue-specific engagement in disease by the presence of specific combinations of surface proteins and their abundance [5]. Anyway, there is always a possibility to suppose the origin of exosomes by their cargo, for example, by miRNA profile, which is discussed later, but considering all of the above identification of exosome fraction of certain miRNA profiles is a non-trivial task. Moreover, the effects of exosomes from different sources might overlap with each other and, for example, might act complementary in eliciting inflammatory reactions, e.g. as has been observed for microvesicles from atherosclerotic plaques [6, 7].

Thirdly, partly due to exosomes' size, there are technical difficulties in identifying exosomal membrane markers especially when there is a complex of these markers. Currently, opportunities for the detection of exosomes are improving due to the new emerged technologies. Imaging flow cytometry is on the edge of these technologies, remaining one of the basic instruments for phenotype description. Imaging flow cytometry overcomes obstacles in traditional flow cytometry by including a CCD camera with a 60× objective, allowing detection of vesicles with sizes below 500 nm through enhanced fluorescence with only a small number of fluorophore-labeled antibodies like two protein targets per exosome [5]. However, this area is growing rapidly, and flow cytometry kits based on beads carrying up to 37 exosomal protein markers on their surface are nowadays available. There are some alternative options for multiplex surface markers recognition on exosomes like proximity-dependent barcoding assay, converting the protein composition to DNA sequence information via bound antibody-DNA conjugates with the following decoding by NGS [5].

And, fourthly, the biological materials which are widely available for sampling are blood, urine, and saliva. Apparently, every of this biomaterial is a stock of everything from everywhere and it is extremely difficult to determine the origin of exosomes, isolated from these biomaterials. A major source of microvesicles in plasma is represented by platelets, other sources of exosomes in blood plasma are endothelial cells, smooth muscle cells, monocytes, lymphocytes, and erythrocytes [6, 8]. Berckmans René et al. in 2001 discovered, that among total exosomes, isolated from human plasma, 82% were platelet exosomes, 15% from erythrocytes, and 3% from leukocytes; in 2019 they discovered, that among total isolated plasma, 52% are platelet EVs, 29% erythrocyte Evs, 20% leucocyte Evs and a low concentration of EVs from (activated) endothelial cells (E-selectin, CD62E) can be detected [9]. The biofluids which allow assuming the specificity of the isolated exosomes are synovial fluid and cerebrospinal fluid (CSF), exosomes from these biomaterials are discussed below.

3. Exosomes from synovial fluid and CFS

The biofluid, which is available for research in a limited number of cases, is synovial fluid. With a large synovial microvesicular pore radius reaching 40 nm, it can be assumed, that the exosomes, isolated from the synovial fluid, are mostly exosomes, produced by fibroblast-like synoviocytes and by chondrocytes, which constitute the synovial membrane and joint cartilage respectively [10].

Huang et al. investigated exosomes from synovial fluids of patients with different joint diseases: gout, rheumatoid arthritis (RA), axial spondyloarthritis (axSpA), and osteoarthritis (OA). The main goal of the experiment was not to identify tissue or cell-specific markers in exosomes but to determine markers, which would primarily allow differentiating these disease states in patients. However, this is valuable research in characterizing tissue specificity of exosomes, which include samples of synovial fluid of total of 100 patients. Twenty-five proteins were found highly expressed in gout uniquely, lysozyme C and protein S100-A9 included, whose bioinformatic analysis was significantly involved in "neutrophil degranulation" and "prion diseases". Along with differentially expressed proteins, there were thirty-nine proteins highly expressed in axSpA uniquely and twenty-eight proteins in RA. In axSpA among others there were RNA-binding protein 8A and protein transport protein Sec24C included, whose bioinformatic analysis was significantly involved in "acute-phase response" and "citrate cycle". In RA, these uniquely expressed proteins included pregnancy zone protein (PZP) and stromelysin-1, whose bioinformatic analysis was significantly involved in "serine-type endopeptidase inhibitor activity" and "complement and coagulation cascade" [11]. Apparently, these molecular events may have distinct functional consequences: exosomes isolated from synovial fibroblasts, which were cultured in conditions mimicking OA, were able to induce MMP-13 and aggrecan expression in articular chondrocytes isolated from healthy synovial joints, suggesting in vitro this would lead to tissue degeneration [12]. Moreover, Esa et al. admit in their review that exosomes produced by both synovial fibroblasts and chondrocytes under OA-like conditions upregulate the release of pro-inflammatory cytokine cascades, including MMP-13, creating a "positive-feedback loop" that drives inflammation within the joint and ultimately leads to the damage of articular cartilage and a loss of structural integrity [13]. By the way, it is interesting to note, that, unlike exosomes from MSCs of different origins, exosomes from healthy individuals or individuals with OA do not differ either in the concentration (OA: 1.18 × 1010 particles/ml, n = 6; non-OA: 1.59 × 1010 particles/ml, n = 6) or in the size (OA: 0.128 μm, n = 6; non-OA: 0.127 μm, n = 6) [14].

Another biofluid that is also available in a limited number of cases is cerebrospinal fluid. Taking into account that CSF is produced by ependymal cells and permeability of blood-brain barrier to hydrophobic molecules and small non-polar molecules, it is possible to assume exosomes, isolated from CSF, are specific for the cells, making up and supporting functioning the central nerve system, such as neurons, astrocytes, microglia, and oligodendrocytes [15]. On the other hand, it should be admitted exosomes can cross BBB in blood-brain direction, which makes them a promising approach for the target delivery of therapeutic agents [15, 16]. The ability of exosomes to cross the blood-brain barrier (BBB) in the opposite direction makes them a highly attractive source of biomarkers originating in the CNS that could be isolated from the blood [17].

Otake et al. detected 14,807 genes in CSF exosomes, of which 4580 genes were commonly detected among four individuals, including neuron-enriched genes such as TUBB3 and CAMK2A. Gene Ontology analysis and pathway analysis with these genes revealed functional enrichment of ubiquitin-proteasome pathway, oxidative stress response, and unfolded protein response in CSF from patients with amyotrophic lateral sclerosis. These pathways are related to pathomechanisms of amyotrophic lateral sclerosis [18]. Along with common exosomal protein markers, expressed on the surface of CSF exosomes and in mRNA exosomal content, there are such proteins as NCAM, L1CAM, SOD1, α-synuclein Aβ42, total tau, TDP-43, and pT181-tau [16, 18]. The presence of SOD1, which is one of the most studied causes of amyotrophic lateral sclerosis, in exosomes secreted from motor-neuron-like NSC-34 cells overexpressing human wild-type or mutant SOD1 provided the first evidence for the secretion and cell-to-cell transmission of SOD1 in the context of ALS [16]. TDP-43 is assumed to facilitate a prion-like spread of its misfolded species [19]. NCAM is a neuronal cell adhesion protein, which is involved in cell-cell and cell-matrix interactions, and L1CAM is an axonal glycoprotein that plays an important role in nervous-system development and its mutations cause neurological syndromes known as CRASH [19, 20].

4. Exosomes from mesenchymal stem cells (MSCs) of different origin

Mesenchymal stem cells (MSCs) are the subject of intense research as they are a potential therapeutic tool for several clinical applications and among others one of the most available options to study stem cells, what is one of the main reasons why exosomes from these cells seem to be mostly described and studied. Thus, exosomes from different variants of mesenchymal stem cells seem to be well described and characterized.

In 2021 González-Cubero et al. described the phenotype of adipose tissue-derived mesenchymal stem cells (ASCs-derived) exosomes: from 37 exosomal surface epitomes 31 were detected and 6 were undetected. Among the detected ones were CD3, CD4, CD19, CD8, HLA-DRDPDQ, CD56, CD105, CD2, CD1c, CD25, CD49e, ROR1, CD209, CD9, SSEA-4, HLA-ABC, CD63, CD40, CD11c, CD81, CD41b, CD86, CD326, CD133/1, CD29, CD69, CD45, CD31, CD20, CD14, while CD3+, CD45+, CD56+, HLA-ABC, and HLA-DRDPDQ were particularly strongly enhanced in samples with ASCs-derived exosomes (99.99% ±0.06%, 55.45% ±6.36%, 88.68% ±4.29%, 84.66% ±5.99%, 59.98% ±7.45%, respectively). However, CD42a, CD44, CD62P, CD142, CD146, and MCSP were undetectable [20]. Like ASCs-derived exosomes, it was shown, that exosomes from BMSC do not express CD146 and CD42a. However, CD1c, CD2, CD3, CD4, CD14, CD20, CD25, CD31, CD40, CD45, CD49e, CD56, CD69, CD133/1, and CD326 also were undetectable in exosomes from BMSC [21].

Moreover, 1 year in 2020 Wang et al. compared the exosomes, isolated from bone marrow-derived MSC (BM-MSC), umbilical cord-derived MSC (UC-MSC), and adipose tissue-derived MSCs (AT-MSC). They found that AT-MSCs produced exosomes more intensively, as far as the concentration of exosomes in the supernatant, collected for the same time period, was higher than that of BM-MSC or UC-MSC exosomes [22]. However, simultaneously in 2020 Xu et al. showed this is not a strict regularity: during the experiment, they got supernatant with the density 2.38 × 1011/mL in exosomes from BMSCs; 1.08 × 1011/mL in exosomes from ADMSCs and 1.75 × 1011/mL in exosomes from UCMSCs [23]. In the research of Wang et al., exosomes from all three different tissue sources were studied with TEM, typical cup-shaped vesicles were observed and no differences in shape among the exosomes were noted [22]. Xu et al. showed there is sometimes possibly a slight difference in the size distribution of exosomes from BMMSCs, ADMSCs, and UCMSCs: in the case of BMMSCs, exosomes were round or dish-shaped with a diameter of 40–100 nm, the average particle diameter of exosomes was 70.3 nm. Exosomes from ADMSCs were uniform in size with a diameter of 30–100 nm with the average particle diameter within 95 nm and the majority of exosomes were 72.8 nm, while the UCMSCs exosomes were round in shape with a diameter of 10–90 nm and most of the particles had diameters of about 80.6 nm [23].

A detailed proteomic analysis revealed 771, 457, and 431 proteins in exosomes from BM-MSC, AT-MSC, and UC-MSC, respectively; comparison of the three types of exosomes revealed 355 common proteins, and 341, 23, and 37 proteins unique to the exosomes from BM-MSC, AT-MSC, and UC-MSC, respectively. In terms of biological process, proteins from BM-MSC exosomes were mainly involved in granulocyte activation and regulation of cell migration, whereas proteins from AT-MSC exosomes were enriched in leukocyte activation involved in immune response and UC-MSC exosomes along with leukocyte activation proteins involved in immune response were enriched in proteins of collagen metabolic process. As for molecular function, AT-MSC exo and UC-MSC exo proteins were both significantly enriched in cell adhesion molecule binding, whereas BM-MSC exo proteins were mostly involved in protein complex binding and integrin binding. Along with protein cargo, Wang et al. examined membrane markers of isolated exosomes and identified some membrane proteins, that are differentially expressed: ATP2B1 and ATP1A1 showed high expression in AT-MSC exosomes, whereas ITGA2 and LRP1 showed low expression. LTGB3 and SLC44A1 showed low expression in UC-MSC exosomes. In contrast, ADAM9, ADAM10, CD81, CACNA2D1, NOTCH2, and HLA-A showed high expression in BM-MSC exosomes [23]. There is a strong data, exosomes of all three sources—BMMSCs, ADMSCs, and UCMSCs—show highly expressed exosomes specific markers CD63, HSP70, CD81, and CD9 [21, 23].

Exosomes from MSCs are known to express another protein, a milk fat globule- epidermal growth factor-factor VIII (MFGE8), a glycoprotein that bridges externalized phosphatidylserine (PS) on the apoptotic cell surface to alphaVbeta3 or alphaVbeta5 integrins on the phagocyte. The expression of this protein has certain functional consequences in exosomes: their administration increases macrophage uptake of apoptotic bodies in the border zone of infarction and is associated with reduced proinflammatory response, increase in neovascularization, lower infarct size, and an improvement in cardiac function [24].

Three years before that in 2017 Mead B. et al. discovered the difference in membrane proteins expression between exosomes from BMSC and fibroblasts: more CD11c+ and CD63+ exosomes were detected on the BMSC exosomes (20.3% ± 8.3%, 81.7% ± 12.3%, respectively) compared to fibroblast exosomes (7.7 ± 0.7, 49.6 ± 2.4, respectively), whereas more CD29+ and CD81+ exosomes were detected on fibroblast exosomes (32.4% ± 0.75%, 39% ± 3.3%, respectively) compared to BMSC exosomes (20.5% ± 1.9%, 15.3% ± 10.6%, respectively) [24]. On the surface of AT-MSCs exosomes along with an abundance of well-known exosomal markers CD63, CD9, and CD81, there was revealed the expression of CD105, an MSC marker, as well as CD44, CD29, CD49e, and melanoma-associated chondroitin sulfate proteoglycan (MCSP). In addition, MSC-exosomes were found to be preferentially distributed in the damaged kidneys of mice with glycerol-induced AKI compared to in the healthy kidneys of control mice [25].

Exosomes from BM-MSCs and ADSCs show similar profiles, which are positive for CD105, CD73, CD90, and CD44; negative for CD45, CD31, and CD34 [26]. Nevertheless, there is a difference in functional capabilities of exosomes derived from BM-MSCs and ADSCs, the latter has a more significant neprilysin (NEP) activity: NEP-specific enzyme activity accounted for 38.3 ± 4.5% of total enzyme activity of ADSCs exosomes while BM-MSCs showed weak or undetectable NEP enzyme activity. Katsuda et al. calculated NEP-specific activity after the subtraction of fluorescence in the presence of thiorphan and they demonstrated that all ADSCs exhibited NEP-specific enzyme activity [27]. This makes ADSCs exosomes a promising approach for Alzheimer's disease treatment. This difference between exosomes from ADSCs and BM-MSCs is also determined in protein expression: immunoblot analysis revealed that the NEP protein expression level in ADSCs was ~4-fold higher than that of BM-MSCs [26].

5. Some membrane and cargo exosomal markers for tissue specificity

As it was already mentioned above, identifying the source of a certain exosome with its membrane markers is a non-trivial task, requiring consideration of the combination of different proteins and their abundance.

Skogberg et al. in their study of exosomes from human thymic epithelial cells (TEC) revealed the typical mTEC-associated cytokeratins K5, K14, and in both cells and exosomes, while the typical cortical thymic epithelial cell (cTEC) associated cytokeratin K8 and, for example, involucrin, a marker for late-stage mTEC differentiation, and CLAUDIN-1 were only identified in cells. Amidst the markers, which were found only in exosomes and not in cells, there were classical exosomal markers such as TSG101, CD82, CD63, MFG-E8, FLOTILIN-1 and immunoproteasome subunits PSMB9 and PSMB10, while PSMB8 was found in both, cells and exosomes. Other proteins, which were identified in cells and in exosomes from these cells, were CP, ALDOC, COL6A1, LAMA2, SRI, HSPG2, TSN, AOC3, SLC34A2, and F13A1 [28].

Mathivanan et al. also revealed some markers, which are specific for colorectal cancer cells (LIM1215) and can be identified both in cells and in exosomes. Amidst others, these are A33 antigen, cadherin-17, carcinoembryonic antigen, and ephrin-B1 and -B2, cell type-specific proteins associated with the gastrointestinal tract. Comparing proteomes of LIM125-derived exosome with previously published proteomes of human urinary exosomes and mast cell-derived exosomes, they found 31 proteins to be common between all of three exosomal proteomes, whereas 79 and 96 proteins were in common between LIM1215-mast cell and LIM1215-urine data sets. The 31 common proteins include Alix, transferrin, actins (α, β, and γ), RAB5B, RAB5C, EH-domain containing 4, heat shock proteins, annexins A6 and A11, and ADP-ribosylation factor 1 among others. Moreover, they found, that LIM125-derived pure exosome proteins are enriched with tetraspanin-containing proteins (p-value 0.0001) when compared with the entire human proteome and were the first to report the presence of phospholipid scramblase 3 in exosomes [29].

Saheera et al. in their recent review admit, exosomes from cardiomyocytes are enriched with proteins, which play critical roles in cardiomyocyte growth and survival like heat shock proteins (Hsp) like Hsp20, Hsp60, and Hsp70. Furthermore, these exosomes are known to be loaded with such inflammatory factors responsible for cardiac remodeling as IL-6 and TNF-α. Among others, these exosomes include GLUT4, GLUT1, and lactate dehydrogenase, different miRNAs, namely miR-320 and miR-126 [29]. The specificity of exosomes is possible to be used in target delivery purposes: the delivery of exosomes, expressing cardiac-targeting peptide on their membrane, in H9C2 cells was 16% greater than that of exosomes, which did not express this peptide, whereas the delivery of the exosomes of these two types was not different in HEK 293 cells exosomes expressing cardiac-targeting peptide (CTP)-Lamp2b on their membrane (CTP-Exo) was generated by introducing vectors encoding CTP-Lamp2b into HEK 293 cells. Moreover, compared with exosomes without cardiac-targeting peptide on its membrane, the in vivo delivery of exosomes to the hearts of mice was increased by 15% with CTP-Exo ($P = 0.035$) [30].

In exosomes from ECC1 cells, which are the most accurate resemblence of the endometrial luminal epithelium, Greening et al. found 14 proteins, which are essential for embryo implantation. As exosomal protein cargo, there were complement decay-accelerating factor (CD55, Rsc 7.1), perlecan (HSPG2, Rsc 5.9), and EGFR (Rsc 5.1), which are highly regulated at the time of blastocyst apposition and attachment [31, 32]. In general, it should be emphasized exosomes participate not only in tissue-specific processes like blastocyst apposition and attachment but in common processes like inflammation, cancer development, and cell senescence. Saheera et al. in their review, dedicated to exosomes' role in cell aging, admit senescence-associated exosomes could transfer many molecules and could accelerate the aging process or associated pathologies in an autocrine, paracrine, and endocrine fashion. Moreover, senescence-associated exosomes can intensify the aging process by cargos transfer between cells that may be recruited to increase the exosome release observed during cellular senescence.

Exosomes from older individuals were shown to have MHC-II expression on monocytes and they are taken up faster by B cells in older individuals when compared to young, and as a result, the levels of circulating exosomes could be reduced [32].

It is worth it to note in some cases exosomes may be one of the features causing graft rejection. Sharma et al. in 2018 revealed a higher expression of some proteins in exosomes isolated from patients with complications compared with patients without complications. They collected serum samples from patients who had undergone lung (n = 30), heart (n = 8), or kidney (n = 15) transplantations. Using western blot along with CD9 identified tissue-associated lung SAgs, collagen V (Col-V) and K-alpha 1 tubulin (Kα1T), heart SAgs, myosin and vimentin, and kidney SAgs, fibronectin and collagen IV (Col-IV). Lung transplant recipients diagnosed with bronchiolitis obliterans syndrome had exosomes with higher expression of Col-V (4.2 fold) and Kα1T (37.1fold) than stable. Heart recipients with coronary artery vasculopathy had a 3.9-fold increase in myosin and a 4.7-fold increase in vimentin compared with stable. Exosomes in kidney transplant recipients diagnosed with transplant glomerulopathy 2-fold increased expression of fibronectin and 2.5-fold increased in Col-IV compared with exosomes from stable patients [33]. This is not a unique case of exosomes involvement in heart pathology processes: exosomes from macrophages exposed to diabetic milieu (high glucose or db/db mice) significantly increase inflammatory and profibrogenic responses in fibroblast (in vitro) and cardiac fibrosis in mice [34].

Some of the features which are specific for exosomes of certain origins are listed in the **Table 1**.

6. Exosomes as a promising approach for drug delivery

Exosome delivery is a novel nanoscale delivery system with many advantages, such as biocompatibility, biodegradability, less toxicity, specificity to the target cells, small size, promotes plasma membrane fusion, among different cells, longer half-life, low-uptake machinery, capability to pass contents from one cell to another cell, low immunogenicity and the unique feature that they have more tendency to accumulate

#	Exosomes' source	Characteristics/effects of certain exosomes in vitro or in vivo	Material/experiment design	Reference
1	Synovial fluid	25 proteins, including lysozyme C and protein S100-A9, uniquely highly expressed in gout patients; 39 proteins including RNA-binding protein 8A and protein transport protein Sec24C uniquely high expressed in axSpA; pregnancy zone protein (PZP) and stromelysin-1 highly expressed in RA	Samples from 100 patients with gout, rheumatoid arthritis (RA), axial spondyloarthritis (axSpA)	[11]
2	Synovial fluid	Induced MMP-13 and aggrecan expression	Exosomes from synovial fibroblasts cultured in OA conditions were added to articular chondrocytes isolated from healthy synovial joints	[12]

#	Exosomes' source	Characteristics/effects of certain exosomes in vitro or in vivo	Material/experiment design	Reference
3	CSF	Exosomes with highly expressed NCAM, L1CAM, SOD1, α-synuclein Aβ42, total tau, TDP-43 and pT181-tau Exosomes with functional enrichment of genes of ubiquitin-proteasome pathway, oxidative stress response, and unfolded protein response in CSF from patients with amyotrophic lateral sclerosis.	CSF from patients including patients with amyoptophic lateral sclerosis	[17, 18]
4	adipose tissue-derived mesenchymal stem cells	ASC-derived exosomes were positive for 31 surface markers including CD3, CD4, CD19, CD8, HLA-DRDPDQ, CD56, CD105, CD2, CD1c, CD25, CD49e, ROR1, CD209, CD9, SSEA-4, HLA-ABC, CD63, CD40, CD11c, CD81, CD41b, CD86, CD326, CD133/1, CD29, CD69, CD45, CD31, CD20, CD14, while CD3+, CD45+, CD56+, HLA-ABC, and HLA-DRDPDQ and negative for CD42a, CD44, CD62P, CD142, CD146, and MCSP	Exosomes isolated from culture media of adipose tissue-derived mesenchymal stem cells	[21]
5	Bone Marrow-MSC, Adipose Tissue-MSC, and Umbilical Cord-MSC	A detailed proteomic analysis revealed 355 common proteins between BM-MSC, AT-MSC, and UC-MSC-derived exosomes, and 341 (out of 771 proteins detected in BM-MSC-derived exosomes), 23 (out of 457 proteins detected in AT-MSC-derived exosomes), and 37 (out of 431 proteins detected in UC-MSC-derived exosomes) proteins unique to the exosomes from BM-MSC, AT-MSC, and UC-MSC, respectively. In AT-MSC exosomes ATP2B1 and ATP1A1 showed high expression; ITGA2 and LRP1 showed low expression. In UC-MSC exosomes LTGB3 and SLC44A1 showed low expression. In BM-MSC exosomes ADAM9, ADAM10, CD81, CACNA2D1, NOTCH2, and HLA-A showed high expression	Exosomes isolated from culture media of Bone Marrow derived MSC, adipose tissue-derived MSC, and umbilical cord- derived MSCs	[22, 23]
6	BM-derived stem cells and fibroblasts	On the exosomes from BMSC there were more CD11c+ and CD63+ (20.3% ± 8.3%, 81.7% ± 12.3%, respectively) compared to fibroblast exosomes (7.7 ± 0.7, 49.6 ± 2.4, respectively), whereas on the fibroblasts derived exosomes there were more CD29+ and CD81+ (32.4% ± 0.75%, 39% ± 3.3%, respectively) compared to BMSC derived exosomes (20.5% ± 1.9%, 15.3% ± 10.6%, respectively).	Exosomes were isolated from cultured media of BM derived MSC and fibroblasts	[24]

#	Exosomes' source	Characteristics/effects of certain exosomes in vitro or in vivo	Material/experiment design	Reference
7	Exosomes from human thymic epithelial cells (TEC)	mTEC exosomes expressed the typical mTEC-associated cytokeratins K5, K14 (like TEC) and were negative for involucrin, cytokeratin K8 and CLAUDIN-1, the typical cortical thymic epithelial cell (cTEC) associated markers. mTEC exosomes were positive classical exosomal markers such as TSG101, CD82, CD63, MFG-E8, FLOTILIN-1 and immunoproteasome subunits PSMB9 and PSMB10 (cells were negative for these markers), while PSMB8 was found in both, cells and exosomes. Such markers as CP, ALDOC, COL6A1, LAMA2, SRI, HSPG2, TSN, AOC3, SLC34A2, F13A1 were identified both in cells and exosomes.	Exosomes were isolated from media of TEC	[28]
8	Exosomes from colorectal cancer cell LIM1215	Exosomes and cells were positive for A33 antigen, cadherin-17, carcinoembryonic antigen, ephrin-B1 and -B2. 31 proteins were be common between exosomal proteomes of LIM1215 cells, mast cells and exosomes from urine, whereas 79 and 96 proteins were in common between LIM1215-mast cell and LIM1215-urine data sets. The 31 common proteins include Alix, transferrin, actins (α, β, and γ), RAB5B, RAB5C, EH-domain containing 4, heat shock proteins, annexins A6 and A11, and ADP-ribosylation factor 1 among others. LIM125-derived pure exosome proteins were enriched with tetraspanin-containing proteins when compared with the entire human proteome and were the first to report the presence of phospholipid scramblase 3 in exosomes.	Exosomes were isolated from culture media of LIM1215 cells	[29]

Table 1.
Some of the surface markers and proteome particularities of the exosomes of a certain origin.

in the cancerous cell than normal cells [35]. Other features making exosome a promising delivery system are innate stability, the ability to cross biological barriers, and enhanced loading capability of biological molecules [36]. It should be noted, due to the preferential homing of exosomes for their source cells, cancer exosomes should not or should be used as drug carriers with particular attention because they may promote tumor invasion or epithelial-mesenchymal transition, or they may transfer tumor resistance genes to tumor cells [37].

Their superior tissue-homing capabilities have been identified such as unidirectional synaptic transfer of microRNA from T cells to antigen-presenting cells. Moreover, depending on the integrin expression pattern of the parent cells, different mammalian tumor exosomes were shown to preferentially target healthy cells in the predicted tissue. As it was mentioned above, cancer exosomes, like exosomes from sarcoma cells, show preferential tumor homing. As for the biodistribution, exosomes accumulate primarily in the liver, lung, spleen, and gastrointestinal tract and this distribution in some cases, like with systemic exosome administration, is not specific [38]. Nevertheless, depending on the origin of exosomes, the biodistribution may be changed: dendritic-cell-derived exosomes are preferentially taken up by the spleen, melanoma-cell-derived exosomes accumulate more prominently in the liver [38]. Despite a shorter half-life compared with liposomes, reaching a maximum of 60 minutes, exosomes were superior in escaping stress-relaxing environments and had a comparatively longer circulation half-life [38, 39].

Among others, there are three relatively simple and effective options for loading cargo into exosomes: electroporation, passive transport of the target during incubation, and sonication. Electroporation is a well-known method for different genetic structures loading into cells has the same principle in exosome loading: pores are created in the exosomal membrane by applying an electric field to a suspension of exosomes facilitating the movement of cargo into the lumen of the exosomes. A very simple and nevertheless effective way of cargo loading is a simple incubation of exosomes with the cargo: curcumin was efficiently loaded into exosomes after only 5 min of incubation at 22°C [40]. Another method to load cargo into exosomes is sonication with the same basic idea as electroporation, which is making pores in the bilipid exosomal membrane and cargo loading into exosomes via these pores. An accurately chosen regimen of sonication does not cause significant changes in the structure and content of exosomal membranes [40]. Thus, the appropriate method for cargo loading should be chosen based on the exosomes concentration, preliminary procedures like method of isolation and exosome storage condition and the loading target. Other methods of loading cargo into exosomes are transfection, freeze-thaw cycles, extrusion, surfactant treatment, and hypotonic dialysis.

Exosomes, being biodegradable nanoparticles, have successfully encapsulated bioactive molecules such as curcumin, paclitaxel, neurotoxin-I, and dexamethasone. Additionally, exosomes are utilized as drug delivery vesicles for multiple disease models of cancers, diabetes, and brain diseases such as Alzheimer's, prions, and Parkinson's [41].

Due to the biocompatibility of exosomes, various routes of administration are possible such as intravenous, intraperitoneal, oral, intranasal, and intratumoral. The exosomes have been considered a transporter of biomolecules, including lipids, proteins, enzymes, transmembrane proteins, cytoskeletal proteins, and genetic material. Exosomes were shown to effectively deliver an antibody-drug conjugate (trastuzumab-emtansine) to cancer cells in HER2-positive cancer [42]. Barok et al. showed that antibody-drug-conjugated exosomes bound to HER2+ cancer cells with growth inhibition and activation of caspases-3 [42]. Another example of successful use of cancer-related exosomes in cancer treatment is loading of modification of inhibitor of apoptosis protein survivin-survivin-T34A, which is a dominant-negative mutant of survivin—into exosomes isolated from melanoma cell lines. These exosomes were shown to effectively induce apoptosis in cancer cells [43, 44]. Kooijmans et al. anchored anti-epidermal growth factor receptor nanobodies to the surfaces of exosome vesicles via glycosylphosphatidylinositol to improve the interactions between exosomes and epidermal growth factor receptor-expressing tumor cells [45].

Elucidation of the mechanisms underlying protein and RNA sorting in exosomes may have great potential for developing various therapeutic applications. Although in clinical trials exosomes are commonly used as diagnostic and/or prognostic and/or predictive markers they are more than viable candidates for targeted drug delivery innovation due to the various benefits mentioned above [41].

7. Conclusion

Working with exosomes isolated from biological fluids we do not havestrong arguments allowing us to firmly assume the tissue origin of the isolated exosomes. This is due to the biogensis features of exosomes and methodological difficulties in performing experiments to identify the tissue specificity of exosomes. All this explains a few data, allowing us to compare membrane proteins and protein and nucleic acids cargo of exosomes of a certain origin except the research on cell lines, which have a wide range of limitations in the extrapolation of obtained data to the corresponding tissue. However, exosomes remain a promising diagnostic approach for different pathologies and gain more interest as therapeutic agents delivery systems because of their biocompatibility, safety, and tissue-homing capabilities. Further research in exosomes biology would provide a big future for the application of these biomolecules for different aspects of clinical medicine.

Conflict of interest

The authors declare no conflict of interest.

Author details

Alisa Petkevich[1*], Aleksandr Abramov[2] and Vadim Pospelov[2]

1 N.N. Blokhin Russian Cancer Research Center, Moscow, Russia

2 Scientific and Practical Center of Specialized Health Care for Children Named After V.F. Voino-Yasenetskiy, Moscow, Russia

*Address all correspondence to: pa.alisa26@gmail.com

References

[1] Leitão AL, Enguita FJ. A structural view of miRNA biogenesis and function. Noncoding RNA. 2022;**8**(1):10. DOI: 10.3390/ncrna8010010

[2] Witwer KW, Théry C. Extracellular vesicles or exosomes? On primacy, precision, and popularity influencing a choice of nomenclature. Journal of Extracellular Vesicles. 2019;**8**(1):1648167. DOI: 10.1080/20013078.2019.1648167

[3] Couch Y, Buzàs EI, Di Vizi D, Gho YS, Harrison P, Hill AF, et al. A brief history of nearly EV-erything - the rise and rise of extracellular vesicles. Journal of Extracellular Vesicles. 2021;**10**(14):e12144. DOI: 10.1002/jev2.12144

[4] Scheuermann S, Lehmann JM, Ramani MR, Reißfelder C, Rückert F, Langejürgen J, et al. TissueGrinder, a novel technology for rapid generation of patient-derived single cell suspensions from solid tumors by mechanical tissue dissociation. Frontiers in Medicine. 2022;**9**:721639. DOI: 10.3389/fmed.2022.721639

[5] Gurung S, Perocheau D, Touramanidou L, Baruteau J. The exosome journey: From biogenesis to uptake and intracellular signalling. Cell Communication and Signaling. 2021;**19**(1):47. DOI: 10.1186/s12964-021-00730-1

[6] Wu D, Yan J, Shen X, Sun Y, Thulin M, Cai Y, et al. Profiling surface proteins on individual exosomes using a proximity barcoding assay. Nature Communications. 2019;**10**(1):3854. DOI: 10.1038/s41467-019-11486-1

[7] Vajen T, Mause SF, Koenen RR. Microvesicles from platelets: Novel drivers of vascular inflammation. Thrombosis and Haemostasis. 2015;**114**(2):228-236. DOI: 10.1160/TH14-11-0962

[8] Hergenreider E et al. Atheroprotective communication between endothelial cells and smooth muscle cells through miRNAs. Nature Cell Biology. 2012;**14**:249-256

[9] Berckmans RJ, Lacroix R, Hau CM, Sturk A, Nieuwland R. Extracellular vesicles and coagulation in blood from healthy humans revisited. Journal of Extracellular Vesicles. 2019;**8**(1):1688936. DOI: 10.1080/20013078.2019.1688936

[10] Simkin PA. The human knee: A window on the microvasculature. Tissue Barriers. 2015;**3**(1-2):e970465. DOI: 10.4161/21688362.2014.970465

[11] Huang Y, Liu Y, Huang Q, Sun S, Ji Z, Huang L, et al. TMT-based quantitative proteomics analysis of synovial fluid-derived exosomes in inflammatory arthritis. Frontiers in Immunology. 2022;**13**:800902. DOI: 10.3389/fimmu.2022.800902

[12] Kato T, Miyaki S, Ishitobi H, Nakamura Y, Nakasa T, Lotz MK, et al. Exosomes from IL-1β stimulated synovial fibroblasts induce osteoarthritic changes in articular chondrocytes. Arthritis Research & Therapy. 2014;**16**(4):R163. DOI: 10.1186/ar4679

[13] Esa A, Connolly KD, Williams R, Archer CW. Extracellular vesicles in the synovial joint: Is there a role in the pathophysiology of osteoarthritis? Malaysian Orthopaedic Journal. 2019;**13**(1):1-7. DOI: 10.5704/MOJ.1903.012

[14] Withrow J, Murphy C, Liu Y, Hunter M, Fulzele S, HamrickM W.

Extracellular vesicles in the pathogenesis of rheumatoid arthritis and osteoarthritis. Arthritis Research & Therapy. 2016;**18**(1):286. DOI: 10.1186/s13075-016-1178-8

[15] Teleanu DM, Chircov C, Grumezescu AM, Volceanov A, Teleanu R. Blood-Brain delivery methods using nanotechnology. Pharmaceutics. 2018;**10**(4):269. DOI: 10.3390/pharmaceutics10040269

[16] Rashed HM, Bayraktar EK, Helal G, Abd-Ellah M, Amero P, et al. Exosomes: From garbage bins to promising therapeutic targets. International Journal of Molecular Sciences. 2017;**18**:E538. DOI: 10.3390/ijms18030538

[17] Hornung S, Dutta S, Bitan G. CNS-derived blood exosomes as a promising source of biomarkers: Opportunities and challenges. Frontiers in Molecular Neuroscience. 2020;**13**:38. DOI: 10.3389/fnmol.2020.00038

[18] Otake K, Kamiguchi H, Hirozane Y. Identification of biomarkers for amyotrophic lateral sclerosis by comprehensive analysis of exosomal mRNAs in human cerebrospinal fluid. BMC Medical Genomics. 2019;**12**(1):7. DOI: 10.1186/s12920-019-0473-z

[19] Shi M, Liu C, Cook TJ, Bullock KM, Zhao Y, Ginghina C, et al. Plasma exosomal α-synuclein is likely CNS-derived and increased in Parkinson's disease. Acta Neuropathologica. 2014;**128**(5):639-650. DOI: 10.1007/s00401-014-1314-y

[20] Bellingham SA, Guo BB, Coleman BM, Hill AF. Exosomes: Vehicles for the transfer of toxic proteins associated with neurodegenerative diseases? Frontiers in Physiology. 2012;**3**:124. DOI: 10.3389/fphys.2012.00124

[21] González-Cubero E, González-Fernández ML, Gutiérrez-Velasco L, Navarro-Ramírez E, Villar-Suárez V. Isolation and characterization of exosomes from adipose tissue-derived mesenchymal stem cells. Journal of Anatomy. 2021;**238**(5):1203-1217. DOI: 10.1111/joa.13365

[22] Wang ZG, He ZY, Liang S, YanC Q, Cheng P, Chen AM. Comprehensive proteomic analysis of exosomes derived from human bone marrow, adipose tissue, and umbilical cord mesenchymal stem cells. Stem Cell Research & Therapy. 2020;**11**(1):511. DOI: 10.1186/s13287-020-02032-8

[23] Xu H, Wang Z, Liu L, Zhang B, Li B. Exosomes derived from adipose tissue, bone marrow, and umbilical cord blood for cardioprotection after myocardial infarction. Journal of Cellular Biochemistry. 2020;**121**(3):2089-2102. DOI: 10.1002/jcb.27399

[24] Mead B, Tomarev S. Bone marrow-derived mesenchymal stem cells-derived exosomes promote survival of retinal ganglion cells through miRNA-dependent mechanisms. Stem Cells Translational Medicine. 2017;**6**(4):1273-1285. DOI: 10.1002/sctm.16-0428

[25] Patil M, Saheera S, Dubey PK, Kahn-Krell A, Kumar GP, Singh S, et al. Novel mechanisms of exosome-mediated phagocytosis of dead cells in injured heart. Circulation Research. 2021;**129**(11):1006-1020. DOI: 10.1161/CIRCRESAHA.120.317900

[26] Lee JH, Ha DH, Go HK, YouG J, Kim HK, Jin RC, et al. Reproducible large-scale isolation of exosomes from adipose tissue-derived mesenchymal stem/stromal cells and their application in acute kidney injury. International Journal of Molecular Sciences.

2020;**21**(13):4774. DOI: 10.3390/ijms21134774

[27] Katsuda T, Tsuchiya R, Kosaka N, Yoshioka Y, Takagaki K, Oki K, et al. Human adipose tissue-derived mesenchymal stem cells secrete functional neprilysin-bound exosomes. Scientific Reports. 2013;**3**:1197. DOI: 10.1038/srep01197

[28] Skogberg G, Lundberg V, Berglund M, Gudmundsdottir J, Telemo E, Lindgren S, et al. Human thymic epithelial primary cells produce exosomes carrying tissue-restricted antigens. Immunology and Cell Biology. 2015;**93**(8):727-734. DOI: 10.1038/icb.2015.33

[29] Mathivanan S, Lim JW, Tauro BJ, Ji H, Moritz RL, Simpson RJ. Proteomics analysis of A33 immunoaffinity-purified exosomes released from the human colon tumor cell line LIM1215 reveals a tissue-specific protein signature. Molecular & Cellular Proteomics. 2010;**9**(2):197-208. DOI: 10.1074/mcp.M900152-MCP200

[30] Saheera S, Jani VP, Witwer KW, Kutty S. Extracellular vesicle interplay in cardiovascular pathophysiology. American Journal of Physiology. Heart and Circulatory Physiology. 2021;**320**(5):H1749-H1761. DOI: 10.1152/ajpheart.00925.2020

[31] Kim H, Yun N, Mun D, Kang JY, Lee SH, Park H, et al. Cardiac-specific delivery by cardiac tissue-targeting peptide-expressing exosomes. Biochemical and Biophysical Research Communications. 2018;**499**(4):803-808. DOI: 10.1016/j.bbrc.2018.03.227

[32] Greening DW, Nguyen HP, Elgass K, Simpson RJ, Salamonsen LA. Human endometrial exosomes contain hormone-specific cargo modulating trophoblast adhesive capacity: Insights into endometrial-embryo interactions. Biology of Reproduction. 2016;**94**(2):38. DOI: biolreprod.115.134890

[33] Sharma M, Ravichandran R, Bansal S, Bremner RM, Smith MA, Mohanakumar T. Tissue-associated self-antigens containing exosomes: Role in allograft rejection. Human Immunology. 2018;**79**(9):653-658. DOI: 10.1016/j.humimm.2018.06.005

[34] Saheera S, Potnuri AG, Krishnamurthy P. Nano-vesicle (Mis) communication in senescence-related pathologies. Cell. 2020;**9**(9):1974. DOI: 10.3390/cells9091974

[35] Govindappa PK, Patil M, Garikipati VNS, Verma SK, Saheera S, Narasimhan G, et al. Targeting exosome-associated human antigen R attenuates fibrosis and inflammation in diabetic heart. FASEB Journal: Official Publication of the Federation of American Societies for Experimental Biology. 2020;**34**(2):2238-2251. DOI: 10.1096/fj.201901995R

[36] Rajput A, Varshney A, Bajaj R, Pokharkar V. Exosomes as new generation vehicles for drug delivery: Biomedical applications and future perspectives. Molecules. 2022;**27**(21):7289. DOI: 10.3390/molecules27217289

[37] Chen H, Wang L, Zeng X, Schwarz H, Nanda HS, Peng X, Zhou Y. Exosomes, a new star for targeted delivery. Frontiers in Cell and Developmental Biology. 2021;**9**:751079. DOI: 10.3389/fcell.2021.751079

[38] Dai J, Su Y, Zhong S, et al. Exosomes: Key players in cancer and potential therapeutic strategy. Signal Transduction and Targeted Therapy. 2020;**5**(1):145. DOI: 10.1038/s41392-020-00261-0

[39] Herrmann IK, Wood MJA, Fuhrmann G. Extracellular vesicles as a

next-generation drug delivery platform. Nature Nanotechnology. 2021;**16**:748-759. DOI: 10.1038/s41565-021-00931-2

[40] Conlan RS, Pisano S, Oliveira MI, Ferrari M, Mendes PI. Exosomes as reconfigurable therapeutic systems. Trends in Molecular Medicine. 2017;**23**(7):636-650. DOI: 10.1016/j.molmed.2017.05.003

[41] Bunggulawa EJ, Wang W, Yin T, et al. Recent advancements in the use of exosomes as drug delivery systems. Journal of Nanbiotechnology. 2018;**16**:81. DOI: 10.1186/s12951-018-0403-9

[42] Barok M, Puhka M, Vereb G, Szollosi J, Isola J, Joensuu H. Cancer-derived exosomes from HER2-positive Cancer cells carry Trastuzumab-Emtansine into Cancer cells leading to growth inhibition and caspase activation. BMC Cancer. 2018;**18**:504. DOI: 10.1186/s12885-018-4418-2

[43] Khan S, Bennit HF, Wall NR. The emerging role of exosomes in Survivin secretion. Histology and Histopathology. 2015;**30**:43-50. DOI: 10.14670/HH-30.43

[44] Huda MN, Nafiujjaman M, Deaguero IG, et al. Potential use of exosomes as diagnostic biomarkers and in targeted drug delivery: Progress in clinical and preclinical applications. ACS Biomaterials Science & Engineering. 2021;**7**(6):2106-2149. DOI: 10.1021/acsbiomaterials.1c00217

[45] Butreddy A, Kommineni N, Dudhipala N. Exosomes as naturally occurring vehicles for delivery of biopharmaceuticals: Insights from drug delivery to clinical perspectives. Nanomaterials (Basel). 2021;**11**(6):1481. DOI: 10.3390/nano11061481

Chapter 7

Perspective Chapter: Exosomes – The Surreptitious Intercellular Messengers in the Body

Naveen Soni, Jitender Jangra, Megha Chaudhary, Gargi Nandi and Bhawana Bissa

Abstract

Exosomes are secret intercellular messengers in the body, carrying crucial information from different organs. Different cargos can be packaged in exosomes including DNA, RNA, and proteins. The type of exosomal cargo can vary according to the tissue type, its pathophysiological state, and circadian rhythm. Therefore, exosomes have an immense potential to be utilized for diagnostic purposes if the conundrum of their cargo can be understood. Recent advances in exosome isolation and characterization have made it possible to define disease-specific cargo carried by these tiny messengers. We attempt to highlight disease-relevant exosomal cargos for diagnostic purposes.

Keywords: exosomes, cancer, neurodegeneration, cardiovascular, miRNA

1. Introduction

Cells are the most unique and well-established micro-machines that assemble and make efficient metabolic molecules and pathways to maintain homeostasis. Exosomes are one of those cellular secretions that carry hidden information about proteins, RNAs, DNAs, and metabolites of secretory cells. Certain amounts of these molecules are packaged in the exosomes during their synthesis and secreted from the cell in a normal process. These exosomes are released in the extracellular environment and get captured by the nearby cells. Exosome content carrying information of parent cells makes the physiological changes in the recipient cell, making them an intercellular messenger of genetic and metabolic information.

Extracellular vesicles are the membrane-enclosed form of cell cargo with dynamic size, variety, and diversity. These can be distributed in three types based on the diameter of the vesicle; microvesicles (100-1000 nm), exosomes (30-150 nm), and apoptotic bodies (50-5000 nm) [1]. Exosomes were first recognized in rat ovum and algae in the 1950s [2, 3]. Soon after this, the detection of EVs was also done in plants and fungi [4, 5]. At that time EVs were not recognized well, instead, they were thought to assist in removing garbage from the cell. Later in 1996, Raposo declared that antigen-specific MHC-2 containing vesicles from B-lymphocytes induces an antigen-specific response in T-cells, clarifying that EVs are not garbage anymore [6]. EVs were also discovered in bat thyroid follicular cells by Nunez and Gershon [7]. This was the first chapter to explain the proximity of multivesicular bodies near the limiting membrane, and their fusion with the membrane to release them into luminal space. EV secretion is the ancient feature, followed by archaea, prokaryotes, and eukaryotes that play a significant role in cell-cell communication [8, 9].

2. Exosome biogenesis

Exosomes like vesicles (ELV) or exosomes are synthesized in the endosomal compartments in a well regulated way, and stress, mutation, and alteration in the microbiological environment may change the generation and secretion of exosomes. This regulation is maintained by the multiple proteins such as RAB, SNAREs, and cytoskeletal proteins [10]. Endosomes are synthesized by the invagination of the cell membranes. A naive endosome is non-judgmental with no decided fate and is called an early endosome. It either can fuse with the available endocytic vesicles containing cargo for export/degradation/recycling or can mature into late endosomes [11, 12]. Late endosomes are slightly more acidic than early endosomes, which might affect exosome production. A study by Logozzi has revealed that when cells are grown in acidic pH, the amount of exosome synthesis also increases as compared to the buffered medium [13]. Within the late endosome, the inward budding of the membrane synthesizes intraluminal vesicles that accumulate cytosolic content such as nucleic acid, proteins, metabolites, ions, and lipids. At this stage, the whole organelle containing ILV is considered as MVBs (Multi Vesicular Bodies). The pre-decided fate of MVB is not clear whether it will fuse with lysosome or autophagosome or exocytose to deliver in luminal space.

Exosomes are synthesized in the MVBs in the form of ILVs. Biogenesis of exosomes necessitates enrichment of CD9 and CD63 tetraspanin molecules and assembly of ESCRT (Endosomal Sorting Complex Required for Transport) complex at the site [14–16]. ESCRT is the preferred route of ILV formation but if ESCRT is necessary for cargo selection and exosome secretion is still controversial. ESCRT consists of four ESCRT protein complexes: ESCRT-0, ESCRT-I, ESCRT-II, and ESCRT-III. Another AAA ATPase Vps4 complex works together with the ESCRT-III to deform and amputee endosomal membrane [17]. These protein complexes show a high degree of cooperativity while sorting cargoes, vesicle budding, and MVB biogenesis [18]. The whole process of cargo selection, vesicle formation, and cargo incorporation occurs simultaneously. ESCRT-0 complex first initiates the recognition of microdomains on the endosomal membrane where ubiquitinated proteins are sequestrated. This occurs through the recognition by the HRS protein of ESCRT-0 to TSG101 of ESCRT-I. This initiates the invagination of the membrane, considering that all the proteins assigned for their secretion/degradation are clustered. ESCRT-0 complex interacts with the ESCRT-I and ESCRT-II and a wide-neck vesicle is formed inside the endosome [19]. Vesicle maturation marks the deubiquitination of clustered proteins. At this stage, ESCRT-0, ESCRT-I, and ESCRT-II units disassociate from the site and ESCRT-III assembles at the site. Snf7 protein, a unit of ESCRT-III, forms an oligomeric assembly and recruits ALIX (ALG-2 interacting protein X) at the site that stabilizes the ESCRT-III and promotes vesicle budding [20]. This complex narrows down the neck of the newly forming vesicle and then interacts with the AAA ATPase Vps4 complex, which is the key energy providing protein in releasing the vesicle from the endosomal membrane. Newly synthesized vesicle containing cargo now disassemble from the endosomal membrane and accumulate in the MVBs.

Another route for exosome production is the ceramide pathway, an ESCRT-Independent pathway. Microdomains present on the endosomal membrane are enriched with sphingomyelinases (SMases). These SMases cleave sphingomyelin lipid of the membrane, remove phosphocholine moiety and incorporate ceramide. These ceramides in the membrane induce lateral phase separation and amalgamate the microdomains of the membrane [21]. Consequently, a negative curvature is formed that promotes budding. Tetraspanins such as CD9, CD63, and CD81 are highly enriched in the exosome membrane and assist in protein sorting and exosome biogenesis. These tetraspanins containing microdomains are the specialized structure involved in an assortment of receptors and signaling molecules in the plasma membrane [22].

3. Exosome secretion

Rab protein is the largest family of small GTPases that governs the switch of GTP hydrolysis. More than 60 members of the Rab family are present in the intracellular membrane, serving as the main regulator of vesicle secretion [23]. Rab GTPases cover a major portion of membrane trafficking by its interaction with SNAREs, motor proteins, and coat proteins. The activation of GTPase activity is regulated by the GEFs (Guanine nucleotide exchange factors). The study also demonstrates that the interaction of SNARE with Rab induces the release of exosomes [24]. Rab proteins are the key molecules that determine the size of exosomes and regulate MVB docking at the plasma membrane, such as Rab27a, and intracellular distribution of MVBs for exosomal traffickings, such as Rab27b [25, 26]. Rab27a and Rab27b interact with their respective effector proteins, Slp4 and Slac2b, respectively, to transfer MVBs from the perinuclear to the periphery area of the cell [25]. Abolishing these interactions leads to decreased exosome release and inhibited breast cancer cell invasion and migration [27]. Additionally, some factors such as HSP90 and lysosome-associated protein transmembrane-4B (LAPTM4B) also transfer MVBs toward the periphery to promote their secretion [28, 29]. KIBRA interacts with Rab27a and enhances its retention, while some other GEFs such as MADD and Fam45a control exocytosis [26, 30, 31]. Rab11 and Rab35 are majorly involved in the endosome recycling pathway, and also assist in exosome secretion and cargo selection. Loss of function in Rab11 and Rab35 results in exosome accumulation in the cells [32]. But a similar study declaring that Rab11a and Rab7 remain uninvolved during the exosome biogenesis process is still controversial. The same study also shows that Rab7 enhances the release of exosomes containing Alix and syntenin in breast cancer cells but its knockdown does not affect exosome release in HeLa cells [25, 33]. Some small GTPases such as Rab2a, Rab5a, and Rab9a also increase exosome secretion [25]. These diversified functions of Rabs modulate the exosome biogenesis machinery and its secretion out of the cells. HRS, STAM1, and TSG101 silencing decrease the exosome release in dendritic cells [34].

4. Exosome cargo

The exosome content is solely dependent on the extracellular environment and intracellular metabolic activities that may vary at any stage of the cell. Exosomes are loaded with RNA, DNA, lipids, and proteins with different concentrations and types. This specificity can be changed from cell to cell even with the same environment. Many studies are ongoing and have been done to get exosome content. For now, few databases are accessible to collect information about the exosome cargo. These are exoRBase, Exocarta, EVpedia, Vesiclepedia, EV-TRACK, and ExoBCD [35–42]. For now, >9700 proteins, >3400 mRNA, >2800 miRNA, and > 1100 lipid data in EVs have been identified [39].

a. DNA: A diverse nature of nucleic acid content is found in the secreted EVs but only a few cases have been studied where genomic and mitochondrial DNA of EV works in cancer detection [43, 44]. Exosome-gDNA-based liquid biopsies for colorectal cancer are often performed [45]. Mammalian cells often discard the mutated portions of DNA and some transposon elements that are harmful to the cell. This fragmented gDNA and mtDNA get accumulated in the cytosol and packaged in exosomes for their secretion out of the cell. A study on pancreatic cancer identified mutated p53 and KRAS DNA in the serum exosomes, revealing it as an important biomarker for early detection of cancer [43, 46, 47]. In the same studies, it was also identified that large double-standard gDNA fragments reflect the mutation status of the tumor, important for molecular mapping. Considering this, exosome DNA databases can be formed for early screening of diseases, DNA modifications, and evaluating drug resistance.

b. RNA (coding, non-coding): Exosomes are enriched with the RNAs specifically functional non-coding RNAs [48]. Out of them, certain miRNAs are found so frequently with high diagnostic potential. Overall, exosomes are enriched with tRNA, 18S, and 28S rRNAs but other RNA species such as mRNA, miRNA, Pre-miRNA, Y-RNA, tRF, lncRNA, sncRNA, *piwi*-RNA, circRNA, and vault RNA are also found [49–52]. RNAs in the EVs were found from as short as 200 bp to >4 kb in length with most of them containing 3'-UTR regions [53]. These RNAs remain protected with the vesicle lipid bilayer or are associated with some RNPs such as RNPs or lipoproteins (HDL and LDL) [54].

   Different mechanisms have been proposed for the loading of RNAs in the EVs. For example, specific sequences within the 3′ UTR act as "zip-code" to export certain specific RNAs in the EVs. These "zip-codes" are about ~25 nt in length, such as the binding site for the miR-1289 carries by another mRNA containing the "CTGCC" sequence on its stem-loop structure [55]. It has also been seen that certain miRNAs carrying four nucleotide sequence motif "GGAG" interact with the hnRNPA2B1, which enhances their sorting in the EVs [56]. In addition, post-transcriptional modifications of miRNAs determine their fate of retention, such as uridylated 3′-end of miRNAs are sorted into the EVs, while adenylated 3′-end keeps them to stay within the cell [57]. Another mechanism is based on the nSmase2 activity, which if, overexpressed, releases more amount of miRNAs by enhancing exosome production [58]. Apart from this, the role of argonaute protein in the loading of RNAs in EVs is still a controversial statement. Some studies support that the knockdown of argonaute protein decreases certain specific miRNAs in the EVs. Whether argonaute is found in the EVs or the MVBs or in the endosomes, is still a complex scenario in the EV research [59, 60].

c. Proteins: The information about the protein cargo within the EVs is still unclear due to the differences in cell types, culture conditions, and isolation procedures. Only a fraction of common EV proteins can be identified that are generally found in the endosomal pathway, like Alix, tetraspanins, and some ESCRT proteins. In addition, proteins for exosome secretion such as Rab27a, Rab11b, and ARF6 are commonly found in the EVs. Interestingly, most of the EVs contain tetraspanins (CD9, CD63, CD81, CD82, CD86), antigen-presenting molecules (MHC-1 and MHC-II), transcription factors (Wnt, Notch, hedgehog), transport and fusion proteins (GTPase and flotillin), heat-shock proteins (Hsp20, Hsp27, Hsp60, Hsp70, Hsp90), cell-surface peptidases (CD13 and CD26), and signaling receptors like EGFR [36, 61–64]. Exosome composition is mostly decided by the cell type it is derived from. A drug-resistant cell secretes exosomes containing MDR-proteins such as ABCB1, ABCC2, ABCG2, and p-glycoproteins to enhance the tumor environment more resistant to drugs [65, 66].

d. Lipids: Exosomes are loaded with certain metabolic active lipids that regularly participate in exosome syntheses, such as sphingomyelins, ceramides, aminophospholipid, cholesterol, and phosphatidyl serine [66]. In addition, a high phosphatidyl serine ratio in the outer layer of exosomes may enhance their uptake by target cell [67]. Overall, the lipid composition of exosomes is ~80% similar to the parent cell but the amount of polyunsaturated glycerophosphoserine and phosphatidyl serine makes it more unique and different [68, 69].

e. Metabolites: Much research is ongoing to capture attention toward the metabolite composition of extracellular vesicles. By targeting urine, serum, or plasma vesicles, more promising results have already been revealed [70–72]. Mostly, exosome lipidomes have been quantified with glycerophospholipids, prenol and sterol lipids, glycerolipids, free fatty acids, and sphingolipids [73, 74]. Some studies also demonstrate that apart from lipids, few amounts of sugar, amino acids, organic acids, carboxylic acids, nucleotides, metabolic intermediates, carnitines, phenolic compounds, and vitamins are also present [75–77].

5. Exosomes in different biological fluids

Exosomes are very small molecules that formed within endosomes *via* different ESCRT-dependent processes [78]. Their sizes range from around 30 nm to 150 nm. These EVs are secreted into the various body fluids, such as blood, urine, saliva, breast milk, ascites effusions, nasal secretions, tears, amniotic, synovial, lymphatic, cerebrospinal, and seminal fluids by the various cell types found within the body, including red blood cells, B cells, T cells, mast cells, platelets, endothelial cells, fibroblasts, adipocytes, epithelial cells [79–85]. Exosomes present in them move through these fluids to other areas or interact with other cells to carry out a variety of biological functions, including the modulation of immune response [86, 87], antigen presentation [88, 89], and the transfer of RNA and proteins [90, 91], intercellular communication, non-classical protein secretion [92], and transmission of pathogenic cargo [93–95]. Exosomes are typically obtained from various body fluids using ultracentrifugation [96] based on the sedimentation principle, which yields a very pure exosomal fraction that is recognized as the gold standard. Size exclusion filtration [97] or chromatography [98] is a different procedure that involves filtering through a number of filters with pores smaller than 100 nm and then centrifuging (100,000 g) to concentrate the exosomes. The biological function and integrity of the exosome are maintained using this method. Using a solid support magnet or flow cytometry, immune affinity capture [99] involves binding specific micro-beads to bio-fluids containing exosomes and separating the exosome-bound micro-beads from the bio-fluids. Exosome isolation is also done using kit-based techniques, such as the precipitation method ExoQuick [100] and the microfluidic technology (ExoChip) [101] based on the immunoaffinity methodology. The sample source and intended use of the exosomes may determine which of these various techniques and procedures to adopt, each of which has advantages and disadvantages of its own. Exosomes contain a variety of nucleic acids to perform various biological functions. The lipid bilayer's DNA, RNA, lipids, proteins, and metabolites keep them stable and allow for long-term storage. Even yet, the microenvironment and the type of cell to which an exosome is delivered determine what is contained within the cargo. As a result, the stability of different biomolecules within the exosome and their enrichment make them appropriate for a range of therapeutic and diagnostic uses. Exosome vesicles are primarily extracted from the serum, plasma, CSF, and urine and are the form that has been examined the most. As of now, exosome vesicles produced from particular fluids have more precise identification and validation than whole body fluid [78]. For instance, Kalra et al. [102] isolated EVs from plasma and demonstrated the depletion of highly abundant plasma proteins [103, 104]. As a result of their cargo and diverse features, exosomes are transformed by cells and may play a role in the progression of various diseases. As a diagnostic biomarker in the early detection and prognosis of diseases, these changed content (proteins or miRNAs) revealing distinct [78] profiles in exosomes are being different from the exosomes released by the normal/healthy cells. Another arm of exosomes is their therapeutic role for different purposes such as vaccination, biological targeting, and drug delivery tools, using a variety of therapeutic materials, including siRNA, antagomirs, g-RNA (siRNA), recombinant proteins, and anti-inflammatory drugs [105].

6. Exosomes in diseases

Exosomes in disease pathophysiology have recently attracted a lot of attention from researchers. Literature studies have shown that due to the potential ability of cell-to-cell communication among homozygous and heterozygous cell types, exosomes acts as a mediator for maintaining healthy physiological conditions [106]. In addition to their regular role, these exosomes are manipulated by the pathogen to infect the host cell activity [107] and act to potentiate stress and damage [106]. Exosomes have been discovered to play a role in the onset and progression of a number of diseases, including cancer, autoimmune disorders, neurodegenerative diseases [108], cardiovascular diseases, liver diseases [109], and genetic diseases, among many others.

6.1 Exosomes in tumor microenvironment, metastasis, and angiogenesis

Cancer is one of the oldest and deadliest diseases in the world. The ability of cancer cells to communicate with other cells is achieved primarily through exosome vesicles to maintain normal physiological conditions and trigger disease progression. These vesicles help cells to communicate between homotypic and heterotypic cells. In homotypic exosome transfer, exosome content and signaling capabilities allow cancer cells to progress and transmit cell growth, transformation, and survival signals to other cancer cells [110]. Various autocrine signaling pathways Akt/PI3K and MAP kinase are involved in its progression [111]. As heterotypic exosome transfer involves all stages of cancer development and progression, tumor spread is driven by its local tumor microenvironment (TME). TME is composed of different cell types, including endothelial cells, fibroblasts, and immune cells. This tumor microenvironment enables a variety of cancer cell-derived exosomes, such as CAF-derived exosomes (CDE) and fibroblast-derived exosomes, to sustain proliferation, evade growth suppression, evade immune recognition, and activate invasion and metastasis cascades. It helps in regulation, resisting cell death, initiation of angiogenesis, promotion of cell proliferation, and deregulation of cell energetics through juxtracrine and paracrine signaling interactions [112, 113].

In cancer metastasis, primary tumor cells migrate to another part of the body where they multiply and form new tumors. There are various stages in this process: vascular invasion, extravasation, tumor latency, and formation of macro- or micro-metastases [114]. The process of metastasis is modulated by EMT, ECM remodeling, activity of the immune system, and alteration in tumor micro-environment [115, 116]. However, exosomes play a significant role during metastasis, as it influences tumor roles and primarily contributes to the formation of the pre-metastatic niche that determines specific organotrophic metastasis [114, 117]. During the invasion, the primary tumor releases various factors (microRNAs, EGFR signaling ligands, EMT inducers, etc.) that promote invasion [118–120]. For example, miR-10b is transported and released by exosomes and promotes the metastatic properties of breast cancer cells [121]. Another, miR-23a inhibits E-cadherin synthesis in lung cancer and melanoma cells, thereby inhibiting the release of TGF-1 supporting EMT-promoting effects [50, 51]. EGFR signaling factors include ligands such as amphiregulin, tissue-type plasminogen activator, and/or annexin II, and significantly increase cancer cell invasion [122]. Exosomes secrete EMT inducers such as vimentin, snail, and twist in urothelial cell lines while reducing E-cadherin and catenin expression through the TGF-1 pathway [123]. These exosomes have properties that drive exosome organotropism in cancer cells, and ITG$\alpha 6\beta 4$ and -$\alpha 6\beta 1$ are associated with lung metastasis, and ITG$\alpha v\beta 5$ is associated with liver metastasis. Related, ITG$\beta 3$ is related to brain metastasis [124]. Exosomes also exhibit stromal cell proliferation, cancer cell migration and survival, and ECM remodeling that increases tumor cell resistance to apoptotic signals. This, along with the effect of chemokines and growth factors, leads to the formation of a new microenvironment for cancer cells, immune cells, and other stromal constituents that is referred to as the PMN [122, 125, 126]. For the initiation of the metastatic process, an adequate blood supply to the tumor facilitates the entry of tumor cells into the bloodstream [127]. Thus, angiogenesis provides an opportunity for tumor growth by supplying cancer with oxygen, nutrients, and metabolite replacement [127]. Exosomes can transport various biomolecules such as microRNAs, DNA fragments, proteins, lipids, and even pharmacological compounds from donor cells to recipient cells [128]. Therefore, noncoding RNAs, especially long noncoding RNAs (lncRNAs) and microRNAs, play important roles in regulating angiogenesis [129]. In addition, exosomes can interact with target cells such as endothelial cells (EC) as well as immune cells to initiate and promote angiogenesis. The uptake of tumor-derived exosomes by normal endothelial cells activates angiogenic signaling pathways and stimulates new blood vessel formation [130]. Exosomes migrate to the cell periphery and invade advanced pseudopods. After complete remodeling, neighboring ECs likely transport exosomes to other ECs and other cells within the TME (tumor microenvironment) *via* nanoparticle structures [131].

6.2 Exosomes in neurodegenerative diseases

The majority of human neurodegenerative diseases, such as Alzheimer's disease, Parkinson's disease, and Huntington's disease, have aggregation of aberrant proteins as a common mechanism [132]. The existence of vesicles in the CSF has proven that these EVs are involved in the pathogenic spread of harmful proteins [132].

Alzheimer's disease is a neurological disorder caused by the disparate modification of Amyloid beta (Aβ) peptide and tau protein. Exosomes carry proteases, APP and its C-terminal fragments (CTFs-APP) that are caused by gamma and β secretase within the early endosomes, ultimately exports Aβ into the exosomes [133]. Exosomes provide a unique pathway for removing Aβ from cells. However, they make Aβ more prone to aggregation and, therefore, could endanger neighboring cells [134]. Another protein called TAU is crucial for accelerating tubulin assembly into microtubules and preserving their structural integrity. Tau's protein biological activity is compromised by hyperphosphorylation, which also results in defective microtubule stabilization and the formation of neurofibrillary tangles that impact neuronal connection and function [135, 136]. The mechanism of exosome-based release of Tau protein helps microglia to spread damaging tau protein [137, 138].

Parkinson's disease is mostly caused by an accumulation of clumped or misfolded alpha-syn nuclei, which affect the cells' ability to function as neurons [139]. Exosomes are thought to protect against neuronal cytotoxicity and prevent intracellular protein aggregation by excreting alpha syn nuclei outside of cells. This could result in an increase in the concentration of harmful alpha syn nuclei in extracellular space. The exosomes can take up both big and small alpha syn structures and cause various forms of downstream mediated toxicity from healthy neuronal cells [140]. These aggregates can kill the other target cells [141–145]. In addition to these, there are several exosomal miRNAs that contribute to the progression of PD pathogenesis. MiR-7 binding to the 3' UTR of SNCA mRNA suppresses transcription, which results in miR-7 loss. This loss of miR-7 is what causes greater -syn upregulation, aggregation, and dopaminergic neuron death in the brain of PD patients [146]. Another mi-RNA, miR-4639-5p has been upregulated, which negatively controlled the post-transcription of DJ-1 to cause significant oxidative stress and neuronal death in PD patients [147]. These all suggest a multi-functional role of exosomes in PD pathogenesis.

6.3 Exosomes in kidney diseases

The role of exosomes in acute and chronic kidney disease is highly specialized. Studies have shown that cell-to-cell communication between different regions of the kidney and organs amplifies kidney damage [148]. This exosome vesicle release contains proteins from different regions of the nephron fragment, including the thick ascending limb of the Henle loop, the distal tubule, and the collecting duct [149]. Due to their different origins, they have different protein content than their origin and serve as biomarkers for certain diseases [150]. The extracellular vesicles release from podocyte mediate communication between glomeruli and renal tubules, whereby alterations in communication outside the vesicles can affect podocytes and cause tubular damage/injury [151]. Studies suggest that there is upregulation of CD2AP mRNA and downregulation of Wilms tumor protein 1 (WT1) in extracellular vesicles are potential biomarkers of podocyte injury. This mechanism contributes to damage amplification, development of tubule-interstitial fibrosis, and progression of CKD [152]. In acute chronic kidney disease, urinary exosomes miRNAs reflect the state of injury and fibrosis by the release of miR-9a, miR-16, miR-200a, and miR-141 [153]. A specific transcriptional repressor for activating transcription factor 3 (ATF3) was increased in sepsis-induced AKI [154]. In chronic kidney diseases such as diabetic nephropathy, there is a high glucose concentration in renal cells that cause changes in exosome composition and trafficking, further modifying and damaging intact cells [155]. Bioinformatics analysis revealed high levels of miR-133b and miR-342 in urinary exosomes of patients with diabetic nephropathy type 2 (T2DN) [156]. In addition, there are specific miRNAs such as miR-let-7i-3p, miR-24-3p, and miR-27b-3p, whose downregulation is involved in Wnt/β-catenin signaling, leading to T2DN pathogenesis [157]. Exosomes overexpress cellular repressors of multiple genes such as envoplakin, villin 1, prominin 1, and E1A-stimulated gene 1 (CREG1), causing autosomal dominant polycystic kidney disease (PKD) with abnormal morphological and proliferative changes [158, 159]. Circulating extracellular vesicles may lead to intra-organ crosstalk that shows an impact on autoimmune kidney diseases such as systemic lupus erythematosus, anti-phospholipid syndrome, and ANCA-associated vasculitis. For instance, circulating extracellular vesicles may encourage coagulation, thrombosis, and immune-mediated renal pathological conditions [160]. Placenta-derived extracellular vesicles carrying anti-angiogenic factors that are released into the maternal circulation in pre-eclampsia may cause proteinuria and glomerular endothelial dysfunction [161].

7. Exosomes in cardiovascular diseases

Cardiovascular diseases are major global diseases that affect the circulatory system [162]. Exosomes produced from the cardiac cells are one of the components in the body that keep cardiac under hypoxia and improve heart function [163]. These exosomes show changes in their states under various cardiovascular pathophysiology conditions and maintain homeostasis primarily during stress signals [164, 165]. Numerous diseases, such as cardiac fibrosis, ischemic heart diseases, heart failure, myocardial infraction, and cardiac hypertrophy, exhibit changes in cargo and protein content and serve as a biomarker for physiological changes [162]. It has been demonstrated that the pattern of fibroblast gene expression is regulated by cardiac cell-derived exosomes [166]. On external stimulation, cardiac fibrosis results in a sustainable remodeling of the extracellular matrix (ECM) through non-canonical Wnt and ERK1/2 pathways, as well as JNK pathways [167]. These pathways are promoted by the WNT-5a-enriched exosomes resulting in IL6 production and fibrosis [168]. Exosomes serve as intercellular communication (regulates intimal integrity) and myocardium remodeling in conditions such as ischemic heart disease and myocardial infarction respectively allowing injured cells to communicate with distant normal cells [162]. Exosomes derived from fibroblasts promote the RAS system and activate angiotensin II in cardiomyocytes that accelerate in cases of cardiac hypertrophy [169].

8. Diagnostic potential of exosomes

Exosomes are small EVs (Extra vesicles) of size 30-150 nm in diameter secreted by both normal cells and diseased cells into the different body fluids such as plasma, saliva, bronchial lavages, urine, and many others [170]. These fluids having exosomes contain different biomolecules including RNA, DNA, proteins for their intercellular communication, and transportation [171, 172]. There is differential expression of exosomal RNA and proteins derived from normal cells and diseased cells [173]. This exosomal protein and nucleic acid emerged as next-generation biomarkers for different pathology conditions such as neurodegenerative diseases, cardiovascular, kidney diseases, cancer, and others.

8.1 Proteins and cargo as diagnostic marker

In cancer cells, the protein content of exosomes varies between healthy cells and diseases, and it resembles a variety of conditions associated with cancer, liver, kidney, and brain diseases [174]. Exosome-specific protein serves as a biomarker for disease pathology. For instance, distinct protein expression of different fluids acts as a biomarker. In breast cancer, serum-derived exosomes show enrichment of ADAM10, metalloprotease, CD9, Annexin-1, and HSP70 [175] proteins, and plasma-derived exosomes show diagnostic potential for fibronectin and developmental endothelial locus-1 (Del-1) [176]. In lung cancer, expression of CD151, CD171, and tetraspanin 8 is higher in serum exosome [177]. Glypican-1 (GPC1)-positive exosomes serve as potential biomarkers in early-stage pancreatic cancer [178] and CD26, CD81, S1C3A1, and CD10 could be used as a potential biomarkers for hepatic damage [179].

Apart from cancer, other diseases also have significant alteration in exosomes profile and lead to different expression of proteins act as a biomarker for diagnostic potential. In neurodegenerative diseases such as Parkinson diseases elevated expression of different proteins such as PrPc (glycoprotein) [180], DJ-1 [181] (plasma neural-derived), OxiDJ-1 [182] (urine-derived), and Tau Protein (neuron-derived) could be a marker for PD diagnosis. Other potential biomarkers such as a decreased expression of C1q derived from serum exosome and more of blood-derived Apolipoprotein A1 (Apo A1), clusterin, complement C1r subcomponent, and fibrinogen gamma chain exosomal expression levels in the plasma of PD subjects may serve as a biomarker for the diagnosis of PD [183, 184]. In Alzheimer's diseases, human serum-derived exosome shows an elevated expression of Cathepsin-D, LAMP-1, ubiquitinylated protein [185]. Downregulation of SNAP-25 [186] marks the synaptic loss during the progression of AD and HSP70 [185, 187] shows dysfunction and neurodegeneration.

The kidneys play a crucial role in the human body's homeostasis regulation and maintenance [188]. The release of exosomes from various parts of the kidney facilitates cell-to-cell communication that has an impact on the physiology of the kidney [189]. The proteins and nucleic acids contained by exosomes carry through the urine serve as a non-invasive diagnostic biomarker for renal diseases. For instance, the protein level of Fuetin-1 and AQP2 have been identified as potential biomarkers for acute kidney injury (AKI) [153, 190]. There is an increased amount of neutrophil gelatinase-associated lipocalin (NGAL) and activating transcription factor 3 used as a marker for early diagnosis in sepsis-induced AKI [154]. The non-invasive biomarker for PKD is demonstrated by the elevated expression of the urinary exosome proteins such as villin-1, periplakin, and envoplakin in ADPKD (autosomal dominant polycystic kidney diseases) [158]. However, increased expression of AQP-2 and AQP-5 in exosomes in chronic diseases like diabetic nephropathy can be used as a biomarker to diagnose T2DN [191].

8.2 Nucleic acid as diagnostic and prognostic biomarker

Exosomes secreted from diseased cells contain different biomolecules than the healthy ones. Therefore, the basic nucleic acid content also varies with the diseases and mainly circulating microRNAs are being focused to carry out effective diagnosis and prognosis of numerous diseases [192]. For example, in breast cancer, the plasma-derived exosomes show the elevated expression of miR-1246 and miR-21 compared to healthy individuals [193, 194]. These serum-derived exosome shows miR-21 levels, which differentiate between metastatic and non-metastatic breast cancer [195]. Apart from these, upregulation of miRNAs, such as miR-223-3p, miR-16, miR-27a/b, miR-152, miR-199a-3p, miR-340, miR-376a, miR-410, and miR-598 [196–198], shows the presence of breast tumor. In non-small cell lung cancer (NSCLC), there is upregulation of different exosome miRNAs subset of 4 miRNAs (miR-378a, miR-379, miR-139-5p, and miR-200b-5p) and six miRNAs (miR-151a-5p, miR-30a-3p, miR-200b-5p, miR-629, miR-100, and miR-154-3p) respectively [199, 200]. Other than this, plasma-derived miRNA-9 and miRNA-15 can distinguish a metastatic and aggressive state of tumor, thus having high potential as a diagnostic marker for NSCLC [201]. However, in the diagnostic marker for hepatocellular carcinoma, there is upregulation of miRNA-21 in the plasma, which distinguishes patients from healthy individuals [202]. On the other hand, the cancer malignancy in hepatoblastoma is mediated by a panel of miRNAs involving miR-21, miR-34a, miR-34b, and miR-34c in plasma which are verified as diagnostic and prognostic tool [203]. High levels of miRNA-10b, miR-21, miR-30c, and miR-181a and decreased let-7a levels are seen in pancreatic ductal adenocarcinoma patients as compared to a healthy individual [204].

In neurodegenerative diseases such as Parkinson's and Alzheimer's disease, blood and peripheral fluids also contain exosomes synthesized from nerve cells that are passed through the BBB (blood-brain barrier). These fluids show different miRNAs expression in patients and healthy controls. miRNAs from serum are the non-invasive and feasible approach to determining biomarkers for neurodegenerative disease. Exosomal miRNAs derived from plasma, CSF, and serum are being either upregulated or downregulated in different pathophysiological conditions. Certain serum-derived miRNAs such as miR-15a-5p, miR-18b-5p, miR-30e-5p, miR-93-5p, miR-106a-5p, miR-143-3p, miR-335-5p, miR-361-5p, and miR-424-5p are upregulated in comparison with healthy individuals and some of the miRNAs such as miR-15b-3p, miR-342-3p, and miR-1306-5p are downregulated in AD patients [205, 206]. CSF-containing exosomes also show potential diagnostic miRNAs such as upregulation of miR-125b-5p and downregulation of miR-16-5p and miR-451a [207]. These differently regulated miRNAs from different fluids improve the early onset and late-onset diagnosis and prognosis of AD. Similarly, in Parkinson's disease, several miRNAs derived from different fluids have differentially regulated miRNAs. Serum-derived exosomes have upregulated miR-24, miR-195, and miR-29a [208]. In plasma-derived exosomes, elevated level of miR-331-5p and let-7e-5p is observed. Some miRNAs like miR-10a-5p, miR-151a-3p, let-7f-5p, and many more are seen upregulated in CSF-derived exosomes [209]. Not only the upregulated miRNAs from different fluids show diagnostic potential but the downregulated miRNAs compared to healthy controls also act as diagnostic markers. For example, in PD patients, CSF-derived exosomal miRNAs show downregulated expression such as miR-27a-3p, miR-423-5p, miR-22-3p, miR-1, miR-22, miR-29, miR-374, miR-119a, miR-28 [210]. Some miRNAs such as miR-505 and miR-19b derived from plasma and serum respectively also show downregulation in PD patients [211].

Kidney diseases include AKI (acute kidney injury), chronic kidney diseases, diabetic nephropathy, polycystic kidney diseases, and various others. Exosomes isolated from urine contain differential biomarkers in form of microRNAs. In the AKI condition, urinary exosomes show various miRNAs for different conditions such as AKI progression including miR-16, miR-24, and miR-200c [212]. Also, miR-210 predicts AKI mortality in ICU patients [213]. In sepsis-induced AKI, there is decreased expression of miR-376b, which acts as a potential biomarker for diagnosis [214]. Certain serum-derived exosomes reportedly decreased miR-24, miR-23a, and miR-145 expression in post-myocardial infarction AKI pathogenesis [215]. There are other serum-derived miRNAs that show a change in expression from healthy and AKI-diseased individuals including miR-101, miR-127, miR-210, miR-126, miR-26b, miR-29a, miR-146a, miR-27a, miR-93, and miR-10a [216]. Other kidney diseases, such as Diabetic Nephropathy, miR-192 is a master miRNA regulator of DN [212, 217]. Expression of miR-130 and miR-145 is upregulated, while miR-155 and miR-424 have reduced levels in diabetic patients with microalbuminuria, acting as a biomarker [218]. miR-415 derived from urinary exosome shows elevated expression in albuminuria and glomerulosclerosis and acts early diagnostic biomarker. miR-126 and the miR-770 family are derived from urine and blood as a promising biomarker for DN progression [212]. Although in diabetic patients, some Urine exosomal miRNAs including miR-192 and miR-21 show upregulated expression while reduced miR-30b levels which altered kidney function [219–222]. In type 2 diabetic nephropathy, the most upregulated miRNAs are MiR-34a and miR-320c which acts as a biomarker, and sediment miR-95 and miR-631 also reflect the severity and prognosis of type 2 DN [223–225]. Apart from these, certain other potential miRNAs biomarkers include miR-15b, miR-636, miR-34a, and miR-4534 in urine [226, 227] and miR-638 in serum. The ratio of albumin–creatinine shows an effect on miR-103a suggesting miR-103a as a dynamic biomarker reflecting pathological status and treatment response [228]. The role of EV miRNAs like miR-3907 upregulation in circulation predicts Autosomal Dominant Polycystic Kidney Disease progression [229]. Diagnosis shows other serum-derived miRNAs including miR-17 family members (miR-20a, miR-93, and miR-106a) show a significant decrease in expression after hemodialysis [230]. Apart from these, in some chronic kidney diseases such as hypertensive nephropathy, Lupus Nephritis, kidney immune diseases, and many others, the role of serum and urine-derived miRNAs show a prominent role in diagnosis, prognosis, and disease progression.

In cardiovascular diseases, circulating EVs miRNAs, miRNA-425, and miRNA-744 acts as a novel biomarkers for cardiac fibrosis [231, 232]. Also, miR-30d is associated with deleterious cardiac remodeling and the expression of fibrosis and

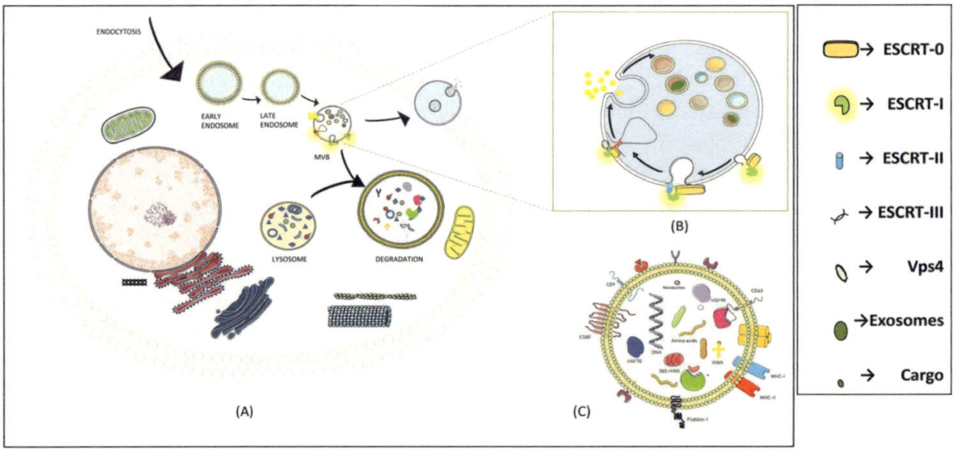

Figure 1.
(A) Multivesicular bodies can either merge with the lysosome or the autophagosome or be secreted out of the cell as a secretome. (B) Major pathways of exosome biogenesis (C) model structure of exosomes/EVs that carry certain proteins and receptors.

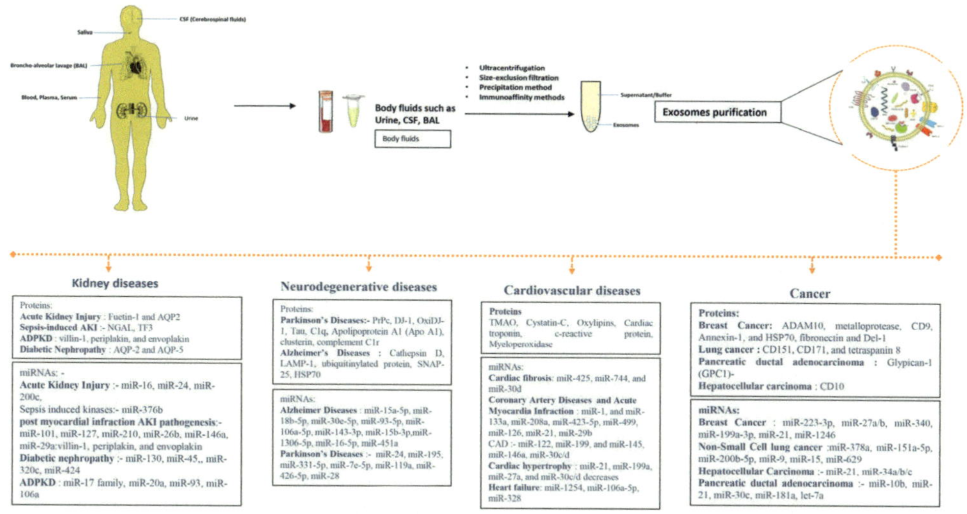

Figure 2.
Schematic representation of exosome isolation and diagnostic importance in different types of disorders.

inflammation-related genes [233]. In both coronary artery diseases and acute myocardial infraction, several exosomal miRNAs including miR-1, miR-133a, miR-208a, miR-423-5p, miR-499, miR-126, miR-21, and miR-29b show increased expression which potentially acts as a diagnostic biomarker as well as a prognostic marker for left ventricle remodeling [234–238]. However certain miRNAs including miR-423-5p [237], miR-499 [235], and miR-29b [239] essentially for AMI. miR-122 andmiR-199a [240] have elevated expression and miR-145 [241], miR-146a [242], miR-30c/d show downregulation that acts as diagnostic marker for CAD [243]. In contrast, miR-21, miR-199a miR-27a, and miR-30c/d show elevated levels, thus having a diagnostic potential of cardiac hypertrophy [244, 245]. However in heart failure diseases, the increased expression of miR-1254, miR-106a-5p, and decreased expression of miR-328 are other potential miRNA molecules apart from miRNA included in AMI, CAD, and cardiac hypertrophy, which act as diagnostic biomarker [246–248] (**Figures 1** and **2**).

Author details

Naveen Soni, Jitender Jangra, Megha Chaudhary, Gargi Nandi and Bhawana Bissa*
Department of Biochemistry, Central University of Rajasthan, Ajmer, Rajasthan, India

*Address all correspondence to: bhawana.bissa@curaj.ac.in

References

[1] Yaker L, Kamel S, Ausseil J, Boullier A. Effects of chronic kidney disease and uremic toxins on extracellular vesicle biology. Toxins. 2020;**12**:811

[2] Sager R, Palade GE. Structure and development of the chloroplast in chlamydomonas: I. the normal green cell. The Journal of Biophysical and Biochemical Cytology. 1957;**3**:463-488

[3] Sotelo JR, Porter KR. An electron microscope study of the rat ovum. The Journal of Biophysical and Biochemical Cytology. 1959;**5**:327-342

[4] Jensen WA. The composition and ultrastructure of the nucellus in cotton. Journal of Ultrastructure Research. 1965;**13**:112-128

[5] Takeo K, Uesaka I, Uehira K, Nishiura M. Fine structure of *Cryptococcus neoformans* grown in vitro as observed by freeze-etching. Journal of Bacteriology. 1973;**113**:1442-1448. DOI: 10.1128/jb.113.3.1442-1448.1973

[6] Raposo G et al. B lymphocytes secrete antigen-presenting vesicles. The Journal of Experimental Medicine. 1996;**183**:1161-1172

[7] Nunez EA, Wallis J, Gershon MD. Secretory processes in follicular cells of the bat thyroid. III. The occurrence of extracellular vesicles and colloid droplets during arousal from hibernation. The American Journal of Anatomy. 1974;**141**:179-201

[8] Deatherage BL, Cookson BT. Membrane vesicle release in bacteria, eukaryotes, and archaea: A conserved yet underappreciated aspect of microbial life. Infection and Immunity. 2012;**80**:(6):1948-1957. DOI: 10.1128/IAI.06014-11. Epub 2012 Mar 12. PMID: 22409932; PMCID: PMC3370574

[9] Doyle LM, Wang MZ. Overview of extracellular vesicles, their origin, composition, purpose, and methods for exosome isolation and analysis. Cell. 2019;**8**:727

[10] Xu M et al. The biogenesis and secretion of exosomes and multivesicular bodies (MVBs): Intercellular shuttles and implications in human diseases. Genes & Diseases. 2022. DOI: 10.1016/j.gendis.2022.03.021

[11] Morelli AE et al. Endocytosis, intracellular sorting, and processing of exosomes by dendritic cells. Blood. 2004;**104**:3257-3266

[12] Stoorvogel W, Strous GJ, Geuze HJ, Oorschot V, Schwartz AL. Late endosomes derive from early endosomes by maturation. Cell. 3 May 1991;**65**(3):417-427. DOI: 10.1016/0092-8674(91)90459-c. PMID: 1850321

[13] Logozzi M, Mizzoni D, Angelini DF, Di Raimo R, Falchi M, Battistini L, et al. Microenvironmental pH and exosome levels interplay in human cancer cell lines of different histotypes. Cancers (Basel). 5 Oct 2018;**10**(10):370. DOI: 10.3390/cancers10100370. PMID: 30301144; PMCID: PMC6210604

[14] Pols MS, Klumperman J. Trafficking and function of the tetraspanin CD63. Experimental Cell Research. 2009;**315**:1584-1592

[15] Wollert T, Hurley JH. Molecular mechanism of multivesicular body biogenesis by ESCRT complexes. Nature. 2010;**464**:864-869

[16] Colombo M et al. Analysis of ESCRT functions in exosome biogenesis,

composition and secretion highlights the heterogeneity of extracellular vesicles. Journal of Cell Science. 2013;**126**:5553-5565

[17] Hill CP, Babst M. Structure and function of the membrane deformation AAA ATPase Vps4. Biochim Biophys Acta. Jan 2012;**1823**(1):172-181. DOI: 10.1016/j.bbamcr.2011.08.017. Epub 2011 Sep 8. PMID: 21925211; PMCID: PMC3245771

[18] Hurley JH. ESCRTs are everywhere. EMBO J. 1 Oct 2015;**34**(19):2398-2407. DOI: 10.15252/embj.201592484. Epub 2015 Aug 25. PMID: 26311197; PMCID: PMC4601661

[19] Henne WM, Buchkovich NJ, Emr SD. The ESCRT pathway. Developmental Cell. 2011;**21**:77-91

[20] Villarroya-Beltri C, Baixauli F, Gutiérrez-Vázquez C, Sánchez-Madrid F, Mittelbrunn M. Sorting IT out: Regulation of exosome loading. Seminars in Cancer Biology. 2014;**28**:3-13

[21] Airola MV, Hannun YA. Sphingolipid metabolism and neutral sphingomyelinases. Handbook of Experimental Pharmacology. 2013;**215**:57-76. DOI: 10.1007/978-3-7091-1368-4_3. PMID: 23579449; PMCID: PMC4043343

[22] Perez-Hernandez D, Gutiérrez-Vázquez C, Jorge I, López-Martín S, Ursa A, Sánchez-Madrid F, et al. The intracellular interactome of tetraspanin-enriched microdomains reveals their function as sorting machineries toward exosomes. Journal Biological Chemistry. 26 Apr 2013;**288**(17):11649-11661. DOI: 10.1074/jbc.M112.445304. Epub 2013 Mar 5. PMID: 23463506; PMCID: PMC3636856

[23] Schwartz SL, Cao C, Pylypenko O, Rak A, Wandinger-Ness A. Rab GTPases at a glance. Journal of Cell Science. 2007 Nov 15;120(Pt 22):3905-3910. DOI: 10.1242/jcs.015909. Erratum in: Journal Cell Sciences. 15 Jan 2008;**121**(Pt 2):246. PMID: 17989088

[24] Pegtel DM, Gould SJ. Exosomes. Annual Review of Biochemistry. 2019;**88**:487-514

[25] Ostrowski M, Carmo NB, Krumeich S, Fanget I, Raposo G, Savina A, et al. Rab27a and Rab27b control different steps of the exosome secretion pathway. Nat Cell Biology. Jan 2010;**12**(1):19-30. sup pp 1-13. DOI: 10.1038/ncb2000. Epub 2009 Dec 6. PMID: 19966785

[26] Song L et al. KIBRA controls exosome secretion via inhibiting the proteasomal degradation of Rab27a. Nature Communications. 2019;**10**:1639

[27] Park J-I et al. BHMPS inhibits breast cancer migration and invasion by disrupting Rab27a-mediated EGFR and fibronectin secretion. Cancers. 2022;**14**:373

[28] Yuyama K, Sun H, Mikami D, Mioka T, Mukai K, Igarashi, Y. Lysosomal-associated transmembrane protein 4B regulates ceramide-induced exosome release. The FASEB Journal (The Journal of the Federation of American Societies for Experimental Biology). 2020;**34**:16022-16033. DOI: 10.1096/fj.202001599R

[29] Lauwers E et al. Hsp90 mediates membrane deformation and exosome release. Molecular Cell. 2018;**71**:689-702.e9

[30] Zhang J et al. DENN domain-containing protein FAM45A regulates the homeostasis of late/multivesicular endosomes. Biochimica et Biophysica Acta (BBA) - Molecular Cell Research. 2019;**1866**:916-929

[31] Imai A, Ishida M, Fukuda M, Nashida T, Shimomura H. MADD/

DENN/Rab3GEP functions as a guanine nucleotide exchange factor for Rab27 during granule exocytosis of rat parotid acinar cells. Archives of Biochemistry and Biophysics. 2013;**536**:31-37

[32] Sato M et al. Regulation of endocytic recycling by C. elegans Rab35 and its regulator RME-4, a coated-pit protein. The EMBO Journal. 2008;**27**:1183-1196

[33] Baietti MF et al. Syndecan-syntenin-ALIX regulates the biogenesis of exosomes. Nature Cell Biology. 2012;**14**:677-685

[34] Tamai K et al. Exosome secretion of dendritic cells is regulated by hrs, an ESCRT-0 protein. Biochemical and Biophysical Research Communications. 2010;**399**:384-390

[35] Kim DK, Kang B, Kim OY, Choi DS, Lee J, Kim SR, et al. EVpedia: An integrated database of high-throughput data for systemic analyses of extracellular vesicles. Journal of Extracellular Vesicles. Mar 2013;**19**:2. DOI: 10.3402/jev.v2i0.20384. PMID: 24009897; PMCID: PMC3760654

[36] Kalra H et al. Vesiclepedia: A compendium for extracellular vesicles with continuous community annotation. PLoS Biology. 2012;**10**:e1001450

[37] Mathivanan S, Simpson RJ. ExoCarta: A compendium of exosomal proteins and RNA. Proteomics. Nov 2009;**9**(21):4997-5000. DOI: 10.1002/pmic.200900351. PMID: 19810033

[38] Simpson RJ, Kalra H, Mathivanan S. ExoCarta as a resource for exosomal research. Journal of Extracellular Vesicles. Apr 2012;**16**:1. DOI: 10.3402/jev.v1i0.18374. PMID: 24009883; PMCID: PMC3760644

[39] Mathivanan S, Fahner CJ, Reid GE, Simpson RJ. ExoCarta 2012: Database of exosomal proteins, RNA and lipids. Nucleic Acids Research. Jan 2012;**40**(Database issue):D1241-1244. DOI: 10.1093/nar/gkr828. Epub 2011 Oct 11. PMID: 21989406; PMCID: PMC3245025

[40] Lai H et al. exoRBase 2.0: An atlas of mRNA, lncRNA and circRNA in extracellular vesicles from human biofluids. Nucleic Acids Research. 2022;**50**:D118-D128

[41] Wang X, Chai Z, Pan G, Hao Y, Li B, Ye T, et al. ExoBCD: A comprehensive database for exosomal biomarker discovery in breast cancer. Briefings in Bioinformatics. 20May 2021;**22**(3):bbaa088. DOI: 10.1093/bib/bbaa088. PMID: 32591816

[42] EV-TRACK Consortium., Van Deun J, Mestdagh P, et al. EV-TRACK: Transparent reporting and centralizing knowledge in extracellular vesicle research. Nat Methods. 2017;**14**:228-232. DOI: 10.1038/nmeth.4185

[43] Thakur B, Zhang H, Becker A, et al. Double-stranded DNA in exosomes: A novel biomarker in cancer detection. Cell Research. 2014;**24**:766-769. DOI: 10.1038/cr.2014.44

[44] Sharma A, Johnson A. Exosome DNA: Critical regulator of tumor immunity and a diagnostic biomarker. Journal of Cellular Physiology. 2020;**235**:1921-1932

[45] Li X, Wang Q, Wang R. Roles of exosome genomic DNA in colorectal cancer. Frontiers in Pharmacology. 2022;**13**

[46] Kahlert C, Melo SA, Protopopov A, Tang J, Seth S, Koch M, et al. Identification of double-stranded genomic DNA spanning all chromosomes with mutated KRAS and p53 DNA

in the serum exosomes of patients with pancreatic cancer. The Journal of Biological Chemistry. 14 Feb 2014;**289**(7):3869-3875. DOI: 10.1074/jbc.C113.532267. Epub 2014 Jan 7. PMID: 24398677; PMCID: PMC3924256

[47] Kalluri R, LeBleu VS. Discovery of double-stranded genomic DNA in circulating exosomes. Cold Spring Harbor Laboratory of Quantitative Biology. 2016;**81**:275-280

[48] Emerging role of exosome-derived long non-coding RNAs in tumor microenvironment - PubMed. Available from: https://pubmed.ncbi.nlm.nih.gov/29678180/

[49] Distinct RNA profiles in subpopulations of extracellular vesicles: apoptotic bodies, microvesicles and exosomes - PubMed. Available from: https://pubmed.ncbi.nlm.nih.gov/24223256/

[50] Characterization of human plasma-derived exosomal RNAs by deep sequencing - PubMed. Available from: https://pubmed.ncbi.nlm.nih.gov/23663360/

[51] Deep sequencing of RNA from immune cell-derived vesicles uncovers the selective incorporation of small non-coding RNA biotypes with potential regulatory functions - PubMed. Available from: https://pubmed.ncbi.nlm.nih.gov/22821563/

[52] Li CCY et al. Glioma microvesicles carry selectively packaged coding and non-coding RNAs which alter gene expression in recipient cells. RNA Biology. 2013;**10**:1333-1344

[53] Batagov AO, Kurochkin IV. Exosomes secreted by human cells transport largely mRNA fragments that are enriched in the 3'-untranslated regions. Biology Direct. 2013;**8**:12

[54] Vickers KC, Palmisano BT, Shoucri BM, Shamburek RD, Remaley AT. MicroRNAs are transported in plasma and delivered to recipient cells by high-density lipoproteins. Nature Cell Biology. 2011;**13**:423-433

[55] Bolukbasi MF et al. miR-1289 and 'Zipcode'-like sequence enrich mRNAs in microvesicles. Molecular Therapy. Nucleic acids. 2012;**1**:e10

[56] Villarroya-Beltri C et al. Sumoylated hnRNPA2B1 controls the sorting of miRNAs into exosomes through binding to specific motifs. Nature Communications. 2013;**4**:2980

[57] Koppers-Lalic D et al. Nontemplated nucleotide additions distinguish the small RNA composition in cells from exosomes. Cell Reports. 2014;**8**:1649-1658

[58] Kosaka N et al. Secretory mechanisms and intercellular transfer of microRNAs in living cells. The Journal of Biological Chemistry. 2010;**285**:17442-17452

[59] Gibbings DJ, Ciaudo C, Erhardt M, Voinnet O. Multivesicular bodies associate with components of miRNA effector complexes and modulate miRNA activity. Nature Cell Biology. 2009;**11**:1143-1149

[60] Li L et al. Argonaute 2 complexes selectively protect the circulating microRNAs in cell-secreted microvesicles. PLoS One. 2012;7:e46957

[61] Robbins PD, Morelli AE. Regulation of immune responses by extracellular vesicles. Nature Reviews. Immunology. 2014;**14**:195-208

[62] Abels ER, Breakefield XO. Introduction to extracellular vesicles: Biogenesis, RNA cargo selection, content, release, and uptake. Cellular

and Molecular Neurobiology. 2016;**36**:301-312

[63] Gupta S, Knowlton AA. HSP60 trafficking in adult cardiac myocytes: Role of the exosomal pathway. American Journal of Physiology. Heart and Circulatory Physiology. 2007;**292**:H3052-H3056

[64] Théry C, Zitvogel L, Amigorena S. Exosomes: Composition, biogenesis and function. Nature Reviews. Immunology. 2002;**2**:569-579

[65] Goler-Baron V, Assaraf YG. Structure and function of ABCG2-rich extracellular vesicles mediating multidrug resistance. PLoS One. 2011;**6**(1):e16007. DOI: 10.1371/journal.pone.0016007

[66] Gong J et al. Microparticle drug sequestration provides a parallel pathway in the acquisition of cancer drug resistance. European Journal of Pharmacology. 2013;**721**:116-125

[67] Selective transfer of exosomes from oligodendrocytes to microglia by macropinocytosis - PubMed. Available from: https://pubmed.ncbi.nlm.nih.gov/21242314/

[68] Bicalho B, Holovati JL, Acker JP. Phospholipidomics reveals differences in glycerophosphoserine profiles of hypothermically stored red blood cells and microvesicles. Biochimica et Biophysica Acta. 2013;**1828**:317-326

[69] Zaborowski MP, Balaj L, Breakefield XO, Lai CP. Extracellular vesicles: Composition, biological relevance, and methods of study. Bioscience. 2015;**65**:783-797

[70] Clinical applications of metabolomics in oncology: A review - PubMed. Available from: https://pubmed.ncbi.nlm.nih.gov/19147747/

[71] Rockel JS, Kapoor M. The metabolome and osteoarthritis: Possible contributions to symptoms and pathology. Metabolites. 2018;**8**:92

[72] Metabolomics biomarkers for detection of colorectal neoplasms: A systematic review - PubMed. Available from: https://pubmed.ncbi.nlm.nih.gov/30060469/

[73] Mast cell- and dendritic cell-derived exosomes display a specific lipid composition and an unusual membrane organization - PubMed. Available from: https://pubmed.ncbi.nlm.nih.gov/14965343/

[74] Distinct lipid compositions of two types of human prostasomes - PubMed. Available from: https://pubmed.ncbi.nlm.nih.gov/23404715/

[75] Enabling metabolomics based biomarker discovery studies using molecular phenotyping of exosome-like vesicles - PubMed. Available from: https://pubmed.ncbi.nlm.nih.gov/26974972/

[76] High-performance chemical isotope labeling liquid chromatography mass spectrometry for exosome metabolomics - PubMed. Available from: https://pubmed.ncbi.nlm.nih.gov/29920066/

[77] Metabolic alterations in urine extracellular vesicles are associated to prostate cancer pathogenesis and progression - PubMed. Available from: https://pubmed.ncbi.nlm.nih.gov/29760869/

[78] Zhang Y, Liu Y, Liu H, Tang WH. Exosomes: Biogenesis, biologic function and clinical potential. Cell & Bioscience. 2019;**9**:19

[79] Zebrowska A, Skowronek A, Wojakowska A, Widlak P, Pietrowska M. Metabolome of exosomes: Focus on vesicles released by cancer cells and present in human body fluids.

International Journal of Molecular Sciences. 2019;**20**:3461

[80] Laulagnier K et al. Mast cell- and dendritic cell-derived exosomes display a specific lipid composition and an unusual membrane organization. The Biochemical Journal. 2004;**380**:161-171

[81] Vlassov AV, Magdaleno S, Setterquist R, Conrad R. Exosomes: Current knowledge of their composition, biological functions, and diagnostic and therapeutic potentials. Biochimica et Biophysica Acta. 2012;**1820**:940-948

[82] Romancino DP et al. Identification and characterization of the nano-sized vesicles released by muscle cells. FEBS Letters. 2013;**587**:1379-1384

[83] Yáñez-Mó M et al. Biological properties of extracellular vesicles and their physiological functions. J. Extracell. Vesicles. 2015;**4**:27066

[84] Wu G et al. Altered microRNA expression profiles of extracellular vesicles in nasal mucus from patients with allergic rhinitis. Allergy Asthma Immunol. Res. 2015;7:449-457

[85] Saunderson SC, Dunn AC, Crocker PR, McLellan AD. CD169 mediates the capture of exosomes in spleen and lymph node. Blood. 2014;**123**:208-216

[86] Zitvogel L et al. Eradication of established murine tumors using a novel cell-free vaccine: Dendritic cell-derived exosomes. Nature Medicine. 1998;**4**:594-600

[87] Théry C et al. Proteomic analysis of dendritic cell-derived exosomes: A secreted subcellular compartment distinct from apoptotic vesicles. Journal of immunology (Baltimore, Md.). 2001;**1950**(166):7309-7318

[88] Karlsson M et al. 'Tolerosomes' are produced by intestinal epithelial cells. European Journal of Immunology. 2001;**31**:2892-2900

[89] Raposo G, Nijman HW, Stoorvogel W, Liejendekker R, Harding CV, Melief CJ, et al. B lymphocytes secrete antigen-presenting vesicles. The Journal of Experimental Medicine. 1 Mar 1996;**183**:1161-1172. DOI: 10.1084/jem.183.3.1161. PMID: 8642258; PMCID: PMC2192324

[90] Hunter MP et al. Detection of microRNA expression in human peripheral blood microvesicles. PLoS One. 2008;**3**:e3694

[91] Valadi H et al. Exosome-mediated transfer of mRNAs and microRNAs is a novel mechanism of genetic exchange between cells. Nature Cell Biology. 2007;**9**:654-659

[92] Amzallag N et al. TSAP6 facilitates the secretion of translationally controlled tumor protein/histamine-releasing factor via a nonclassical pathway. The Journal of Biological Chemistry. 2004;**279**:46104-46112

[93] Fevrier B et al. Cells release prions in association with exosomes. Proceedings of the National Academy of Sciences of the United States of America. 2004;**101**:9683-9688

[94] Robertson C et al. Cellular prion protein is released on exosomes from activated platelets. Blood. 2006;**107**:3907-3911

[95] Nguyen DG, Booth A, Gould SJ, Hildreth JEK. Evidence that HIV budding in primary macrophages occurs through the exosome release pathway. The Journal of Biological Chemistry. 2003;**278**:52347-52354

[96] Li Y et al. Circular RNA is enriched and stable in exosomes: A promising

biomarker for cancer diagnosis. Cell Research. 2015;**25**:981-984

[97] György B et al. Membrane vesicles, current state-of-the-art: Emerging role of extracellular vesicles. Cellular and Molecular Life Sciences. 2011;**68**:2667-2688

[98] Isolation of biologically-active exosomes from human plasma - PubMed. Available from: https://pubmed.ncbi.nlm.nih.gov/24952243/

[99] Théry C, Amigorena S, Raposo G, Clayton A. Isolation and characterization of exosomes from cell culture supernatants and biological fluids. Current Protocols in Cell Biology. 2006. Chapter 3:Unit 3.22. DOI: 10.1002/0471143030.cb0322s30. PMID: 18228490

[100] Qu L et al. Exosome-transmitted lncARSR promotes sunitinib resistance in renal cancer by acting as a competing endogenous RNA. Cancer Cell. 2016;**29**:653-668

[101] Song J et al. PBMC and exosome-derived Hotair is a critical regulator and potent marker for rheumatoid arthritis. Clinical and Experimental Medicine. 2015;**15**:121-126

[102] Kalra H et al. Comparative proteomics evaluation of plasma exosome isolation techniques and assessment of the stability of exosomes in normal human blood plasma. Proteomics. 2013;**13**:3354-3364

[103] Properzi F, Logozzi M, Fais S. Exosomes: The future of biomarkers in medicine. Biomarkers in Medicine. 2013;**7**:769-778

[104] Mathivanan S, Ji H, Simpson RJ. Exosomes: Extracellular organelles important in intercellular communication. Journal of Proteomics. 2010;**73**:1907-1920

[105] Batrakova EV, Kim MS. Using exosomes, naturally-equipped nanocarriers, for drug delivery. Journal of Controlled Release. 2015;**219**:396-405

[106] Isola AL, Chen S. Exosomes: The messengers of health and disease. Current Neuropharmacology. 2017;**15**:157

[107] Trypanosoma cruzi immune evasion mediated by host cell-derived microvesicles - PubMed. Available from: https://pubmed.ncbi.nlm.nih.gov/22262654/

[108] The role of exosomes in the processing of proteins associated with neurodegenerative diseases – SpringerLink. Available from: https://link.springer.com/article/10.1007/s00249-007-0246-z.

[109] Exosomes in the pathogenesis, diagnostics and therapeutics of liver diseases - ScienceDirect. Available from: https://www.sciencedirect.com/science/article/pii/S0168827813002079

[110] Li I, Nabet BY. Exosomes in the tumor microenvironment as mediators of cancer therapy resistance. Molecular Cancer. 2019;**18**:32

[111] Qu JL, Qu XJ, Zhao MF, Teng YE, Zhang Y, Hou KZ, et al. Gastric cancer exosomes promote tumour cell proliferation through PI3K/Akt and MAPK/ERK activation. Dig. Liver Dis. Dec 2009;**41**(12):875-880. DOI: 10.1016/j.dld.2009.04.006. Epub 2009 May 26. PMID: 19473897

[112] Friedl P, Alexander S. Cancer invasion and the microenvironment: Plasticity and reciprocity. Cell. 2011;**147**:992-1009

[113] Hallmarks of cancer: The next generation - PubMed. Available from: https://pubmed.ncbi.nlm.nih.gov/21376230/

[114] Tian W, Liu S, Li B. Potential role of exosomes in cancer metastasis. BioMed Research International. 2019;**2019**:1-12

[115] Paget's 'seed and soil' theory of cancer metastasis: An idea whose time has come - PubMed. Available from: https://pubmed.ncbi.nlm.nih.gov/30339548/

[116] Peinado H et al. Pre-metastatic niches: Organ-specific homes for metastases. Nature Reviews. Cancer. 2017;**17**:302-317

[117] Steeg PS. Targeting metastasis. Nature Reviews. Cancer. 2016;**16**:201-218

[118] The multiple roles of exosomes in metastasis - PubMed. Available from: https://pubmed.ncbi.nlm.nih.gov/28031234/

[119] Exosomes released from breast cancer carcinomas stimulate cell movement - PubMed. Available from: https://pubmed.ncbi.nlm.nih.gov/25798887/

[120] Frontiers — Functions and therapeutic roles of exosomes in cancer. Available from: https://www.frontiersin.org/articles/10.3389/fonc.2014.00127/full

[121] Exosome-mediated transfer of miR-10b promotes cell invasion in breast cancer - PubMed. Available from: https://pubmed.ncbi.nlm.nih.gov/25428807/

[122] Molecular principles of metastasis: A hallmark of cancer revisited – Signal transduction and targeted therapy. Available from: https://www.nature.com/articles/s41392-020-0134-x

[123] The role of exosomes in cancer metastasis - PubMed. Available from: https://pubmed.ncbi.nlm.nih.gov/28215970/

[124] Tumour exosome integrins determine organotropic metastasis - PubMed. Available from: https://pubmed.ncbi.nlm.nih.gov/26524530/.

[125] Mu W, Rana S, Zöller M. Host matrix modulation by tumor exosomes promotes motility and invasiveness. Neoplasia (New York, N.Y.). 2013;**15**:875-887

[126] Fabbri, M. et al. MicroRNAs bind to toll-like receptors to induce prometastatic inflammatory response. Proceedings of the National Academy of Sciences of the United States of America 109, E2110–E2116 (2012). Available from: https://www.google.com/search?q=Fabbri%2C+M.+et+al.+MicroRNAs+bind+to+Toll-like+receptors+to+induce+prometastatic+inflammatory+response.+Proc.+Natl+Acad.+Sci.+USA+109%2C+E2110%E2%80%93E2116+(2012)&oq=Fabbri%2C+M.+et+al.+MicroRNAs+bind+to+Toll-like+receptors+to+induce+prometastatic+inflammatory+response.+Proc.+Natl+Acad.+Sci.+USA+109%2C+E2110%E2%80%93E2116+(2012)&aqs=chrome..69i57.803j0j7&sourceid=chrome&ie=UTF-8

[127] Olejarz W, Kubiak-Tomaszewska G, Chrzanowska A, Lorenc T. Exosomes in angiogenesis and anti-angiogenic therapy in cancers. International Journal of Molecular Sciences. 2020;**21**:5840

[128] Communication in tiny packages: Exosomes as means of tumor-stroma communication - PubMed. Available from: https://pubmed.ncbi.nlm.nih.gov/31926290/

[129] Zhao Z. Mechanisms of lncRNA/microRNA interactions Available from:. https://scholar.google.com/scholar_lookup?title=Mechanisms+of+lncRNA/microRNA+interactions+in+angiogenesis&author=Zhao,+Z.&author=Sun,+W.&author=Guo,+Z.&author=Zhang,+J.&author=Yu,+H.&author=Liu,+B.&publication_year=2020&journal=Life+Sci.&volume=254&pages=116900&doi=10.1016/j.lfs.2019.116900

[130] Whiteside TL. Tumor-derived exosomes and their role in cancer

progression. Advances in Clinical Chemistry. 2016;**74**:103-141

[131] Internalization of Exosomes through Receptor-Mediated Endocytosis – Molecular Cancer Research – American Association for Cancer Research. Available from: https://aacrjournals.org/mcr/article/17/2/337/90046/Internalization-of-Exosomes-through-Receptor

[132] Schiera G, Di Liegro CM, Di Liegro I. Extracellular membrane vesicles as vehicles for brain cell-to-cell interactions in physiological as well as pathological conditions. BioMed Research International. 2015;**2015**:152926

[133] Sharples RA, Vella LJ, Nisbet RM, Naylor R, Perez K, Barnham KJ, et al. Inhibition of gamma-secretase causes increased secretion of amyloid precursor protein C-terminal fragments in association with exosomes. FASEB J. May 2008;**22**(5):1469-1478. DOI: 10.1096/fj.07-9357com. Epub 2008 Jan 2. PMID: 18171695

[134] Yuyama K, Sun H, Mitsutake S, Igarashi Y. Sphingolipid-modulated exosome secretion promotes clearance of amyloid-β by microglia. Journal of Biological Chemistry. 30 Mar 2012;**287**(14):10977-10989. DOI: 10.1074/jbc.M111.324616. Epub 2012 Feb 2. PMID: 22303002; PMCID: PMC3322859

[135] Vandendriessche C, Bruggeman A, Van Cauwenberghe C, Vandenbroucke RE. Extracellular vesicles in Alzheimer's and Parkinson's disease: Small entities with large consequences. Cell. 2020;**9**:2485

[136] Familial Alzheimer's disease mutations at position 22 of the amyloid β-peptide sequence differentially affect synaptic loss, tau phosphorylation and neuronal cell death in an ex vivo system. PLoS One

[137] Frontiers – The Role of Microglia in the Spread of Tau: Relevance for Tauopathies. Available from: https://www.frontiersin.org/articles/10.3389/fncel.2018.00172/full

[138] Depletion of microglia and inhibition of exosome synthesis halt tau propagation - PMC. Available from: https://www.ncbi.nlm.nih.gov/pmc/articles/PMC4694577/

[139] Cell biology and pathophysiology of α-synuclein. Available from: http://perspectivesinmedicine.cshlp.org/content/8/3/a024091

[140] Alvarez-Erviti L, Seow Y, Schapira AH, Gardiner C, Sargent IL, Wood MJ, Cooper JM. Lysosomal dysfunction increases exosome-mediated alpha-synuclein release and transmission. Neurobiol Dis. Jun 2011;**42**(3):360-367. DOI: 10.1016/j.nbd.2011.01.029. Epub 2011 Feb 18. PMID: 21303699; PMCID: PMC3107939

[141] Desplats. Inclusion formation and neuronal cell death. Available from: https://scholar.google.com/scholar_lookup?journal=Proc+Natl+Acad+Sci+U+S+A&title=Inclusion+formation+and+neuronal+cell+death+through+neuron-to-neuron+transmission+of+alpha-synuclein&author=P+Desplats&author=HJ+Lee&author=EJ+Bae&author=C+Patrick&author=E+Rockenstein&volume=106&publication_year=2009&pages=13010-13015&pmid=19651612&

[142] Hansen C et al. α-Synuclein propagates from mouse brain to grafted dopaminergic neurons and seeds aggregation in cultured human cells. The Journal of Clinical Investigation. 2011;**121**:715-725

[143] Fan RZ, Guo M, Luo S, Cui M, Tieu K. Exosome release and neuropathology induced by α-synuclein:

New insights into protective mechanisms of Drp1 inhibition. Acta Neuropathologica Communications. 2019;7:184

[144] Guo M et al. Microglial exosomes facilitate α-synuclein transmission in Parkinson's disease. Brain: A Journal of Neurology. 2020;**143**:1476-1497

[145] Harischandra DS et al. Manganese promotes the aggregation and prion-like cell-to-cell exosomal transmission of α-synuclein. Science Signaling. 2019;**12**:eaau4543

[146] McMillan KJ et al. Loss of MicroRNA-7 regulation leads to α-synuclein accumulation and dopaminergic neuronal loss in vivo. Molecular Therapy. 2017;**25**:2404-2414

[147] Chen Y et al. MicroRNA-4639 is a regulator of DJ-1 expression and a potential early diagnostic marker for Parkinson's disease. Frontiers in Aging Neuroscience. 2017;**9**:232

[148] (PDF) Glomerular endothelial derived vesicles mediate podocyte dysfunction: A potential role for miRNA. Available from: https://www.researchgate.net/publication/340218215_Glomerular_endothelial_derived_vesicles_mediate_podocyte_dysfunction_A_potential_role_for_miRNA

[149] Urinary extracellular vesicles as biomarkers of kidney disease: From diagnostics to therapeutics - PMC. Available from: https://www.ncbi.nlm.nih.gov/pmc/articles/PMC7277956/

[150] Reduced urinary release of AQP1- and AQP2-bearing extracellular vesicles in patients with advanced chronic kidney disease - Oshikawa-Hori - 2021 - Physiological Reports - Wiley Online Library. Available from: https://physoc.onlinelibrary.wiley.com/doi/full/10.14814/phy2.15005

[151] Hill N et al. Glomerular endothelial derived vesicles mediate podocyte dysfunction: A potential role for miRNA. PLoS One. 2020;**15**:e0224852

[152] Grange C, Bussolati B. Extracellular vesicles in kidney disease. Nature Reviews. Nephrology. 2022;**18**:499-513

[153] Sonoda H et al. miRNA profiling of urinary exosomes to assess the progression of acute kidney injury. Scientific Reports. 2019;**9**:4692

[154] Panich T et al. Urinary exosomal activating transcriptional factor 3 as the early diagnostic biomarker for sepsis-induced acute kidney injury. BMC Nephrology. 2017;**18**:10

[155] da Silva Novaes A, Borges FT, Maquigussa E, Varela VA, Dias MVS, Boim MA. Influence of high glucose on mesangial cell-derived exosome composition, secretion and cell communication. Sci Rep. 18 Apr 2019;**9**(1):6270. DOI: 10.1038/s41598-019-42746-1. Erratum in: Sci Rep. 2020 Jan 29;**10**(1):1730. PMID: 31000742; PMCID: PMC6472340

[156] Clinical verification of a novel urinary microRNA panal: 133b, −342 and −30 as biomarkers for diabetic nephropathy identified by bioinformatics analysis - PubMed. Available from: https://pubmed.ncbi.nlm.nih.gov/27470555/

[157] Prabu P et al. MicroRNAs from urinary extracellular vesicles are non-invasive early biomarkers of diabetic nephropathy in type 2 diabetes patients with the 'Asian Indian phenotype'. Diabetes & Metabolism. 2019;**45**:276-285

[158] Salih M et al. Proteomics of urinary vesicles links plakins and complement to polycystic kidney disease. Journal of the American Society of Nephrology. 2016;**27**:3079-3092

[159] Bruschi M et al. Proteomic analysis of urinary microvesicles and exosomes in medullary sponge kidney disease and autosomal dominant polycystic kidney disease. Clinical Journal of the American Society of Nephrology. 2019;**14**:834-843

[160] Mazzariol M, Camussi G, Brizzi MF. Extracellular vesicles tune the immune system in renal disease: A focus on systemic lupus erythematosus, antiphospholipid syndrome, thrombotic microangiopathy and ANCA-Vasculitis. International Journal of Molecular Sciences. 2021;**22**:4194

[161] Salomon C et al. A gestational profile of placental exosomes in maternal plasma and their effects on endothelial cell migration. PLoS One. 2014;**9**:e98667

[162] Liu Q, Piao H, Wang Y, Zheng D, Wang W. Circulating exosomes in cardiovascular disease: Novel carriers of biological information. Biomedicine & Pharmacotherapy. 2021;**135**:111148

[163] Cardiac myocyte exosomes: stability, HSP60, and proteomics - PubMed. Available from: https://pubmed.ncbi.nlm.nih.gov/23376832/

[164] Zhang X et al. Exosomes in cancer: Small particle, big player. Journal of Hematology & Oncology. 2015;**8**:83

[165] Bellin G et al. Exosome in cardiovascular diseases: A complex world full of hope. Cell. 2019;**8**:166

[166] Rezaie J et al. Cardioprotective role of extracellular vesicles: A highlight on exosome beneficial effects in cardiovascular diseases. Journal of Cellular Physiology. 2019;**234**:21732-21745

[167] Interstitial fibrosis and growth factors - PubMed. Available from: https://pubmed.ncbi.nlm.nih.gov/10931794/

[168] Stem cell-derived exosomes, autophagy, extracellular matrix turnover, and miRNAs in cardiac regeneration during stem cell therapy - PubMed. Available from: https://pubmed.ncbi.nlm.nih.gov/27807762/

[169] Exosomes secreted by cardiosphere-derived cells reduce scarring, attenuate adverse remodelling, and improve function in acute and chronic porcine myocardial infarction - PubMed. Available from: https://pubmed.ncbi.nlm.nih.gov/28158410/

[170] Kanninen KM, Bister N, Koistinaho J, Malm T. Exosomes as new diagnostic tools in CNS diseases. Biochim Biophys Acta. Mar 2016;**1862**(3):403-410. DOI: 10.1016/j.bbadis.2015.09.020. Epub 2015 Oct 20. PMID: 26432482

[171] Beach: Exosomes: An overview of biogenesis, composition. Available from: https://scholar.google.com/scholar_lookup?journal=J+Ovarian+Res&title=Exosomes:+an+overview+of+biogenesis,+composition+and+role+in+ovarian+cancer&author=A+Beach&author=HG+Zhang&author=MZ+Ratajczak&author=SS+Kakar&volume=7&publication_year=2014&pages=14&pmid=24460816&

[172] Li M et al. Analysis of the RNA content of the exosomes derived from blood serum and urine and its potential as biomarkers. Philosophical Transactions of the Royal Society of London. Series B, Biological Sciences. 2014;**369**:20130502

[173] The Complete Exosome Workflow Solution: From Isolation to Characterization of RNA Cargo - PMC. Available from: https://www.ncbi.nlm.nih.gov/pmc/articles/PMC3800616/

[174] Potential use of exosomes as diagnostic biomarkers and in targeted drug delivery: Progress in clinical and

preclinical applications - PubMed. Available from: https://pubmed.ncbi.nlm.nih.gov/33988964/

[175] The proteomic analysis of breast cell line exosomes reveals disease patterns and potential biomarkers - PubMed. Available from: https://pubmed.ncbi.nlm.nih.gov/32782317/

[176] Moon P-G et al. Fibronectin on circulating extracellular vesicles as a liquid biopsy to detect breast cancer. Oncotarget. 2016;**7**:40189-40199

[177] Sandfeld-Paulsen B et al. Exosomal proteins as diagnostic biomarkers in lung cancer. Journal of Thoracic Oncology: Official Publication of the International Association for the Study of Lung Cancer. 2016;**11**:1701-1710

[178] Glypican-1 identifies cancer exosomes and detects early pancreatic cancer - PubMed. Available from: https://pubmed.ncbi.nlm.nih.gov/26106858/

[179] Exosomes in cancer development, metastasis, and drug resistance: A comprehensive review - PubMed. Available from: https://pubmed.ncbi.nlm.nih.gov/23709120/

[180] Leng B et al. Plasma exosomal prion protein levels are correlated with cognitive decline in PD patients. Neuroscience Letters. 2020;**723**:134866

[181] Frontiers – Increased DJ-1 and α-synuclein in plasma neural-derived exosomes as potential markers for Parkinsons disease. Available from: https://www.frontiersin.org/articles/10.3389/fnagi.2018.00438/full

[182] Oxidized DJ-1 levels in urine samples as a putative biomarker for Parkinson's Disease - PMC. Available from: https://www.ncbi.nlm.nih.gov/pmc/articles/PMC5985070/

[183] Quantification of brain-derived extracellular vesicles in plasma as a biomarker to diagnose Parkinson's and related diseases - PubMed. Available from: https://pubmed.ncbi.nlm.nih.gov/30502924/

[184] Kitamura Y et al. Proteomic profiling of exosomal proteins for blood-based biomarkers in Parkinson's disease. Neuroscience. 2018;**392**:121-128

[185] Goetzl EJ et al. Altered lysosomal proteins in neural-derived plasma exosomes in preclinical Alzheimer disease. Neurology. 2015;**85**:40-47

[186] Agliardi C. SNAP-25 in serum is carried by exosomes. Available from: https://scholar.google.com/scholar_lookup?journal=Mol.+Neurobiol.&title=SNAP-25+in+Serum+Is+Carried+by+Exosomes+of+Neuronal+Origin+and+Is+a+Potential+Biomarker+of+Alzheimer%E2%80%99s+Disease.&author=C.+Agliardi&author=F.+R.+Guerini&author=M.+Zanzottera&author=A.+Bianchi&author=R.+Nemni&volume=56&publication_year=2019&pages=5792-5798&pmid=30680692&doi=10.1007/s12035-019-1501-x&

[187] Chanteloup G. Exosomal HSP70 for monitoring of frontotempor Available from: https://scholar.google.com/scholar_lookup?journal=J.+Alzheimers+Dis.&title=Exosomal+HSP70+for+Monitoring+of+Frontotemporal+Dementia+and+Alzheimer%E2%80%99s+Disease:+Clinical+and+FDG-PET+Correlation.&author=G.+Chanteloup&author=M.+Cordonnier&author=T.+Moreno-Ramos&author=V.+Pytel&author=J.+Matias-Guiu&volume=71&publication_year=2019&pages=1263-1269&pmid=31498123&doi=10.3233/JAD-190545&

[188] Thongboonkerd V. Roles for exosome in various kidney diseases and

disorders. Frontiers in Pharmacology. 2020;**10**:1655

[189] Ståhl A, Johansson K, Mossberg M, Kahn R, Karpman D. Exosomes and microvesicles in normal physiology, pathophysiology, and renal diseases. Pediatric Nephrology (Berlin, Germany). 2019;**34**:11-30

[190] Exosomal Fetuin-A identified by proteomics: A novel urinary biomarker for detecting acute kidney injury - PMC. Available from: https://www.ncbi.nlm.nih.gov/pmc/articles/PMC2277342/

[191] Urinary Excretion of Kidney Aquaporins as Possible Diagnostic Biomarker of Diabetic Nephropathy - PMC. Available from: https://www.ncbi.nlm.nih.gov/pmc/articles/PMC5299189/

[192] Zhang Y et al. Harnessing the therapeutic potential of extracellular vesicles for cancer treatment. Seminars in Cancer Biology. 2021;**74**:92-104

[193] Plasma exosome microRNAs are indicative of breast cancer – Breast Cancer Research – Full Text. Available from: https://breast-cancer-research.biomedcentral.com/articles/10.1186/s13058-016-0753-x

[194] Zhai LY, et al. In Situ detection of plasma exosomal microrna-1246 for breast cancer diagnostics by a Au nanoflare probe. ACS Applied Materials & Interfaces. 2018;**10**:39478-39486

[195] Exosomal miRNA profile as complementary tool in the diagnostic and prediction of treatment response in localized breast cancer under neoadjuvant chemotherapy - PubMed. Available from: https://pubmed.ncbi.nlm.nih.gov/30728048/

[196] Yoshikawa M et al. Exosome-encapsulated microRNA-223-3p as a minimally invasive biomarker for the early detection of invasive breast cancer. Oncology Letters. 2018;**15**:9584-9592

[197] Ni Q, Stevic I, Pan C, et al. Different signatures of miR-16, miR-30b and miR-93 in exosomes from breast cancer and DCIS patients. Scientific Reports. 2018;**8**:12974. Available from: https://www.nature.com/articles/s41598-018-31108-y

[198] Stevic I, Müller V, Weber K, et al. Specific microRNA signatures in exosomes of triple-negative and HER2-positive breast cancer patients undergoing neoadjuvant therapy within the GeparSixto trial. BMC Medicine. 2018;**16**:179. DOI: 10.1186/s12916-018-1163-y

[199] Cazzoli R et al. microRNAs derived from circulating exosomes as noninvasive biomarkers for screening and diagnosing lung cancer. Journal of Thoracic Oncology: Official Publication of the International Association for the Study of Lung Cancer. 2013;**8**:1156-1162

[200] Jin X et al. Evaluation of tumor-derived exosomal miRNA as potential diagnostic biomarkers for early-stage non-small cell lung cancer using next-generation sequencing. Clinical Cancer Research : An Official Journal of the American Association for Cancer Research. 2017;**23**:5311-5319

[201] Exosome-derived microRNA: Efficacy in Cancer - PMC. Available from: https://www.ncbi.nlm.nih.gov/pmc/articles/PMC8460558/

[202] Liu W, Chen S, Liu B. Diagnostic and prognostic values of serum exosomal microRNA-21 in children with hepatoblastoma: A Chinese population-based study. Pediatric Surgery International. 2016;**32**:1059-1065

[203] Jiao C, Jiao X, Zhu A, Ge J, Xu X. Exosomal miR-34s panel as potential

novel diagnostic and prognostic biomarker in patients with hepatoblastoma. Journal of Pediatric Surgery. 2017;**52**:618-624

[204] Lai X et al. A microRNA signature in circulating exosomes is superior to exosomal glypican-1 levels for diagnosing pancreatic cancer. Cancer Letters. 2017;**393**:86-93

[205] Cheng L et al. Prognostic serum miRNA biomarkers associated with Alzheimer's disease shows concordance with neuropsychological and neuroimaging assessment. Molecular Psychiatry. 2015;**20**:1188-1196

[206] Manna I, De Benedittis S, Quattrone A, Maisano D, Iaccino E, Quattrone A. Exosomal miRNAs as potential diagnostic biomarkers in Alzheimer's disease. Pharmaceuticals (Basel). 2020;**13**(9):243. DOI: 10.3390/ph13090243. PMID: 32932746; PMCID: PMC7559720

[207] McKeever PM et al. MicroRNA expression levels are altered in the cerebrospinal fluid of patients with young-onset Alzheimers disease. Molecular Neurobiology. 2018;**55**:8826-8841

[208] Altered microRNA profiles in cerebrospinal fluid exosome in Parkinson disease and Alzheimer disease - PMC. Available from: https://www.ncbi.nlm.nih.gov/pmc/articles/PMC4741914/

[209] Dos Santos MCT et al. miRNA-based signatures in cerebrospinal fluid as potential diagnostic tools for early stage Parkinson's disease. Oncotarget. 2018;**9**:17455-17465

[210] Margis R, Margis R, Rieder CRM. Identification of blood microRNAs associated to Parkinsonĭs disease. Journal of Biotechnology. 2011;**152**:96-101

[211] Ramaswamy P, Yadav R, Pal PK, Christopher R. Clinical application of circulating MicroRNAs in Parkinson's disease: The challenges and opportunities as diagnostic biomarker. Annals of Indian Academy of Neurology. 2020;**23**:84

[212] The extracellular miRNA fingerprint of kidney disease: A narrative review - Miguel - ExRNA. Available from: https://exrna.amegroups.com/article/view/64320/html

[213] Circulating miR-210 predicts survival in critically ill patients with acute kidney injury - PubMed. Available from: https://pubmed.ncbi.nlm.nih.gov/21700819/

[214] JCI Insight - The negative feedback loop of NF-κB/miR-376b/NFKBIZ in septic acute kidney injury. Available from: https://insight.jci.org/articles/view/142272

[215] Fan PC, Chen CC, Peng CC, et al. A circulating miRNA signature for early diagnosis of acute kidney injury following acute myocardial infarction. Journal of Translational Medicine. 2019;**17**:139. DOI: 10.1186/s12967-019-1890-7

[216] Aguado-Fraile E, Ramos E, Conde E, Rodríguez M, Martín-Gómez L, Lietor A, et al. A pilot study identifying a set of microRNAs as precise diagnostic biomarkers of acute kidney injury. PLoS One. 2015;**10**(6):e0127175. DOI: 10.1371/journal.pone.0127175

[217] miR-192 Mediates TGF-β/Smad3-Driven Renal Fibrosis - PMC. Available from: https://www.ncbi.nlm.nih.gov/pmc/articles/PMC2938591/

[218] Barutta F, Tricarico M, Corbelli A, et al. Urinary exosomal microRNAs in incipient diabetic nephropathy. PLoS One. 2013;**8**:e73798 Available from:

https://www.google.com/search?q=.Barutta+F%2C+Tricarico+M%2C+Corbelli+A%2C+et+al.+Urinary+exosomal+microRNAs+in+incipient+diabetic+nephropathy.+PLoS+One+2013%3B8%3Ae73798.&oq=.Barutta+F%2C+Tricarico+M%2C+Corbelli+A%2C+et+al.+Urinary+exosomal+microRNAs+in+incipient+diabetic+nephropathy.+PLoS+One+2013%3B8%3Ae73798.&aqs=chrome..69i57.554j0j4&sourceid=chrome&ie=UTF-8

[219] The expression of miR-192 and its significance in diabetic nephropathy patients with different urine albumin creatinine ratio - PMC. Available from: https://www.ncbi.nlm.nih.gov/pmc/articles/PMC4736386/

[220] miRNAs in urine extracellular vesicles as predictors of early-stage diabetic nephropathy - PubMed. Available from: https://pubmed.ncbi.nlm.nih.gov/26942205/

[221] Serum miR-21 may be a potential diagnostic biomarker for diabetic nephropathy - PubMed. Available from: https://pubmed.ncbi.nlm.nih.gov/26575121/

[222] Zang J, Maxwell AP, Simpson DA, et al. Differential expression of urinary exosomal MicroRNAs miR-21-5p and miR-30b-5p in individuals with diabetic kidney disease. Scientific Reports. 2019;**9**:10900. DOI: 10.1038/s41598-019-47504-x

[223] Han Q, Zhang Y, Jiao T, et al. Urinary sediment microRNAs can be used as potential noninvasive biomarkers for diagnosis, reflecting the severity and prognosis of diabetic nephropathy. Nutrition & Diabetes. 2021;**11**:24. DOI: 10.1038/s41387-021-00166-z

[224] MicroRNA-135a is involved in podocyte injury in a transient receptor potential channel 1-dependent manner. Available from: https://www.spandidos-publications.com/10.3892/ijmm.2017.3152

[225] Delić D et al. Urinary exosomal miRNA signature in type II diabetic nephropathy patients. PLoS One. 2016;**11**:e0150154

[226] Eissa S, Matboli M, Aboushahba R, Bekhet MM, Soliman Y. Urinary exosomal microRNA panel unravels novel biomarkers for diagnosis of type 2 diabetic kidney disease. Journal of Diabetes and its Complications. 2016;**30**:1585-1592

[227] Urinary exosomal MiRNA-4534 as a novel diagnostic biomarker for diabetic kidney disease - PubMed. Available from: https://pubmed.ncbi.nlm.nih.gov/32982978/

[228] Atala A. Re: Circulating miR-103a-3p contributes to angiotensin II-induced renal inflammation and fibrosis via a SNRK/NF-κB/p65 regulatory axis. The Journal of Urology. 2020;**203**:34-35

[229] Serum microRNA profiles in patients with autosomal dominant polycystic kidney disease show systematic dysregulation partially reversible by hemodialysis - PubMed. Available from: https://pubmed.ncbi.nlm.nih.gov/34900055/

[230] Serum micro-RNA profiles in patients with autosomal dominant polycystic kidney disease according to hypertension and renal function - PubMed. Available from: https://pubmed.ncbi.nlm.nih.gov/28558802/

[231] Fan J, Ren M, He Y. Diagnostic and Therapeutic Properties of Exosomes in Cardiac Fibrosis. Frontiers in Cell and Development Biology. 4 Jul 2022;**10**:931082. DOI: 10.3389/fcell.2022.931082. PMID: 35859903; PMCID: PMC9289295

[232] Wang L, Liu J, Xu B, Liu Y-L, Liu Z. Reduced exosome miR-425 and miR-744 in the plasma represents the progression of fibrosis and heart failure. The Kaohsiung Journal of Medical Sciences. 2018;**34**:626-633

[233] Li J et al. Mir-30d regulates cardiac remodeling by intracellular and paracrine signaling. Circulation Research. 2021;**128**:e1-e23

[234] Cheng Y et al. A translational study of circulating cell-free microRNA-1 in acute myocardial infarction. Clinical Science (London, England). 2010;**1979**(119):87-95

[235] D'Alessandra Y et al. Circulating microRNAs are new and sensitive biomarkers of myocardial infarction. European Heart Journal. 2010;**31**:2765-2773

[236] Widera C et al. Diagnostic and prognostic impact of six circulating microRNAs in acute coronary syndrome. Journal of Molecular and Cellular Cardiology. 2011;**51**:872-875

[237] Olivieri F et al. Diagnostic potential of circulating miR-499-5p in elderly patients with acute non ST-elevation myocardial infarction. International Journal of Cardiology. 2013;**167**:531-536

[238] Diagnostic and prognostic value of miR-1 and miR-29b on adverse ventricular remodeling after acute myocardial infarction - The SITAGRAMI-miR analysis - PubMed. Available from: https://pubmed.ncbi.nlm.nih.gov/28663047/

[239] MicroRNA29: a mechanistic contributor and potential biomarker in atrial fibrillation - PubMed. Available from: https://pubmed.ncbi.nlm.nih.gov/23459615/

[240] D'Alessandra Y, Carena MC, Spazzafumo L, Martinelli F, Bassetti B, Devanna P, et al. Diagnostic potential of plasmatic MicroRNA signatures in stable and unstable angina. PLoS One. 2013;**8**(11):e80345. DOI: 10.1371/journal.pone.0080345

[241] Fichtlscherer S et al. Circulating microRNAs in patients with coronary artery disease. Circulation Research. 2010;**107**:677-684

[242] Wagner J et al. Characterization of levels and cellular transfer of circulating lipoprotein-bound microRNAs. Arteriosclerosis, Thrombosis, and Vascular Biology. 2013;**33**:1392-1400

[243] Chen X, Luo Q. Potential clinical applications of exosomes in the diagnosis, treatment, and prognosis of cardiovascular diseases: A narrative review. Annals of Translational Medicine. 2022;**10**:372-372

[244] Fang L, Ellims AH, Moore Xl, et al. Circulating microRNAs as biomarkers for diffuse myocardial fibrosis in patients with hypertrophic cardiomyopathy. Journal of Translational Medicine. 2015;**13**:314. DOI: 10.1186/s12967-015-0672-0

[245] Roncarati R et al. Circulating miR-29a, among other up-regulated microRNAs, is the only biomarker for both hypertrophy and fibrosis in patients with hypertrophic cardiomyopathy. Journal of the American College of Cardiology. 2014;**63**:920-927

[246] Prognostic value of circulating microRNAs on heart failure-related morbidity and mortality in two large diverse cohorts of general heart failure patients - PubMed. Available from: https://pubmed.ncbi.nlm.nih.gov/28949058/

[247] Serially measured circulating microRNAs and adverse clinical outcomes in patients with acute heart

failure - PubMed. Available from: https://pubmed.ncbi.nlm.nih.gov/28948688/

[248] Ovchinnikova ES et al. Signature of circulating microRNAs in patients with acute heart failure. European Journal of Heart Failure. 2016;**18**:414-423

Chapter 8

Perspective Chapter: Clinical Application of Exosome Components

Mengyuan Hou, Jingwu Li, Zhiwu Wang and Yankun Liu

Abstract

Exosomes belong to a subpopulation of EVs that carry different functional molecular cargoes, including proteins, nucleic acids, metabolites, and lipids. Notably, evidence has demonstrated that exosomes participate in bidirectional cell–cell communication and act as critical molecular vehicles in regulating numerous physiological and pathological processes. Since the specific contents within exosomes carry the information from their cells of origin, this property permits exosomes to act as valuable biomarkers. This chapter summarizes the potential use of exosome components in diagnosing, prognosis, or monitoring and treating multiple cancers and other non-neoplastic diseases. We also discuss the deficiency of basic applications, including the limitations of research methods and different research institutions and the differences generated by specimen sources. Thus, a better understanding of the problem of exosome detection may pave the way to promising exosome-based clinical applications.

Keywords: exosomes, cancer, dieases, diagnosis, prognosis, therapy

1. Introduction

Exosomes are a subpopulation of EVs secreted by the endocytosis process, with a diameter ranging from 30 to 150 nm [1]. Exosomes are naturally secreted by all kinds of cells and carry diverse functional molecular cargoes, including proteins, lipids, nucleic acids, enzymes, and metabolites to promote intercellular communication. As one of the types of cargo of exosomes, nucleic acids include DNA, messenger, and noncoding RNA. Among all the molecular cargoes, proteins, and nucleic acids are the most abundant contents in exosomes [2]. They have biological functions and are selectively packaged into exosomes. As exosomes are naturally secreted by all kinds of cells and are commonly detected in bodily fluids, including blood, urine, saliva, and cerebrospinal fluid [3], the application potential of exosomes in clinical tumor diagnosis and therapy is promising. In this chapter, we will discuss the bioactive exosomal contents, focusing on proteins, noncoding RNAs, and DNA to better clarify their roles in disease development and the potential application of exosome cargoes (**Figure 1**).

IntechOpen

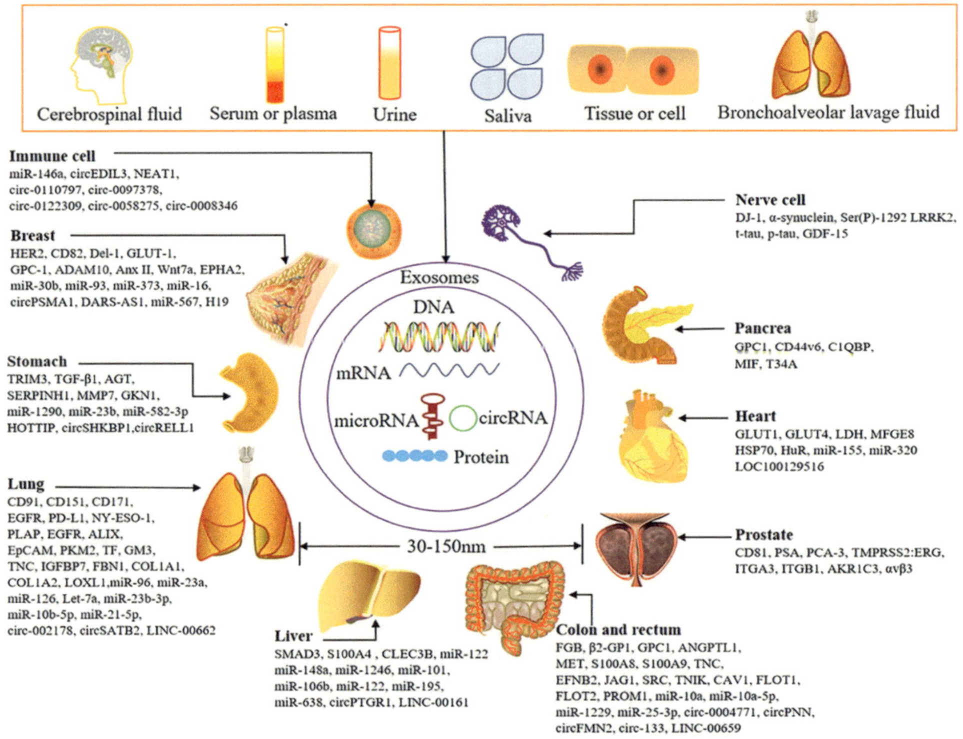

Figure 1.
Application of exosome components in diseases.

2. Exosome protein

With the recent development of isolation methods of exosomes and the applications of protein spectrum, the roles of exosome proteins in the diagnosis, prognosis, and treatment of diseases have been demonstrated in many medical fields, especially for cancer [4]. Exosomal proteins include (1) Membrane transport and fusion-related proteins, such as annexin (Anx II), Rab-GTPase, and heat shock proteins (HSPs), including Hsp60, Hsp70, and Hsp90; (2) Four-transmembrane cross-linked proteins, namely CD9, CD63, CD81, CD82, CD106, Tspan8, intercellular adhesion molecule-1 (ICAM-1); (3) Multi-vesicular bodies (MVBs)-related proteins, for instance, ALIX and TSG101; (4) Other proteins, like integrins, actin, and myosin [5].

2.1 Application of exosomal proteins in tumors: Diagnosis, prognosis, and treatment

2.1.1 Lung cancer

Numerous studies have focused on the clinical application of protein components in circulating exosomes from lung cancer patients. Yet, blood derivatives are the biofluids of choice for metabolomic clinical studies due to their low invasiveness and wealth of biological information [6]. Of note, some exosomal surface proteins, like CD91, CD151, and CD171, have been investigated to be used as biomarkers for early diagnosis of lung cancer [7, 8]. Of these, exosomal CD91 showed a high sensitivity for diagnosing stage I and II lung adenocarcinoma (LUAD) patients [7]. Notably, exosomal CD151 and CD171 have been demonstrated to be upregulated in LUAD and can distinguish the subgroups of lung cancer [8]. Besides that, as a diagnostic biomarker, exosomal epidermal growth factor receptor (EGFR) and programmed death-ligand 1 (PD-L1) are considered to be the compact surface plasmon resonance (SPR) biosensor in lung cancer diagnosis [9]. Moreover, plasma exosomal proteins have also been reported to be served as prognostic and therapeutic biomarkers. As such, New York esophageal squamous cell carcinoma-1 (NY-ESO-1), placental alkaline phosphatase (PLAP), EGFR, ALIX (ALG-2-interacting protein X), and epithelial cell adhesion molecule (EpCAM) in circulating exosomes have been detected by extracellular vesicle array and correlated with overall survival (OS) of non-small cell lung cancer (NSCLC), which are recognized to be potential prognostic biomarkers for NSCLC [10]. Wang et al. also revealed that hypoxia-induced exosomes delivering pyruvate kinase M2 (PKM2) transmit cisplatin resistance to sensitive NSCLC cells. Additionally, Wang et al. found that exosomal PKM2 might be a potential biomarker and therapeutic target for cisplatin resistance in NSCLC [11]. Therefore, these exosomal proteins for lung cancer diagnosis, prognosis, and treatment must be further validated in larger cohorts.

2.1.2 Gastric cancer

Gastric cancer (GC) is one of the most malignant cancers worldwide [12]. Importantly, exosomal proteins are specific diagnostic, prognostic, and therapeutic biomarkers for GC [13]. Various methods, such as liquid chromatography–tandem mass spectrometry (LC–MS/MS), have detected the proteomic profile of exosomes from the serum of GC patients. For example, a study reported that tripartite motif-containing protein 3 (TRIM3) protein in GC patients' serum exosomes was lower than in healthy donors using LC–MS/MS [14]. The higher exosomal transforming growth factor beta 1 (TGF-β1) expression of GC has been analyzed to be associated with tumor-node-metastasis (TNM) stage and lupus nephritis (LN) metastasis by enzyme-linked immunosorbent assay (ELISA) [15]. In addition, the high expression of exosomal TGF-β1 correlated with forkhead box protein 3^+ ($FOXP3^+$) Treg cells in draining LNs, and the high percentage of $FOXP3^+$ Treg cells correlated with tumor size, Bormann type, tumor depth, and lymph node metastasis [15]. Furthermore, exosomal angiotensinogen (AGT), serpin family H member 1 (SERPINH1), and matrix metallopeptidase 7 (MMP7) have been demonstrated to perform well in predicting OS and be non-invasive prognostic biomarkers of GC [16]. Gastrokine 1 (GKN1) has also been identified to be secreted from HFE-145 gastric epithelial cells and can reduce tumor growth and tumor volume, which could be served as a therapeutic target for GC [17]. Likewise, these effective therapeutic proteins can be encapsulated into the exosomes and might prevent GC progression [18]. Thus, these exosomal proteins contribute to the development of GC.

2.1.3 Breast cancer

Exosomal proteins play an essential role in diagnosis evaluation and prognosis prediction of breast cancer (BC) [19]. Notably, it has been demonstrated that the exosomal human epidermal growth factor receptor 2 (HER2) was significantly increased in BC patients compared with healthy donors [20]. In addition, exosomal

CD82 was significantly decreased in BC tissues compared with healthy donors and benign breast disease tissues [21]. Likewise, exosomes in preoperative plasma contained a higher level of developmental endothelial locus-1 (Del-1) than the postoperative plasma, and the high Del-1 level in postoperation was associated with early relapse [22]. Another report identified 1107 exosomal proteins between metastatic BC cell lines MDA-MB-231 and non-cancerous epithelial breast cell lines MCF-10A [23]. Moreso, 87 proteins were associated with BC, and 16 were correlated to BC metastasis [23]. Among them, exosomal glucose transporter 1 (GLUT-1), glypican 1 (GPC-1), and a disintegrin and metalloproteinase 10 (ADAM10) may be served as BC potential biomarkers [23]. Exosomes carrying proteins, including Anx II, Wnt7a, and ephrin type-A receptor 2 (EPHA2) could stimulate BC's invasive, angiogenesis, and metastasis abilities [24–26]. Exosomal Anx II has stimulated angiogenesis and BC metastasis [24]. Further, exosomal Wnt7a has been found to promote lung metastasis of BC [25]. Exosomal EPHA2 has also been found to activate the AMP-activated protein kinase (AMPK) signal pathway via the Ephrin A1-EPHA2 forward signal that promoted the angiogenesis and metastasis of BC [26]. Therefore, these exosome proteins may serve as potential BC therapeutic targets.

2.1.4 Colorectal cancer

Due to carcinoembryonic antigen (CEA), carbohydrate antigen 19-9 (CA19-9), and CA24-2 having poor specificity for the diagnosis of colorectal cancer (CRC) [27], novel biomarkers need to be explored to diagnose CRC development. In recent years, exosomal proteins have been explored for their potential clinical values to serve as tissue and/or liquid biopsy biomarkers to diagnose early CRC. For example, Sun et al. extracted the exosomes in tissues and plasma. They validated that the fibrinogen beta chain (FGB) levels and beta-2-glycoprotein1 (β2-GP1) levels of exosomes in CRC tissue were significantly higher than those in paracancerous tissues [28]. Notably, the areas under the receiver operating characteristic (ROC) curve of plasma exosomal FGB and β2-GP1 as CRC biomarkers were 0.871 and 0.834, respectively, higher than those of CEA (0.723) and CA19-9 (0.614) [28]. Another oncogenic biomarker, exosomal GPC1 protein, was increased in tumor tissue and plasma of CRC patients [29]. However, GPC1 was also highly expressed in other tumor exosomes, which posed a challenge to the specificity of GPC1 in diagnosing CRC. In addition, some exosomal proteins were also proved to be carcinostatic biomarkers. For example, Jiang et al. verified that the level of exosomal angiopoietin-like protein 1 (ANGPTL1) was significantly decreased in CRC tissues compared with paired normal tissues and inhibited CRC metastasis to the liver [30]. Likewise, an exosome protein profile result demonstrated that the adherence-related proteins were enriched in the primary CRC cell (SW480) exosomes [31]. The metastatic factors (MET, S100 calcium-binding protein A8 (S100A8), S100A9, Tenascin-C(TNC)), signal transduction molecules (Ephrin B2 (EFNB2), Jagged1 (JAG1), SRC, Traf2- and Nck-interacting kinase (TNIK)), and lipid raft and lipid raft-associated components (Caveolin-1 (CAV1), Flotillin-1 (FLOT1), Flotillin-2 (FLOT2), Prominin 1(PROM1)) were enriched in the metastatic CRC cell (SW620) exosomes, which were associated with tumor progression and poor prognosis [31]. Interestingly, most exosomal proteins correlate with epithelial mesenchymal transition (EMT), migration, invasion, and angiogenesis. Therefore, exosomal proteins may be biomarkers for predicting CRC metastasis.

2.1.5 Pancreatic cancer

Pancreatic cancer (PC) is one of the most lethal malignant neoplasms worldwide [32]. Existing tumor markers, such as CA19–9, cannot reasonably predict the occurrence and progression of PC, while exosomal proteins may play decisive roles in the occurrence and development of PC [33]. Excitingly, exosomal GPC1 has also been found in PC. Notably, the area under the ROC curve of GPC1 circulating exosomes (from the serum of pancreatic ductal adenocarcinoma (PDAC), benign pancreatic disease patients, and healthy donors) was 1.0, and the sensitivity and specificity of exosomal GPC1 were 100% [33]. Moreover, the level of circulating GPC1 exosomes was associated with tumor burden and the OS of PC patients [33]. Besides that, Xie et al. also observed that the high expression of exosomal CD44v6 (CD44 variant isoform 6) and C1QBP (complement C1q binding protein) was associated with a poor prognosis and a higher risk of postoperative liver metastasis of PDAC [34]. Costa-Silva et al. also found that exosomal migration inhibitory factor (MIF) was highly expressed in PDAC patients, which promoted liver pre-metastatic niche formation and metastasis [35]. The expression of exosomal MIF in PDAC liver metastasis was significantly higher than those without liver metastasis [35]. Furthermore, exosome survivin-T34A (T34A) enhances the sensitivity of gemcitabine to PC cells [36]. Importantly, these biomarkers illustrate their potential value in predicting the occurrence and development of PC.

2.1.6 Liver cancer

Hepatocellular carcinoma (HCC) is one of the most common forms of cancer [37]. Although serum α-fetoprotein (AFP) has been widely applied as a biomarker for diagnosis and dynamic monitoring of HCC, it is not elevated in each HCC patient [38]. As a result, exosomal proteins have been searched for diagnosis, prognosis, and treatment of HCC. Fu et al. reported that high exosomal small mother against decapentaplegic family member 3 (SMAD3) protein level was positively related to tumor size and TNM stage and correlated negatively with disease-free survival (DFS) [39]. Sun et al. also found that HCC patients with high plasma exosomal S100A4 had a poor prognosis, which promoted HCC cell metastasis by activating the signal transducer and activator of transcription 3 (STAT3)/OPN signal pathway [40]. Moreso, down-regulated C-Type Lectin Domain Family 3 Member B (CLEC3B) in HCC-derived exosomes promoted migration, invasion, and EMT of HCC cells via AMPK and vascular endothelial growth factor (VEGF) signals. Furthermore, the downregulation of CLEC3B in exosomes suppressed VEGF secretion in both HCC cells and endothelial cells (ECs), eventually inhibiting angiogenesis [41]. Therefore, these studies suggest that exosomal proteins play different roles in HCC development.

2.1.7 Prostate cancer

Prostate cancer (PCa) is a life-threatening disease among men worldwide [42]. Notably, prostate-specific antigen (PSA) has often been used as a diagnostic biomarker for PCa [43]. However, due to PSA's lack of sensitivity and specificity, new biomarkers are urgently needed to assist in diagnosing, prognosis, and treating PCa [43]. A study reported that plasmatic exosomes expressing CD81 and PSA reached 100% specificity and sensitivity in distinguishing PCa patients from healthy donors [44]. Except for the blood exosomes, urine exosomal prostate cancer antigen 3 (PCA3) and transmembrane protease serine 2:ERG (TMPRSS2:ERG) derived from PCa patients can also be used as non-invasive diagnostic biomarkers and monitor cancer patients' PCa status [45]. Another study reported that the urine exosomes integrin alpha-3 (ITGA3) and integrins beta-1 (ITGB1) in metastatic PCa patients were higher than PCa and benign prostatic hyperplasia (BPH) [46]. Plasma exosomal aldo-keto reductase family 1 member C3 (AKR1C3) have also been demonstrated to be associated with the OS of PCa patient, which is recognized to be a potential prognostic biomarker for PCa [47]. Furthermore, Krishn et al. demonstrated that αvβ3 integrin was transferred to β3-negative recipient cells by exosomes derived from PCa patient plasma and can be identified as a therapeutic target for PCa [48].

2.2 Application of exosomal proteins in other diseases: Diagnosis, prognosis, and treatment

2.2.1 Cardiovascular disease

In recent years, many studies have paid more attention to the roles of exosomal proteins in cardiovascular diseases (CVD). Notably, exosomal proteins from different cell origination play critical roles in cardiac cell development [49]. For instance, GLUT1, GLUT4, and lactate dehydrogenase (LDH) functioned in ECs for glucose transport and metabolism in cardiac cell-derived exosomes [50]. Proteins carried by exosomes using *in vitro* cultures of neonatal cardiac fibroblasts under normoxic conditions are known to be associated with the extracellular matrix, cytoskeleton, mitochondrial, and nucleotide-binding [51]. Exosomal milk fat globule epidermal growth factor VIII (MFGE8) could activate phagocytic signaling and efficiently clear dead cells, promoting cardiac recovery after injury [52]. Additionally, *ex vivo*, *in vivo*, and *in vitro* studies using settings of ischemia-reperfusion found that exosomal HSP70 transmitted cardioprotective signals to the heart by activating the toll-like receptor 4 (TLR4) downstream signal pathway [53]. Exosomal-associated human antigen R (HuR) has also been recently reported to increase inflammatory and profibrogenic responses *in vitro* and *in vivo* using diabetic heart models [54]. Thus, exosomal HuR might be a therapeutic target to alleviate cardiac inflammation and fibrosis in diabetes [54]. Hence, exosomal proteins can affect CVD by regulating metabolism, macrophage engulfment, and inflammatory and profibrogenic responses.

2.2.2 Respiratory system disease

Exosomes released from severe acute respiratory syndrome coronavirus 2 (SARS-CoV-2) infection induced tissue factor (TF) expression that may drive thrombosis [55]. The EVs TF activity was related to disease severity and mortality and could be a prognostic biomarker and therapeutic for coronavirus disease 2019 (COVID-19) [55]. Monosialodihexosyl ganglioside (GM3)-enriched exosomes may contribute to the pathological processes related to COVID-19 and provide the most significant repository on the plasma lipidome and metabolome distinct to COVID-19 [56]. Moreso, *in vitro* studies have demonstrated that EV proteins, such as TNC, insulin-like-growth-factor-binding protein 7 (IGFBP7), fibrillin-1 (FBN1), alpha-2 collagen chain (I) (COL1A2), alpha-1 collagen chain (I) (COL1A1), and lysyl oxidase homolog 1 (LOXL1), secreted by fibroblasts might contribute to idiopathic pulmonary fibrosis (IPF) [57]. Furthermore, exosomes also transferred proteins to distant recipient cells and were expected to be a new drug delivery system and a novel therapeutic target [58].

2.2.3 Nervous system diseases

Parkinson's disease (PD) and Alzheimer's (AD) are classic chronic neurodegenerative diseases [59]. Previous studies have reported few specific blood biomarkers in diagnosing PD and AD [60]. This is, to some extent, likely attributed to the lack of biomarker specificity [60]. For example, exosomal DJ-1 and α-synuclein in plasma failed to distinguish between PD patients and healthy donors [60]. However, the two proteins in plasma neural-derived exosomes could distinguish PD patients and healthy donors [60]. Besides the circulating specimen, the urine exosomal Ser(P)-1292 LRRK2 (leucine-rich repeat kinase 2) was considered a biomarker associated with PD progression [61]. In addition, the t-tau and p-tau levels derived from neuron exosomes of mild-AD groups were significantly higher than age-matched controls and mild cognitive impairment groups [62]. Likewise, exosomal growth differentiation factor-15 (GDF-15) derived from bone mesenchymal stem cells (MSCs) was confirmed to alleviate SH-SY5Y cell damage of AD by activating AKT/GSK-3β/β-catenin pathway [63]. Thus, exosomal proteins from different specimen sources may be used as potential biomarkers for diagnosis and prognosis of nervous system diseases.

3. Exosome RNA

Exosomal RNAs include miRNAs, circRNAs, lncRNAs, and mRNAs [64]. Additionally, evidence has established that exosomes play a significant role in tumorigenesis and tumor progression by transferring miRNAs, circRNAs, and LncRNAs [1]. These exosomal RNAs are biomarkers and therapeutic targets for human diseases, particularly malignant tumors.

3.1 Application of exosomal RNAs in tumors: diagnosis, prognosis, and treatment

3.1.1 Lung cancer

It has been reported that free RNA molecules secreted by tumor cells will degenerate in the bloodstream [65]. The exceptions are cell-free microRNAs that can be detected in cancer patients' blood plasma or serum [65]. Relevant RNA molecular information, such as exosomes, may also be obtained in EVs [66]. The existing literature also shows that exosomal RNAs play critical roles in different stages of the development cascade of cancer. For instance, serum exosomal miR-96 and miR-23a were upregulated in lung cancer and could be used as a biomarker for diagnosing lung cancer [67, 68]. Besides circulating exosomal miRNAs, exosomes released from bronchoalveolar lavage fluid could also serve as biomarkers for early lung cancer diagnosis. For instance, exosomal miR-126 and Let-7a from bronchoalveolar lavage fluid were significantly higher in LUAD patients than in healthy donors [69]. Exosomal miRNAs could be used as a prognostic biomarker for NSCLC development, such as miR-23b-3p, miR-10b-5p, and miR-21-5p were found to be independently associated with poor OS of NSCLC [70]. Moreso, exosomal circ-002178 was enriched in plasma exosomes from LUAD patients and could be delivered into $CD8^+$ T cells to induce PD1 expression [71]. Exosomes from NSCLC patient serum were enriched with circSATB2, which has high sensitivity and specificity for clinical detection and is related to lung cancer metastasis [72]. Furthermore, Lv et al. verified that exosomal long intergenic non-coding 00662 (LINC-00662) promoted proliferation, invasion, and migration of NSCLC by the miR-320d/E2F1 axis, indicating that LINC-00662 may be a potential therapeutic target for lung cancer [73].

3.1.2 Gastric cancer

As discussed earlier, several circulating RNAs are excellent as potential diagnostic markers of GC. Circulating exosomal miR-1290 has been reported to be upregulated in various malignant cancers, including GC [74], LUAD [75], epithelial ovarian cancer [76], and PCa [77]. Kumata et al. observed that the miR-23b in exosomes from the plasma of GC patients was significantly lower than that of the healthy donors [78]. Many studies have also confirmed that exosomal circRNAs act as molecular sponges of miRNAs to regulate the proliferation, invasion, metastasis, and angiogenesis of GC cells [79–81]. Moreso, the circSHKBP1, elevated in GC tissues and serum, promoted GC progression by sponging miR-582-3p to increase HuR expression and suppress HSP90 degradation [79]. In contrast, exosomal circRELL1 has been reported to inhibit the progression of GC via the circRELL1/miR-637/EPHB3 axis [80]. Furthermore, exosomal lncRNA HOTTIP was also found to be a GC diagnostic biomarker associated with poor OS of GC patients [82]. In summary, these exosomal RNAs may serve as potential biomarkers for GC.

3.1.3 Liver cancer

Much evidence has demonstrated that exosomal RNAs are involved in the growth, metastasis, and angiogenesis of HCC cells and could be used as diagnostic and prognostic biomarkers and therapeutic tools in HCC [83, 84]. Notably, exosomal miRNAs have been studied as the potential diagnostic biomarker for HCC. For example, serum exosomal miR-122, miR-148a, and miR-1246 were significantly higher in HCC patients than in liver cirrhosis and healthy donors [85]. Interestingly, exosomal miR-101, miR-106b, miR-122, and miR-195 were significantly lower in HCC serum than in chronic hepatitis B (CHB) [86]. A study also reported that high serum exosomal miR-638 was associated with HCC recurrence, suggesting the potential of exosomal miR-638 as a reliable biomarker for prognostic monitoring [87]. Another study reported that serum exosomal circPTGR1 was upregulated in HCC patients and associated with the TNM stage and OS. Moreover, exosomal circPTGR1 has promoted the proliferation, invasion, and migration of HCC via the miR-449a-MET axis [88]. Beyond miRNAs, some lncRNAs in exosomes may also be served as the promising diagnostic marker for HCC. Sun et al. indicated that the serum exosomal LINC-00161 was higher in HCC patients than in healthy donors, suggesting that LINC-00161 could be a potential diagnostic biomarker for HCC [89].

3.1.4 Breast cancer

Most BC patients are hormone-dependent [90]. Increasing evidence demonstrated that exosomes play an essential role in breast tumorigenesis and progression by transferring miRNAs and LncRNAs [1]. Triple-negative breast cancer (TNBC) refers to the expression of estrogen receptor (ER), progesterone receptor (PR), and HER2 being negative in BC tissue [91]. Notably, miR-30b was associated with recurrence, and miR-93 was abundant in ductal carcinoma in situ (DCIS) [92]. Circulating exosomal miR-373 has been enriched in TNBC, and serum exosomal miR-373 was higher in ER-negative and PR-negative patients than in patients with hormone-receptor-positive patients [93]. In contrast, exosomal miRNAs, such as miR-16, were particularly enriched in estrogen-positive BC patients [92]. These studies remind us that the expression level of miRNAs in exosomes may contribute to the luminal classification of BC. Beyond miRNAs, circPSMA1 in exosomes acted as a "miRNAs sponge" to absorb miR-637 [94]. It could transmit migration and proliferation capacity to recipient cells to promote TNBC cell proliferation, migration, and metastasis via the miR-637/Akt1/β-catenin (cyclin D1) axis [94]. The lncRNA DARS-AS1 delivered by exosomes has been found to effectively inhibit TNBC cell growth and liver metastasis [95]. Thus, different RNA types can play different roles in TNBC development. To date, drug resistance is a significant obstacle to BC treatment [96]. Many pieces of evidence have demonstrated that exosomes regulate drug resistance for BC by delivering RNA. For instance, Han et al. demonstrated that miR-567 delivered by exosomes increased the sensitivity of BC cells to trastuzumab [97]. Similarly, lncRNA H19 could be transferred via exosomes to sensitive cells, leading to doxorubicin resistance in BC [98]. Thus, these studies strongly suggest that exosomal RNAs are known to act as biomarkers for BC development and drug resistance.

3.1.5 Colorectal cancer

Exosomes carry and deliver specific molecules and have been found to mediate crosstalk between primary cancer sites and metastatic cancer loci [31, 84]. Exosomal miR-10a derived from SW480 cells inhibits human lung fibroblast migration and inflammatory factors releases, transferring the metastasis suppression signal to primary CRC [99]. Further studies have established a pair of human liver fibroblast cell lines to confirm the regulation function of miR-10a-5p between primary CRC and metastatic liver loci [100]. As mentioned above, abnormal expression of exosomal RNAs in peripheral blood can also be considered emerging diagnostic, prognostic, and therapeutic biomarkers of CRC. For instance, exosomal miR-1229 is significantly upregulated in the serum exosomes from CRC patients and was associated with tumor size, TNM stage, lymphatic metastasis, and poor OS [101]. Zeng et al. also found that miR-25-3p could form a pre-metastatic niche via stimulating angiogenesis and vascular permeability in CRC [102]. Circulating exosomal circRNAs could also serve as strong diagnostic biomarkers for CRC. Serum exosomal circ-0004771, circPNN, and circFMN2 levels were significantly upregulated in CRC patients [103–105]. Exosomal circ-133 was also significantly upregulated in the plasma of CRC patients and associated with hypoxia and cell metastasis by miR-133a/GEF-H1/RhoA axis [106]. Moreover, the mechanisms for targeting dysfunctional exosomal LncRNAs are being developed to treat CRC. For example, exosomal LINC-00659 has been found to promote CRC cells proliferation, invasion, migration, and EMT by miR-342-3p/ANXA2 pathway, suggesting that LINC-00659 could work as a potential biomarker for selecting a suitable treatment strategy [107]. Essential to the development of improved therapeutic strategies is a mechanistic understanding of exosome-mediated cell communications. Furthermore, MSCs -derived exosomes have been used as carriers to deliver anticancer agents in CRC [108]. Notably, this therapeutic effect is based on direct cell–cell communications and indirect communications mediating by cell secretome [109].

3.2 Application of exosomal RNAs in other diseases: Diagnosis, prognosis, and treatment

3.2.1 Cardiovascular disease

As mentioned earlier, exosomal RNAs secreted from senescent cells are considered to be associated with CVD and vascular aging [110]. miR-155 contained in exosomes is transferred from smooth muscle cells to endothelial cells to induce endothelial injury and promote atherosclerosis [111]. In diabetic cardiomyopathy, miR-320 is enriched in diabetic patients and could inhibit Hsp20 in endothelial cells, exerting an anti-angiogenic function [112]. Additionally, exosomal LOC100129516 has been found to ultimately alleviate the progression of atherosclerosis and decrease the cholesterol level via the PPARγ/LXRα/ABCA1 pathway [113]. Therefore, these studies suggest that the pathologic role of exosomes involves RNA delivery and could contribute to developing diabetic cardiomyopathy via different cell signals.

3.2.2 Autoimmune disease

Autoimmune diseases may be related to genetic, environmental, hormonal, and immunological factors [114]. Mounting evidence indicates that exosomes play an important role in autoimmune diseases, such as systemic lupus erythematosus (SLE), rheumatoid arthritis (RA), and ankylosing spondylitis (AS). For example, it was demonstrated that urinary exosome miR-146a level was significantly increased in SLE patients compared with healthy donors. Its expression level was closely related to renal injury index, like proteinuria, histological features, and lupus activity [115]. It was also verified that exosomal circEDIL3 suppresses inflammation-induced angiogenesis and ameliorates RA via the miR-485-3p/PIAS3/STAT3 pathway [116]. In addition, the expression of serum exosomal nuclear paraspeckle assembly transcript 1 (NEAT1) in RA patients was higher than that of healthy donors. Moreover, NEAT1 has promoted the progression of RA by downregulating miR-144-3p and upregulating Rho-associated protein kinase 2 (ROCK2), suggesting that NEAT1 may be a potential biomarker and therapeutic target for RA [117]. The levels of exosomal circRNAs, like circ-0110797, circ-0097378, circ-0122309, circ-0058275, and circ-0008346 in AS, were significantly down-regulated compared with healthy donors, providing more optional biomarkers for the early diagnosis of AS [118].

4. Exosome DNA

Circulating tumor DNA (ctDNA) fragments are released by tumor cells into the bloodstream. The information on genomic alterations identified in tumors, including point mutations, rearrangements, amplifications, and even gene copy variations, could be identified by analyzing ctDNA molecules [119]. Although cancer detection by monitoring ctDNA is an area of active investigation, identifying very low amounts of ctDNA in blood samples with variable amounts of free DNA (cfDNA) remains challenging. To date, the studies focused on exosome DNA (exoDNA) are fewer than those on exosome RNA and protein [120]. It is revealed that a variety of cancer-derived DNA markers in exosomes by high throughput genome and transcriptome comparative analyses, including copy number, point mutation, insertion, deletion, and gene fusion. ExoDNA has great potential for disease diagnosis, prognosis assessment, and treatment monitoring. For instance, methylation tests of exoDNA and/or cfDNA derived from the gastric fluid can be used to diagnose GC. In fact, the difference between exoDNA and cfDNA is that the former derives from living cells, the latter from dead ones [121]. Urine from bladder cancer patients contained significant amounts of exoDNA compared with healthy donors [122]. Bernard et al. studied that the increased level of exoDNA was significantly associated with disease progression. Moreover, PC patients with metastases and detectable ctDNA at baseline status had poor progression-free survival (PFS) and OS compared with patients without detectable ctDNA [123]. Degli Esposti et al. also demonstrated that neuroblastoma patients with high tumor mutation load values in exoDNA had a worse outcome than those with lower values [124]. Importantly, the advantage of exoDNA is that they are stable enough to be analyzed retrospectively from frozen bio-banked samples [125]. Meanwhile, exoDNA widely exists in various body fluids and can be easily collected [126]. Therefore, exoDNA may be an ideal liquid biopsy method and a novel tumor marker. However, due to the uncertainty of technical methods and high cost, research on exoDNA is relatively limited.

5. Problems and prospects of exosomes

Exosomes can be isolated from multiple sources, including cell culture medium, body fluids, and tumor tissues [28, 127, 128]. Thus, the components of exosomes have potential applications in diagnosis and prognosis for cancer and other diseases. Nevertheless, the basic application of exosomes is at an early stage and restricts their clinical application. Furthermore, considering that the tissue collection method is a non-invasive procedure, patient compliance may also limit the clinical application of exosomes.

5.1 Various isolation methods of exosomes

Exosomes can be extracted by differential ultracentrifugation (UC), density gradient fractionation, polymeric precipitation, microfluidics techniques, and immunoaffinity isolation [129]. The major problem is the different methods will cause significant differences in the composition and content of exosomes. In addition, the low amounts of components in exosomes led to difficulties in quantification. To date, differential UC is the most commonly used isolation method to harvest highly purified exosomes from a cell culture medium [130]. Polymeric precipitation requires little hands-on time but produces the highest contamination [131]. Additionally, immunoaffinity isolation is based on the characteristic surface proteins on certain exosomes [132]. Antibodies conjugated with beads can select the desired exosomes (immuno-enrichment) or trap unwanted exosomes (immuno-depletion) [129]. This selection process makes it possible to clarify unique exosome populations while undoubtedly leading to lower yields [129]. Each method has advantages and limitations and varies in the quantification of exosome size [133]. As exosomes diagnostic and prognostic platforms become available, there will be requirements for clinical application and manufacturing standards development.

5.2 Differences in research institutions

A biomarker that can be used in clinical applications should meet the following premise: There should be no statistically significant differences between different detection institutions, detection methods, and researchers. However, it is not the case in the current situation of studying exosomes. For example, a report indicated that surface protein CD47 in circulating exosomes was higher in healthy than BC patients [134]. However, exosomal CD47 in BC patients was reported to be significantly higher than those in healthy controls [19]. Thus, the standards of specimen source, collection, and process in different institutions should first be well established.

5.3 The differences generated by sources of specimen

Specimens for clinical application could be obtained from blood, tissues, and other biological fluids, like urine, hydrothorax, ascites, and cerebrospinal fluid [6, 28]. Among all these specimens, serum and plasma are the most suitable for reflecting healthy or diseased conditions, genetic variations, environmental factors, lifestyle, nutrition habits, and drugs [6]. They can also provide important information at a systemic level [6]. Nevertheless, the exosomal contents from plasma and serum simultaneously and place have been identified to differ in the stability and composition of metabolome and lipoproteome [6]. Thus, the criterion should be established for using different specimens, and collection tubes, even among the same blood matrix.

6. Conclusions

In summary, technological improvements and our understanding of exosomal proteins, nucleic acids, and their exosomal content profiles may provide diagnostic, prognostic, and therapeutic clues for diseases in the future.

Acknowledgements

This work was supported by the Natural Science Foundation of Hebei Province [no: H 2021105019] and the Key Laboratory of Precision Medical Testing in Tangshan [no: 2021TS009b]. The authors thank AiMi Academic Services (www.aimieditor.com) for English language editing and review services. The authors thank Professor Zhengang Wu reviewed and revised the manuscript before submission.

Conflict of interest

The authors declare no conflict of interest.

Author details

Mengyuan Hou[1], Jingwu Li[2], Zhiwu Wang[3] and Yankun Liu[4*]

1 North China University of Technology, Tangshan, China

2 Cancer Institute, Tangshan People's Hospital, Tangshan, China

3 Department of Chemoradiotherapy, Tangshan People's Hospital, Tangshan, China

4 Department of Medical Molecular Diagnosis, Tangshan People's Hospital, Tangshan, China

*Address all correspondence to: rmyy_lyk@163.com

References

[1] Lakshmi S, Hughes TA, Priya S. Exosomes and exosomal RNAs in breast cancer: A status update. European Journal of Cancer. 2021;**144**:252-268. DOI: 10.1016/j.ejca.2020.11.033

[2] Wang X, Tian L, Lu J, Ng IO. Exosomes and cancer - Diagnostic and prognostic biomarkers and therapeutic vehicle. Oncogene. 2022;**11**(1):54. DOI: 10.1038/s41389-022-00431-5

[3] Zhang Y, Liu Y, Liu H, Tang WH. Exosomes: Biogenesis, biologic function and clinical potential. Cell & Bioscience. 2019;**9**:19. DOI: 10.1186/s13578-019-0282-2

[4] Wang X, Huang J, Chen W, Li G, Li Z, Lei J. The updated role of exosomal proteins in the diagnosis, prognosis, and treatment of cancer. Experimental & Molecular Medicine. 2022;**54**(9):1390-1400. DOI: 10.1038/s12276-022-00855-4

[5] Dai J, Su Y, Zhong S, Cong L, Liu B, Yang J, et al. Exosomes: Key players in cancer and potential therapeutic strategy. Signal Transduction and Targeted Therapy. 2020;**5**(1):145. DOI: 10.1038/s41392-020-00261-0

[6] Vignoli A, Tenori L, Morsiani C, Turano P, Capri M, Luchinat C. Serum or plasma (and which plasma), that is the question. Journal of Proteome Research. 2022;**21**(4):1061-1072. DOI: 10.1021/acs.jproteome.1c00935

[7] Ueda K, Ishikawa N, Tatsuguchi A, Saichi N, Fujii R, Nakagawa H. Antibody-coupled monolithic silica microtips for highthroughput molecular profiling of circulating exosomes. Scientific Reports. 2014;**4**:6232. DOI: 10.1038/srep06232

[8] Sandfeld-Paulsen B, Jakobsen KR, Bæk R, Folkersen BH, Rasmussen TR, Meldgaard P, et al. Exosomal proteins as diagnostic biomarkers in lung cancer. Journal of Thoracic Oncology. 2016;**11**(10):1701-1710. DOI: 10.1016/j.jtho.2016.05.034

[9] Liu C, Zeng X, An Z, Yang Y, Eisenbaum M, Gu X, et al. Sensitive detection of exosomal proteins via a compact surface plasmon resonance biosensor for cancer diagnosis. ACS Sensors. 2018;**3**(8):1471-1479. DOI: 10.1021/acssensors.8b00230

[10] Sandfeld-Paulsen B, Aggerholm-Pedersen N, Bæk R, Jakobsen KR, Meldgaard P, Folkersen BH, et al. Exosomal proteins as prognostic biomarkers in non-small cell lung cancer. Molecular Oncology. 2016;**10**(10):1595-1602. DOI: 10.1016/j.molonc.2016.10.003

[11] Wang D, Zhao C, Xu F, Zhang A, Jin M, Zhang K, et al. Cisplatin-resistant NSCLC cells induced by hypoxia transmit resistance to sensitive cells through exosomal PKM2. Theranostics. 2021;**11**(6):2860-2875. DOI: 10.7150/thno.51797

[12] Machlowska J, Baj J, Sitarz M, Maciejewski R, Sitarz R. Gastric cancer: Epidemiology, risk factors, classification, genomic characteristics and treatment strategies. International Journal of Molecular Sciences. 2020;**21**(11):4012. DOI: 10.3390/ijms21114012

[13] Su H, Ren W, Zhang D. Research progress on exosomal proteins as diagnostic markers of gastric cancer (review article). Clinical and Experimental Medicine. 2022. DOI: 10.1007/s10238-022-00793-5

[14] Fu H, Yang H, Zhang X, Wang B, Mao J, Li X, et al. Exosomal TRIM3 is a novel marker and therapy target for gastric cancer. Journal of Experimental & Clinical Cancer Research. 2018;**37**(1):162. DOI: 10.1186/s13046-018-0825-0

[15] Yen EY, Miaw SC, Yu JS, Lai IR. Exosomal TGF-β1 is correlated with lymphatic metastasis of gastric cancers. American Journal of Cancer Research. 2017;**7**(11):2199-2208 DOI:

[16] Liu L, Pang H, He Q, Pan B, Sun X, Shan J, et al. A novel strategy to identify candidate diagnostic and prognostic biomarkers for gastric cancer. Cancer Cell International. 2021;**21**(1):335. DOI: 10.1186/s12935-021-02007-6

[17] Yoon JH, Ham IH, Kim O, Ashktorab H, Smoot DT, Nam SW, et al. Gastrokine 1 protein is a potential theragnostic target for gastric cancer. Gastric Cancer. 2018;**21**(6):956-967. DOI: 10.1007/s10120-018-0828-8

[18] Gutierrez-Millan C, Calvo Díaz C, Lanao JM, Colino CI. Advances in exosomes-based drug delivery systems. Macromolecular Bioscience. 2021;**21**(1):e2000269. DOI: 10.1002/mabi.202000269

[19] Wang M, Ji S, Shao G, Zhang J, Zhao K, Wang Z, et al. Effect of exosome biomarkers for diagnosis and prognosis of breast cancer patients. Clinical & Translational Oncology. 2018;**20**(7):906-911. DOI: 10.1007/s12094-017-1805-0

[20] Vinduska V, Gallops CE, O'Connor R, Wang Y, Huang X. Exosomal surface protein detection with quantum dots and immunomagnetic capture for cancer detection. Nanomaterials (Basel). 2021;**11**(7):1853. DOI: 10.3390/nano11071853

[21] Wang X, Zhong W, Bu J, Li Y, Li R, Nie R, et al. Exosomal protein CD82 as a diagnostic biomarker for precision medicine for breast cancer. Molecular Carcinogenesis. 2019;**58**(5):674-685. DOI: 10.1002/mc.22960

[22] Lee SJ, Lee J, Jung JH, Park HY, Moon PG, Chae YS, et al. Exosomal Del-1 as a potent diagnostic marker for breast cancer: Prospective cohort study. Clinical Breast Cancer. 2021;**21**(6):e748-ee56. DOI: 10.1016/j.clbc.2021.02.002

[23] Risha Y, Minic Z, Ghobadloo SM, Berezovski MV. The proteomic analysis of breast cell line exosomes reveals disease patterns and potential biomarkers. Scientific Reports. 2020;**10**(1):13572. DOI: 10.1038/s41598-020-70393-4

[24] Maji S, Chaudhary P, Akopova I, Nguyen PM, Hare RJ, Gryczynski I, et al. Exosomal annexin II promotes angiogenesis and breast cancer metastasis. Molecular Cancer Research. 2017;**15**(1):93-105. DOI: 10.1158/1541-7786.Mcr-16-0163

[25] Li C, Yoshimura T, Tian M, Wang Y, Kondo T, Yamamoto KI, et al. Exosomal Wnt7a from a low metastatic subclone promotes lung metastasis of a highly metastatic subclone in the murine 4t1 breast cancer. Breast Cancer Research. 2022;**24**(1):60. DOI: 10.1186/s13058-022-01557-5

[26] Han B, Zhang H, Tian R, Liu H, Wang Z, Wang Z, et al. Exosomal EPHA2 derived from highly metastatic breast cancer cells promotes angiogenesis by activating the AMPK signaling pathway through Ephrin A1-EPHA2 forward signaling. Theranostics. 2022;**12**(9):4127-4146. DOI: 10.7150/thno.72404

[27] Rao H, Wu H, Huang Q, Yu Z, Zhong Z. Clinical value of serum CEA, CA24-2 and CA19-9 in patients with colorectal cancer. Clinical Laboratory.

2021;**67**(4):10.7754. DOI: 10.7754/Clin.Lab.2020.200828

[28] Sun Z, Ji S, Wu J, Tian J, Quan W, Shang A, et al. Proteomics-based identification of candidate exosomal glycoprotein biomarkers and their value for diagnosing colorectal cancer. Frontiers in Oncology. 2021;**11**:725211. DOI: 10.3389/fonc.2021.725211

[29] Li J, Chen Y, Guo X, Zhou L, Jia Z, Peng Z, et al. GPC1 exosome and its regulatory miRNAs are specific markers for the detection and target therapy of colorectal cancer. Journal of Cellular and Molecular Medicine. 2017;**21**(5):838-847. DOI: 10.1111/jcmm.12941

[30] Jiang K, Chen H, Fang Y, Chen L, Zhong C, Bu T, et al. Exosomal ANGPTL1 attenuates colorectal cancer liver metastasis by regulating Kupffer cell secretion pattern and impeding MMP9 induced vascular leakiness. Journal of Experimental & Clinical Cancer Research. 2021;**40**(1):21. DOI: 10.1186/s13046-020-01816-3

[31] Ji H, Greening DW, Barnes TW, Lim JW, Tauro BJ, Rai A, et al. Proteome profiling of exosomes derived from human primary and metastatic colorectal cancer cells reveal differential expression of key metastatic factors and signal transduction components. Proteomics. 2013;**13**(10-11):1672-1686. DOI: 10.1002/pmic.201200562

[32] Pan Y, Tang H, Li Q, Chen G, Li D. Exosomes and their roles in the chemoresistance of pancreatic cancer. Cancer Medicine. 2022;**11**(24):4979-4988. DOI: 10.1002/cam4.4830

[33] Melo SA, Luecke LB, Kahlert C, Fernandez AF, Gammon ST, Kaye J, et al. Glypican-1 identifies cancer exosomes and detects early pancreatic cancer. Nature. 2015;**523**(7559):177-182. DOI: 10.1038/nature14581

[34] Xie Z, Gao Y, Ho C, Li L, Jin C, Wang X, et al. Exosome-delivered CD44v6/C1QBP complex drives pancreatic cancer liver metastasis by promoting fibrotic liver microenvironment. Gut. 2022;**71**(3):568-579. DOI: 10.1136/gutjnl-2020-323014

[35] Costa-Silva B, Aiello NM, Ocean AJ, Singh S, Zhang H, Thakur BK, et al. Pancreatic cancer exosomes initiate pre-metastatic niche formation in the liver. Nature Cell Biology. 2015;**17**(6):816-826. DOI: 10.1038/ncb3169

[36] Aspe JR, Diaz Osterman CJ, Jutzy JM, Deshields S, Whang S, Wall NR. Enhancement of Gemcitabine sensitivity in pancreatic adenocarcinoma by novel exosome-mediated delivery of the Survivin-T34A mutant. Journal of Extracellular Vesicles. 2014;**3**:10.3402. DOI: 10.3402/jev.v3.23244

[37] Wu X, Li J, Gassa A, Buchner D, Alakus H, Dong Q, et al. Circulating tumor DNA as an emerging liquid biopsy biomarker for early diagnosis and therapeutic monitoring in hepatocellular carcinoma. International Journal of Biological Sciences. 2020;**16**(9):1551-1562. DOI: 10.7150/ijbs.44024

[38] Kim KH, Lee SY, Kim DG, Lee SY, Kim JY, Yoo JS. Absolute quantification of N-glycosylation of alpha-fetoprotein using parallel reaction monitoring with stable isotope-labeled n-glycopeptide as an internal standard. Analytical Chemistry. 2020;**92**(18):12588-12595. DOI: 10.1021/acs.analchem.0c02563

[39] Fu Q, Zhang Q, Lou Y, Yang J, Nie G, Chen Q, et al. Primary tumor-derived exosomes facilitate metastasis by regulating adhesion of circulating tumor cells via SMAD3 in liver cancer.

Oncogene. 2018;**37**(47):6105-6118. DOI: 10.1038/s41388-018-0391-0

[40] Sun H, Wang C, Hu B, Gao X, Zou T, Luo Q, et al. Exosomal S100A4 derived from highly metastatic hepatocellular carcinoma cells promotes metastasis by activating STAT3. Signal Transduction and Targeted Therapy. 2021;**6**(1):187. DOI: 10.1038/s41392-021-00579-3

[41] Dai W, Wang Y, Yang T, Wang J, Wu W, Gu J. Downregulation of exosomal CLEC3B in hepatocellular carcinoma promotes metastasis and angiogenesis via AMPK and VEGF signals. Cell Communication and Signaling: CCS. 2019;**17**(1):113. DOI: 10.1186/s12964-019-0423-6

[42] Akoto T, Saini S. Role of exosomes in prostate cancer metastasis. International Journal of Molecular Sciences. 2021;**22**(7):3528. DOI: 10.3390/ijms22073528

[43] Tsaur I, Thurn K, Juengel E, Gust KM, Borgmann H, Mager R, et al. sE-cadherin serves as a diagnostic and predictive parameter in prostate cancer patients. Journal of Experimental & Clinical Cancer Research. 2015;**34**(1):43. DOI: 10.1186/s13046-015-0161-6

[44] Logozzi M, Angelini DF, Giuliani A, Mizzoni D, Di Raimo R, Maggi M, et al. Increased plasmatic levels of PSA-expressing exosomes distinguish prostate cancer patients from benign prostatic hyperplasia: A prospective study. Cancers (Basel). 2019;**11**(10):1449. DOI: 10.3390/cancers11101449

[45] Nilsson J, Skog J, Nordstrand A, Baranov V, Mincheva-Nilsson L, Breakefield XO, et al. Prostate cancer-derived urine exosomes: a novel approach to biomarkers for prostate cancer. British Journal of Cancer. 2009;**100**(10):1603-1607. DOI: 10.1038/sj.bjc.6605058

[46] Bijnsdorp IV, Geldof AA, Lavaei M, Piersma SR, van Moorselaar RJ, Jimenez CR. Exosomal ITGA3 interferes with non-cancerous prostate cell functions and is increased in urine exosomes of metastatic prostate cancer patients. Journal of Extracellular Vesicles. 2013;**2**:10.3402. DOI: 10.3402/jev.v2i0.22097

[47] Zhu S, Ni Y, Wang Z, Zhang X, Zhang Y, Zhao F, et al. Plasma exosomal AKR1C3 mRNA expression is a predictive and prognostic biomarker in patients with metastatic castration-resistant prostate cancer. The Oncologist. 2022;**27**(11):e870-e8e7. DOI: 10.1093/oncolo/oyac177

[48] Krishn SR, Singh A, Bowler N, Duffy AN, Friedman A, Fedele C, et al. Prostate cancer sheds the αvβ3 integrin in vivo through exosomes. Matrix Biology. 2019;**77**:41-57. DOI: 10.1016/j.matbio.2018.08.004

[49] Saheera S, Jani VP, Witwer KW, Kutty S. Extracellular vesicle interplay in cardiovascular pathophysiology. American Journal of Physiology. Heart and Circulatory Physiology. 2021;**320**(5):H1749-H1h61. DOI: 10.1152/ajpheart.00925.2020

[50] Garcia NA, Moncayo-Arlandi J, Sepulveda P, Diez-Juan A. Cardiomyocyte exosomes regulate glycolytic flux in endothelium by direct transfer of GLUT transporters and glycolytic enzymes. Cardiovascular Research. 2016;**109**(3):397-408. DOI: 10.1093/cvr/cvv260

[51] Cosme J, Guo H, Hadipour-Lakmehsari S, Emili A, Gramolini AO. Hypoxia-induced changes in the fibroblast secretome, exosome, and whole-cell proteome using cultured, cardiac-derived cells isolated from neonatal mice. Journal of Proteome

Research. 2017;**16**(8):2836-2847. DOI: 10.1021/acs.jproteome.7b00144

[52] Patil M, Saheera S, Dubey PK, Kahn-Krell A, Kumar Govindappa P, Singh S, et al. Novel mechanisms of exosome-mediated phagocytosis of dead cells in injured heart. Circulation Research. 2021;**129**(11):1006-1020. DOI: 10.1161/circresaha.120.317900

[53] Vicencio JM, Yellon DM, Sivaraman V, Das D, Boi-Doku C, Arjun S, et al. Plasma exosomes protect the myocardium from ischemia-reperfusion injury. Journal of the American College of Cardiology. 2015;**65**(15):1525-1536. DOI: 10.1016/j.jacc.2015.02.026

[54] Govindappa PK, Patil M, Garikipati VNS, Verma SK, Saheera S, Narasimhan G, et al. Targeting exosome-associated human antigen R attenuates fibrosis and inflammation in diabetic heart. The FASEB Journal. 2020;**34**(2):2238-2251. DOI: 10.1096/fj.201901995R

[55] Rosell A, Havervall S, von Meijenfeldt F, Hisada Y, Aguilera K, Grover SP, et al. Patients with COVID-19 have elevated levels of circulating extracellular vesicle tissue factor activity that is associated with severity and mortality-brief report. Arteriosclerosis, Thrombosis, and Vascular Biology. 2021;**41**(2):878-882. DOI: 10.1161/atvbaha.120.315547

[56] Song JW, Lam SM, Fan X, Cao WJ, Wang SY, Tian H, et al. Omics-driven systems interrogation of metabolic dysregulation in COVID-19 pathogenesis. Cell Metabolism. 2020;**32**(2):188-202.e5. DOI: 10.1016/j.cmet.2020.06.016

[57] Velázquez-Enríquez JM, Santos-ÁlvarezJC,Ramírez-HernándezAA, Reyes-Jiménez E, López-Martínez A, Pina-Canseco S, et al. Proteomic analysis reveals key proteins in extracellular vesicles cargo associated with idiopathic pulmonary fibrosis in vitro. Biomedicine. 2021;**9**(8):1058. DOI: 10.3390/biomedicines9081058

[58] Kubo H. Extracellular vesicles in lung disease. Chest. 2018;**153**(1):210-216. DOI: 10.1016/j.chest.2017.06.026

[59] Mayo S, Benito-León J, Peña-Bautista C, Baquero M, Cháfer-Pericás C. Recent evidence in epigenomics and proteomics biomarkers for early and minimally invasive diagnosis of Alzheimer's and Parkinson's Diseases. Current Neuropharmacology. 2021;**19**(8):1273-1303. DOI: 10.2174/1570159x19666201223154009

[60] Zhao ZH, Chen ZT, Zhou RL, Zhang X, Ye QY, Wang YZ. Increased DJ-1 and α-synuclein in plasma neural-derived exosomes as potential markers for Parkinson's disease. Frontiers in Aging Neuroscience. 2018;**10**:438. DOI: 10.3389/fnagi.2018.00438

[61] Fraser KB, Rawlins AB, Clark RG, Alcalay RN, Standaert DG, Liu N, et al. Ser(P)-1292 LRRK2 in urinary exosomes is elevated in idiopathic Parkinson's disease. Movement Disorders. 2016;**31**(10):1543-1550. DOI: 10.1002/mds.26686

[62] Nam E, Lee YB, Moon C, Chang KA. Serum tau proteins as potential biomarkers for the assessment of Alzheimer's disease progression. International Journal of Molecular Sciences. 2020;**21**(14):5007. DOI: 10.3390/ijms21145007

[63] Xiong WP, Yao WQ, Wang B, Liu K. BMSCs-exosomes containing GDF-15 alleviated SH-SY5Y cell injury model of Alzheimer's disease via AKT/GSK-3β/β-catenin. Brain Research

Bulletin. 2021;**177**:92-102. DOI: 10.1016/j.brainresbull.2021.09.008

[64] Zheng D, Huo M, Li B, Wang W, Piao H, Wang Y, et al. The role of exosomes and exosomal MicroRNA in cardiovascular disease. Frontiers in Cell and Development Biology. 2020;**8**:616161. DOI: 10.3389/fcell.2020.616161

[65] Schwarzenbach H, Nishida N, Calin GA, Pantel K. Clinical relevance of circulating cell-free microRNAs in cancer. Nature Reviews. Clinical Oncology. 2014;**11**(3):145-156. DOI: 10.1038/nrclinonc.2014.5

[66] Joosse SA, Pantel K. Tumor-educated platelets as liquid biopsy in cancer patients. Cancer Cell. 2015;**28**(5):552-554. DOI: 10.1016/j.ccell.2015.10.007

[67] Wu H, Zhou J, Mei S, Wu D, Mu Z, Chen B, et al. Circulating exosomal microRNA-96 promotes cell proliferation, migration and drug resistance by targeting LMO7. Journal of Cellular and Molecular Medicine. 2017;**21**(6):1228-1236. DOI: 10.1111/jcmm.13056

[68] Hsu YL, Hung JY, Chang WA, Lin YS, Pan YC, Tsai PH, et al. Hypoxic lung cancer-secreted exosomal miR-23a increased angiogenesis and vascular permeability by targeting prolyl hydroxylase and tight junction protein ZO-1. Oncogene. 2017;**36**(34):4929-4942. DOI: 10.1038/onc.2017.105

[69] Kim JE, Eom JS, Kim WY, Jo EJ, Mok J, Lee K, et al. Diagnostic value of microRNAs derived from exosomes in bronchoalveolar lavage fluid of early-stage lung adenocarcinoma: A pilot study. Thoracic Cancer. 2018;**9**(8):911-915. DOI: 10.1111/1759-7714.12756

[70] Liu Q, Yu Z, Yuan S, Xie W, Li C, Hu Z, et al. Circulating exosomal microRNAs as prognostic biomarkers for non-small-cell lung cancer. Oncotarget. 2017;**8**(8):13048-13058. DOI: 10.18632/oncotarget.14369

[71] Wang J, Zhao X, Wang Y, Ren F, Sun D, Yan Y, et al. circRNA-002178 act as a ceRNA to promote PDL1/PD1 expression in lung adenocarcinoma. Cell Death & Disease. 2020;**11**(1):32. DOI: 10.1038/s41419-020-2230-9

[72] Zhang N, Nan A, Chen L, Li X, Jia Y, Qiu M, et al. Circular RNA circSATB2 promotes progression of non-small cell lung cancer cells. Molecular Cancer. 2020;**19**(1):101. DOI: 10.1186/s12943-020-01221-6

[73] Lv X, Lian Y, Liu Z, Xiao J, Zhang D, Yin X. Exosomal long non-coding RNA LINC00662 promotes non-small cell lung cancer progression by miR-320d/E2F1 axis. Aging (Albany NY). 2021;**13**(4):6010-6024. DOI: 10.18632/aging.202522

[74] Huang J, Shen M, Yan M, Cui Y, Gao Z, Meng X. Exosome-mediated transfer of miR-1290 promotes cell proliferation and invasion in gastric cancer via NKD1. Acta Biochimica et Biophysica Sinica (Shanghai). 2019;**51**(9):900-907. DOI: 10.1093/abbs/gmz077

[75] Wu Y, Wei J, Zhang W, Xie M, Wang X, Xu J. Serum exosomal miR-1290 is a potential biomarker for lung adenocarcinoma. Oncotargets and Therapy. 2020;**13**:7809-7818. DOI: 10.2147/ott.S263934

[76] Jeon H, Seo SM, Kim TW, Ryu J, Kong H, Jang SH, et al. Circulating exosomal miR-1290 for diagnosis of epithelial ovarian cancer. Current Issues in Molecular Biology. 2022;**44**(1):288-300. DOI: 10.3390/cimb44010021

[77] Wang S, Du P, Cao Y, Ma J, Yang X, Yu Z, et al. Cancer associated fibroblasts secreted exosomal miR-1290 contributes to prostate cancer cell growth and metastasis via targeting GSK3β. cell Death Discovery. 2022;**8**(1):371. DOI: 10.1038/s41420-022-01163-6

[78] Kumata Y, Iinuma H, Suzuki Y, Tsukahara D, Midorikawa H, Igarashi Y, et al. Exosome-encapsulated microRNA-23b as a minimally invasive liquid biomarker for the prediction of recurrence and prognosis of gastric cancer patients in each tumor stage. Oncology Reports. 2018;**40**(1):319-330. DOI: 10.3892/or.2018.6418

[79] Xie M, Yu T, Jing X, Ma L, Fan Y, Yang F, et al. Exosomal circSHKBP1 promotes gastric cancer progression via regulating the miR-582-3p/HUR/VEGF axis and suppressing HSP90 degradation. Molecular Cancer. 2020;**19**(1):112. DOI: 10.1186/s12943-020-01208-3

[80] Sang H, Zhang W, Peng L, Wei S, Zhu X, Huang K, et al. Exosomal circRELL1 serves as a miR-637 sponge to modulate gastric cancer progression via regulating autophagy activation. Cell Death & Disease. 2022;**13**(1):56. DOI: 10.1038/s41419-021-04364-6

[81] Lu J, Wang YH, Yoon C, Huang XY, Xu Y, Xie JW, et al. Circular RNA circ-RanGAP1 regulates VEGFA expression by targeting miR-877-3p to facilitate gastric cancer invasion and metastasis. Cancer Letters. 2020;**471**:38-48. DOI: 10.1016/j.canlet.2019.11.038

[82] Zhao R, Zhang Y, Zhang X, Yang Y, Zheng X, Li X, et al. Exosomal long noncoding RNA HOTTIP as potential novel diagnostic and prognostic biomarker test for gastric cancer. Molecular Cancer. 2018;**17**(1):68. DOI: 10.1186/s12943-018-0817-x

[83] Li X, Li C, Zhang L, Wu M, Cao K, Jiang F, et al. The significance of exosomes in the development and treatment of hepatocellular carcinoma. Molecular Cancer. 2020;**19**(1):1. DOI: 10.1186/s12943-019-1085-0

[84] Fang T, Lv H, Lv G, Li T, Wang C, Han Q, et al. Tumor-derived exosomal miR-1247-3p induces cancer-associated fibroblast activation to foster lung metastasis of liver cancer. Nature Communications. 2018;**9**(1):191. DOI: 10.1038/s41467-017-02583-0

[85] Wang Y, Zhang C, Zhang P, Guo G, Jiang T, Zhao X, et al. Serum exosomal microRNAs combined with alpha-fetoprotein as diagnostic markers of hepatocellular carcinoma. Cancer Medicine. 2018;**7**(5):1670-1679. DOI: 10.1002/cam4.1390

[86] Sohn W, Kim J, Kang SH, Yang SR, Cho JY, Cho HC, et al. Serum exosomal microRNAs as novel biomarkers for hepatocellular carcinoma. Experimental & Molecular Medicine. 2015;**47**(9):e184. DOI: 10.1038/emm.2015.68

[87] Yokota Y, Noda T, Okumura Y, Kobayashi S, Iwagami Y, Yamada D, et al. Serum exosomal miR-638 is a prognostic marker of HCC via downregulation of VE-cadherin and ZO-1 of endothelial cells. Cancer Science. 2021;**112**(3):1275-1288. DOI: 10.1111/cas.14807

[88] Wang G, Liu W, Zou Y, Wang G, Deng Y, Luo J, et al. Three isoforms of exosomal circPTGR1 promote hepatocellular carcinoma metastasis via the miR449a-MET pathway. eBioMedicine. 2019;**40**:432-445. DOI: 10.1016/j.ebiom.2018.12.062

[89] Sun L, Su Y, Liu X, Xu M, Chen X, Zhu Y, et al. Serum and exosome long non coding RNAs as potential biomarkers for hepatocellular carcinoma. Journal of

Cancer. 2018;**9**(15):2631-2639. DOI: 10.7150/jca.24978

[90] Jozwik KM, Carroll JS. Pioneer factors in hormone-dependent cancers. Nature Reviews. Cancer. 2012;**12**(6):381-385. DOI: 10.1038/nrc3263

[91] Liedtke C, Mazouni C, Hess KR, André F, Tordai A, Mejia JA, et al. Response to neoadjuvant therapy and long-term survival in patients with triple-negative breast cancer. Journal of Clinical Oncology. 2008;**26**(8):1275-1281. DOI: 10.1200/jco.2007.14.4147

[92] Ni Q, Stevic I, Pan C, Müller V, Oliveira-Ferrer L, Pantel K, et al. Different signatures of miR-16, miR-30b and miR-93 in exosomes from breast cancer and DCIS patients. Scientific Reports. 2018;**8**(1):12974. DOI: 10.1038/s41598-018-31108-y

[93] Eichelser C, Stückrath I, Müller V, Milde-Langosch K, Wikman H, Pantel K, et al. Increased serum levels of circulating exosomal microRNA-373 in receptor-negative breast cancer patients. Oncotarget. 2014;**5**(20):9650-9663. DOI: 10.18632/oncotarget.2520

[94] Yang SJ, Wang DD, Zhong SL, Chen WQ, Wang FL, Zhang J, et al. Tumor-derived exosomal circPSMA1 facilitates the tumorigenesis, metastasis, and migration in triple-negative breast cancer (TNBC) through miR-637/Akt1/β-catenin (cyclin D1) axis. Cell Death & Disease. 2021;**12**(5):420. DOI: 10.1038/s41419-021-03680-1

[95] Liu X, Zhang G, Yu T, He J, Liu J, Chai X, et al. Exosomes deliver lncRNA DARS-AS1 siRNA to inhibit chronic unpredictable mild stress-induced TNBC metastasis. Cancer Letters. 2022;**543**:215781. DOI: 10.1016/j.canlet.2022.215781

[96] He J, Fortunati E, Liu DX, Li Y. Pleiotropic roles of ABC transporters in breast cancer. International Journal of Molecular Sciences. 2021;**22**(6):3199. DOI: 10.3390/ijms22063199

[97] Han M, Hu J, Lu P, Cao H, Yu C, Li X, et al. Exosome-transmitted miR-567 reverses trastuzumab resistance by inhibiting ATG5 in breast cancer. Cell Death & Disease. 2020;**11**(1):43. DOI: 10.1038/s41419-020-2250-5

[98] Wang X, Pei X, Guo G, Qian X, Dou D, Zhang Z, et al. Exosome-mediated transfer of long noncoding RNA H19 induces doxorubicin resistance in breast cancer. Journal of Cellular Physiology. 2020;**235**(10):6896-6904. DOI: 10.1002/jcp.29585

[99] Wang J, Liu Y, Li Y, Zheng X, Gan J, Wan Z, et al. Exosomal-miR-10a derived from colorectal cancer cells suppresses migration of human lung fibroblasts, and expression of IL-6, IL-8 and IL-1β. Molecular Medicine Reports. 2021;**23**(1):84. DOI: 10.3892/mmr.2020.11723

[100] Zheng X, Li JW, Liu YK, Ma YF, Gan JH, Han SG, et al. microRNA-10a-5p overexpression suppresses malignancy of colon cancer by regulating human liver cancer fibroblasts. Neoplasma. 2021;**68**(6):1157-1168. DOI: 10.4149/neo_2021_210226N250

[101] Hu HY, Yu CH, Zhang HH, Zhang SZ, Yu WY, Yang Y, et al. Exosomal miR-1229 derived from colorectal cancer cells promotes angiogenesis by targeting HIPK2. International Journal of Biological Macromolecules. 2019;**132**:470-477. DOI: 10.1016/j.ijbiomac.2019.03.221

[102] Zeng Z, Li Y, Pan Y, Lan X, Song F, Sun J, et al. Cancer-derived exosomal miR-25-3p promotes pre-metastatic niche formation by inducing vascular

permeability and angiogenesis. Nature Communications. 2018;**9**(1):5395. DOI: 10.1038/s41467-018-07810-w

[103] Pan B, Qin J, Liu X, He B, Wang X, Pan Y, et al. Identification of serum exosomal hsa-circ-0004771 as a novel diagnostic biomarker of colorectal cancer. Frontiers in Genetics. 2019;**10**:1096. DOI: 10.3389/fgene.2019.01096

[104] Xie Y, Li J, Li P, Li N, Zhang Y, Binang H, et al. RNA-Seq profiling of serum exosomal circular RNAs reveals circ-PNN as a potential biomarker for human colorectal cancer. Frontiers in Oncology. 2020;**10**:982. DOI: 10.3389/fonc.2020.00982

[105] Li Y, Li C, Xu R, Wang Y, Li D, Zhang B. A novel circFMN2 promotes tumor proliferation in CRC by regulating the miR-1182/hTERT signaling pathways. Clinical Science (London, England). 2019;**133**(24):2463-2479. DOI: 10.1042/cs20190715

[106] Yang H, Zhang H, Yang Y, Wang X, Deng T, Liu R, et al. Hypoxia induced exosomal circRNA promotes metastasis of colorectal cancer via targeting GEF-H1/RhoA axis. Theranostics. 2020;**10**(18):8211-8226. DOI: 10.7150/thno.44419

[107] Zhou L, Li J, Tang Y, Yang M. Exosomal LncRNA LINC00659 transferred from cancer-associated fibroblasts promotes colorectal cancer cell progression via miR-342-3p/ANXA2 axis. Journal of Translational Medicine. 2021;**19**(1):8. DOI: 10.1186/s12967-020-02648-7

[108] Karami Fath M, Anjomrooz M, Taha SR, Shariat Zadeh M, Sahraei M, Atbaei R, et al. The therapeutic effect of exosomes from mesenchymal stem cells on colorectal cancer: Toward cell-free therapy. Pathology, Research and Practice. 2022;**237**:154024. DOI: 10.1016/j.prp.2022.154024

[109] Vakhshiteh F, Atyabi F, Ostad SN. Mesenchymal stem cell exosomes: A two-edged sword in cancer therapy. International Journal of Nanomedicine. 2019;**14**:2847-2859. DOI: 10.2147/ijn.S200036

[110] Saheera S, Potnuri AG, Krishnamurthy P. Nano-vesicle (mis) communication in senescence-related pathologies. Cell. 2020;**9**(9):1974. DOI: 10.3390/cells9091974

[111] Zheng B, Yin WN, Suzuki T, Zhang XH, Zhang Y, Song LL, et al. Exosome-mediated miR-155 transfer from smooth muscle cells to endothelial cells induces endothelial injury and promotes atherosclerosis. Molecular Therapy. 2017;**25**(6):1279-1294. DOI: 10.1016/j.ymthe.2017.03.031

[112] Wang X, Huang W, Liu G, Cai W, Millard RW, Wang Y, et al. Cardiomyocytes mediate anti-angiogenesis in type 2 diabetic rats through the exosomal transfer of miR-320 into endothelial cells. Journal of Molecular and Cellular Cardiology. 2014;**74**:139-150. DOI: 10.1016/j.yjmcc.2014.05.001

[113] Sun L, He X, Zhang T, Han Y, Tao G. Knockdown of mesenchymal stem cell-derived exosomal LOC100129516 suppresses the symptoms of atherosclerosis via upregulation of the PPARγ/LXRα/ABCA1 signaling pathway. International Journal of Molecular Medicine. 2021;**48**(6):208. DOI: 10.3892/ijmm.2021.5041

[114] Stojanovich L, Marisavljevich D. Stress as a trigger of autoimmune disease. Autoimmunity Reviews. 2008;**7**(3):209-213. DOI: 10.1016/j.autrev.2007.11.007

[115] Perez-Hernandez J, Martinez-Arroyo O, Ortega A, Galera M, Solis-Salguero MA, Chaves FJ, et al. Urinary exosomal miR-146a as a marker of albuminuria, activity changes and disease flares in lupus nephritis. Journal of Nephrology. 2021;**34**(4):1157-1167. DOI: 10.1007/s40620-020-00832-y

[116] Zhang J, Zhang Y, Ma Y, Luo L, Chu M, Zhang Z. Therapeutic potential of exosomal circRNA derived from synovial mesenchymal cells via targeting circEDIL3/miR-485-3p/PIAS3/STAT3/VEGF functional module in rheumatoid arthritis. International Journal of Nanomedicine. 2021;**16**:7977-7994. DOI: 10.2147/ijn.S333465

[117] Liu R, Jiang C, Li J, Li X, Zhao L, Yun H, et al. Serum-derived exosomes containing NEAT1 promote the occurrence of rheumatoid arthritis through regulation of miR-144-3p/ROCK2 axis. Therapeutic Advances in Chronic Disease. 2021;**12**:2040622321991705. DOI: 10.1177/2040622321991705

[118] Zhang L, Qu L, Zhang Y, Xu Z, Tang H. Differential expression of circular RNAs in plasma exosomes from patients with ankylosing spondylitis. Cell Biology International. 2022;**46**(4):649-659. DOI: 10.1002/cbin.11760

[119] Kwan EM, Wyatt AW, Chi KN. Towards clinical implementation of circulating tumor DNA in metastatic prostate cancer: Opportunities for integration and pitfalls to interpretation. Frontiers in Oncology. 2022;**12**:1054497. DOI: 10.3389/fonc.2022.1054497

[120] Bardelli A, Pantel K. Liquid biopsies, what we do not know (yet). Cancer Cell. 2017;**31**(2):172-179. DOI: 10.1016/j.ccell.2017.01.002

[121] Yamamoto H, Watanabe Y, Oikawa R, Morita R, Yoshida Y, Maehata T, et al. BARHL2 methylation using gastric wash DNA or gastric juice exosomal DNA is a useful marker for early detection of gastric cancer in an H. pylori-independent manner. Clinical and Translational Gastroenterology. 2016;**7**(7):e184. DOI: 10.1038/ctg.2016.40

[122] Zhou X, Kurywchak P, Wolf-Dennen K, Che SPY, Sulakhe D, D'Souza M, et al. Unique somatic variants in DNA from urine exosomes of individuals with bladder cancer. Molecular Therapy. Methods & Clinical Development. 2021;**22**:360-376. DOI: 10.1016/j.omtm.2021.05.010

[123] Bernard V, Kim DU, San Lucas FA, Castillo J, Allenson K, Mulu FC, et al. Circulating nucleic acids are associated with outcomes of patients with pancreatic cancer. Gastroenterology. 2019;**156**(1):108-18.e4. DOI: 10.1053/j.gastro.2018.09.022

[124] Degli, Esposti C, Iadarola B, Maestri S, Beltrami C, Lavezzari D, Morini M, et al. Exosomes from plasma of neuroblastoma patients contain doublestranded DNA reflecting the mutational status of parental tumor cells. International Journal of Molecular Sciences. 2021;**22**(7):3667. DOI: 10.3390/ijms22073667

[125] Yu W, Hurley J, Roberts D, Chakrabortty SK, Enderle D, Noerholm M, et al. Exosome-based liquid biopsies in cancer: Opportunities and challenges. Annals of Oncology. 2021;**32**(4):466-477. DOI: 10.1016/j.annonc.2021.01.074

[126] Müller Bark J, Kulasinghe A, Amenábar JM, Punyadeera C. Exosomes in cancer. Advances in Clinical Chemistry. 2021;**101**:1-40. DOI: 10.1016/bs.acc.2020.06.006

[127] Purushothaman A. Exosomes from cell culture-conditioned medium: Isolation by ultracentrifugation and characterization. Methods in Molecular Biology. 1952;**2019**:233-244. DOI: 10.1007/978-1-4939-9133-4_19

[128] Yu D, Li Y, Wang M, Gu J, Xu W, Cai H, et al. Exosomes as a new frontier of cancer liquid biopsy. Molecular Cancer. 2022;**21**(1):56. DOI: 10.1186/s12943-022-01509-9

[129] Witwer KW, Buzás EI, Bemis LT, Bora A, Lässer C, Lötvall J, et al. Standardization of sample collection, isolation and analysis methods in extracellular vesicle research. Journal of Extracellular Vesicles. 2013;**2**:10.3402. DOI: 10.3402/jev.v2i0.20360

[130] Théry C, Amigorena S, Raposo G, Clayton A. Isolation and characterization of exosomes from cell culture supernatants and biological fluids. Current Protocols in Cell Biology. 2006;Chapter 3:Unit 3.22. DOI: 10.1002/0471143030.cb0322s30

[131] Alvarez ML, Khosroheidari M, Kanchi Ravi R, DiStefano JK. Comparison of protein, microRNA, and mRNA yields using different methods of urinary exosome isolation for the discovery of kidney disease biomarkers. Kidney International. 2012;**82**(9):1024-1032. DOI: 10.1038/ki.2012.256

[132] Kim G, Yoo CE, Kim M, Kang HJ, Park D, Lee M, et al. Noble polymeric surface conjugated with zwitterionic moieties and antibodies for the isolation of exosomes from human serum. Bioconjugate Chemistry. 2012;**23**(10):2114-2120. DOI: 10.1021/bc300339b

[133] Xu R, Greening DW, Zhu HJ, Takahashi N, Simpson RJ. Extracellular vesicle isolation and characterization: Toward clinical application. The Journal of Clinical Investigation. 2016;**126**(4):1152-1162. DOI: 10.1172/jci81129

[134] Kibria G, Ramos EK, Lee KE, Bedoyan S, Huang S, Samaeekia R, et al. A rapid, automated surface protein profiling of single circulating exosomes in human blood. Scientific Reports. 2016;**6**:36502. DOI: 10.1038/srep36502

Chapter 9

Perspective Chapter: Development of Exosomes for Esthetic Use

Byong Seung Cho and Diane Irvine Duncan

Abstract

While there are thousands of peer-reviewed papers on exosomes, most of the work has been done in the medical field. Studies and clinical trials on exosome-related products for the esthetic industry have just begun to be a regular occurrence. One of the reasons for this is a lack of regulatory approval for any exosome use. The FDA does not regulate topical cosmetic use, while only a few exosomes are registered on the International Cosmetic Ingredient Dictionary (ICID) of the Personal Care Product Council (PCPC), so most esthetic providers are utilizing exosomes in this manner. Clinical uses for exosomes in esthetic practice include the treatment of burns, active acne, atopic dermatitis, and chronic skin irritations. When used in combination with energy-based device treatment, exosomes reduce inflammation and redness, improve the rapidity of healing for laser and microneedling patients, and reduce the tendency for fibrosis and thick hypertrophic scar formation when used topically. Byong Cho is the CEO & CTO of ExoCoBio, one of the four largest exosome companies globally. He has developed a large research, development, and GMP manufacturing facility just south of Seoul, Korea. His topic, the development of exosomes for clinical esthetic use, will take us through the process of developing a safe and cost-effective biological regenerative product while staying in line with regulatory limitations.

Keywords: regenerative, esthetic, exosome, secretome, scar treatment, resurfacing, hair restoration, burn treatment

1. Introduction

I first learned about exosomes in early 2016. I heard the word "exosome" for the first time from a close friend and professor of biology. After that, for several months, I did basic research and study on papers and patents related to exosomes [1]. Through this, I found that exosomes can develop a completely new biotech technology, and in particular, I became very interested in "stem cell-derived exosomes" for regeneration and dermatological applications. During 6 months in 2016, I was able to secure basic knowledge about it. In addition, it was identified that stem cell exosomes have great potential as a next-generation regeneration plus anti-inflammation technology. Further, I became very interested in Dr. Sai Kiang Lim, and her brilliant discovery, who discovered stem cell-derived exosomes for the first time in the world [2].

Additional factors that made me interested in exosomes in 2016 include my background. I had more than 15 years of experience in investing in biotechnology and commercialization in venture capital. After putting together 2 biotech startups in early 2002, I was the first venture capital investor in Asia who supported the commercialization of botulinum toxin technology. I have continued to have a deep interest and experience in the field of medical esthetics since then, and I thought that I found "something new" about the commercialization potential of stem cell-derived exosomes. I have been continuously trying to find and commercialize new technologies in the field of "regenerative medicine or aesthetics" for more than 10 years before knowing about exosomes.

My vision was to fill an unmet need for our global aging population. While there are botulinum toxins, dermal fillers, & energy-based devices, not all of them would be appropriate for very senior people. We would need something new—a regenerative esthetics or regenerative medicine treatment option that might be able to reverse certain aspects of aging. Also, stem cell-derived exosomes can be used to treat incurable or very difficult skin diseases like dermatitis, psoriasis, scleroderma, skin fibrosis, and so on, based on the dual and synergistic function of regeneration and anti-inflammation. This premise of exosome therapy could certainly expand the field of regenerative dermatology.

2. As a pioneer in the field, what were your first steps in developing exosomes?

After learning about exosomes, the most important tasks for me were (1) establishing a business plan, (2) licensing and developing exosome technology, (3) financing to create a successful exosome startup, (4) registering adipose stem cell-derived exosomes as a cosmetic ingredient, and (5) finding a partner for marketing and sales in the US.

While exploring numerous scientific papers and patents on exosomes around the world [3, 4], I sought what kind of business to do with exosomes. In particular, the biggest challenge was to determine whether stem cell exosomes would become a major technology in the field of "regenerative medicine or regenerative aesthetics" in the future. And, since then I had no exosome technology on my own, and to license stem cell exosome technology, I read all the publications of Dr. SK Lim and directly contacted her to discuss technology licensing and to have her as a scientific advisor for 6 months in 2016. While studying other scientists' technologies and patents [5, 6], I was able to build a solid business plan at the time of ExoCoBio's establishment. Of course, since exosome technology is in its infancy, and I thought there would be many changes in the future, I planned to develop various types of exosome-based esthetic technologies and products in my 5-year business plan (**Figure 1**).

In the commercialization of new technology such as exosomes, the most important thing was a series of financing to support the business plan. With my early ideas, I made lots of calls to my VC friends to pre-market the business plan for 6 months. At that time, I had about 15 years of experience in the venture capital industry and successful commercialization and IPO (Initial Public Offering) of two biotech companies. With this background, I felt I could incorporate ExoCoBio in Jan 2017. Just after 3 months, I was able to raise about USD 12 million in March 2017 through Series A financing and angel financing from multiple venture capital firms and individuals. It was the biggest financing as Series A funding for a biotech startup in South Korea.

Our first office was small. After setting up my business plan and team building, ExoCoBio was incorporated in a tiny office of about 270 SqFt outside Seoul,

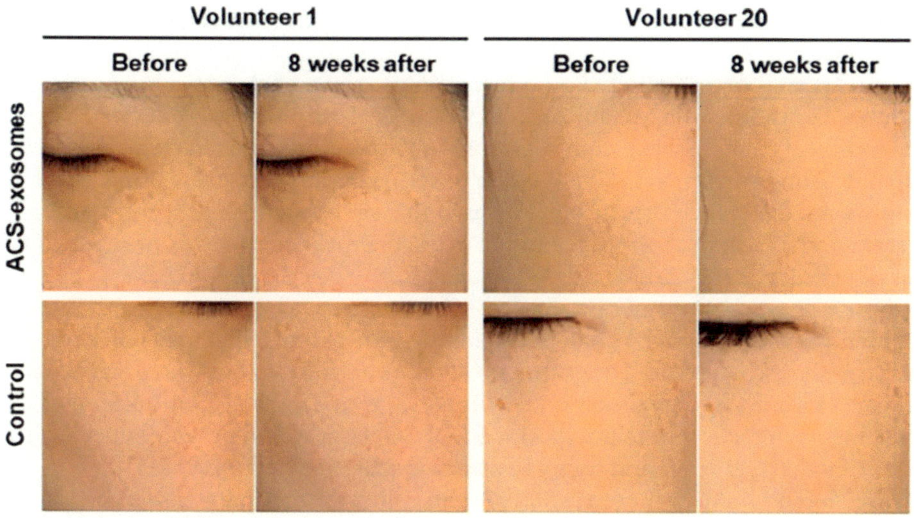

Figure 1.
Clinical evaluation of the skin brightening effect of ASC-exosomes.

South Korea, in Jan 2017. The company successfully raised about $2 million from individual investors to get the first office and ExoCoBio got a small and humble laboratory in a university to start to develop our own manufacturing process of cell culture, TFF process, in vitro tests, and others.

One of the most significant jobs in 2017 was to register our own exosomes based on adipose stem cells (ASCE) to the ICID of the PCPC in the US. Since I knew that cosmetic registration was critical to commercialize this new exosome technology, and, I wanted to be the first in the world, the registration process was started immediately after the financing around April 2017. It took about 9 months which was longer than expected, because there was no predicate ever of cosmetic exosomes. With all the efforts, ExoCoBio became the first to have the International Nomenclature Cosmetic Ingredient (INCI) name and, still now, ExoCoBio has proudly the biggest number of exosome registration in the ICID.

The last job to develop a successful exosome business in 2017 was to find a partner who can do market this new technology and sell our products even before we have an actual product of ASCE 2 years ago. So, I was introduced to BENEV Inc. in California, US, which had about 20 years of experience in growth factor-based esthetic products worldwide. When I first met Mr. Ethan Min at his office in May 2017, in Mission Viejo, CA, we did talk a lot about our experiences and business plan including the product concept for several hours. Very fortunately, we had the same mind! He gave me important insight into the future of regenerative esthetics based on exosomes and then we initiated to collaborate to be the first and to create a new industry.

3. Were there any sources (say bone marrow) that you tried and discarded? Why choose ADSCs for cosmetic use?

This is a very good question. It seems that many scientists and doctors have a misunderstanding about the source and quality of exosomes, especially about adipose stem cell-derived exosomes (ASCE).

So far, ExoCoBio has been focusing on adipose stem cell-derived exosome technology.

In 2019, ExoCoBio conducted an internal comparison of three types of stem cell exosomes. In other words, we cultured three types of adipose tissue-derived stem cells, umbilical cord-derived stem cells, and Wharton Jelly-derived stem cells and isolated exosomes from each. Then, when in vitro efficacy tests were done, there was no significant difference in efficacy. Through this series of internal studies, it was determined that adipose stem cell exosomes are the most commercially superior in terms of efficacy and cost.

Adipose stem cell exosomes produced by ExoCoBio have been proven with 8 scientific publications [7–12] and 48 patents including 8 US patents, that they will be the most effective in the esthetic field. For example, our clinical trial demonstrated that skin with acne scars was improved by the combined use of exosome derived from adipose tissue-derived mesenchymal stem cells with fractional CO_2 laser would provide synergistic effects on both the efficacy and safety of atrophic acne scar treatments [11].

As of March 11, 2023, there are 5609 "stem cell exosome" papers searched in Pubmed, including 625 "adipocyte stem cell exosome" papers, which is a significant proportion. I believe absolutely that ASCE has been scientifically validated. ExoCoBio is the only company that has performed a double-blinded, randomized, and split-face clinical study based on any kind of stem cell exosomes in the world. Also, according to a paper published by Xu, H. et al. in 2019 (41), it is known that adipose stem cell exosomes have the highest regenerative effect and contain the most growth factors for cardioprotection and anti-apoptotic effects than other exosome sources (**Figure 2**).

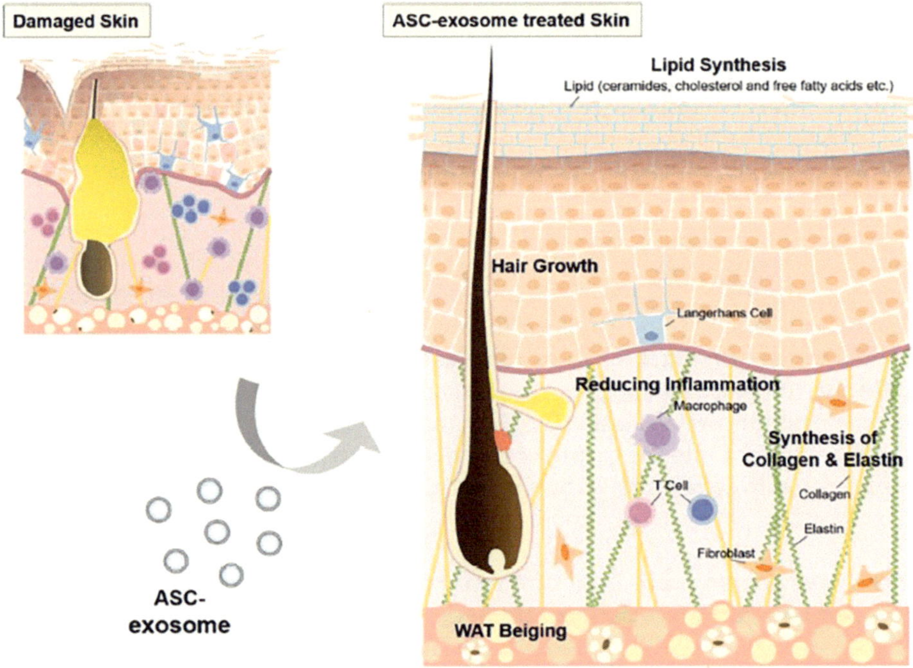

Figure 2.
Effects of ASC-exosomes on skin.

Some important discoveries made in the field of stem cells over the past 20 years, and as a result, several pros and cons were found. Exosomes derived from stem cell has been studied and the results of published articles demonstrated that exosome can overcome the cons of stem cell [13]. Stem cells and exosomes are different in many ways. In addition, adipose stem cell exosomes have the following advantages:

- Stem cells and stem cell exosomes are fundamentally different. Stem cells are live cells, but stem cell-derived exosomes are not live. In terms of the risk of adverse effects, since exosomes are not living cells, there is a much lower risk of adverse effects, such as immune rejection, tumor formation, and infection, which can occur with stem cell transplantation.

- There are a variety of stem cells, but each seems to have different characteristics. In particular, in terms of anti-inflammatory effect, adipose stem cells and their exosomes are judged to be the most excellent [14]. According to our unpublished findings, ASCE contains a huge number of miRNA-let-7, as the most abundant miRNA among about 200 types of miRNAs inside exosomes. Actually, miRNA-let-7 is the most well-known anti-inflammatory as well as an anti-cancer miRNA [15].

- The largest organ in the human body is the "skin" [16]. The skin is the most important organ that protects us from the external environment. In addition, "subcutaneous fat" is the organ with the biggest number of stem cells in our body [14]. Therefore, adipose stem cells, as one of the most critical parts of our skin, constantly secrete exosomes to protect us and keep our skin healthy and young.

- In addition, when researchers compare and analyze the three types of stem cells, adipose stem cells are usually compared after being collected from adults. In this case, of course, the cell passage number, which is the number of times that the culture has been sub-cultured, is high, so it is not fair to compare these with younger stem cell populations. If we compare these with umbilical cord-derived stem cells, for example, at passage 5, we think we should compare adipose stem cells with the same passage number. However, since most papers compare stem cells with different passage numbers, it is presumed that there are significant errors in comparative data.

- Moreover, exosomes seem to have significantly different efficacy depending on the way they are produced. ExoCoBio has been continuously developing and upgrading the patented ExoSCRT™ technology (KR Patent No. 10–1,895,916) for mass manufacturing of exosomes at the highest and consistent quality in compliance with the Good Manufacturing Practice (GMP), with 4 master cell banks created which store autologous adipose tissue-derived stem cell at passage 2 with stem cell positive markers and without negative markers.

- Lastly, adipose stem cells are the most accessible cell source of the lowest cost. Through this, it is possible to produce exosomes at the most affordable price.

4. Were there any processes production wise that you tried and changed?

In my view, there are a few important decisions to make or still to develop something to have better exosomes. ExoCoBio has tried to improve some parts in the last few years.

First, we need to think about the purity and impurities of exosomes. This is also related to regulatory affairs. During the last two decades or more, multiple clinical studies [17, 18] have shown that stem cells, including allogeneic stem cell treatments, are generally safe. So, it is very natural that stem cell-derived exosomes are believed to be generally safe, even though we need to do an extensive toxicological evaluation in the future. How many impurities can a product contain and retain safety? For example, any blood-derived exosomes may naturally contain lots of lipoproteins or proteins aggregate during the isolation process. Though not toxic, the presence of these may dilute the efficacy of the exosome product.

Second, the choice of a storage buffer is very important to maintain the potency of exosomes in the long term. For many companies and scientists, exosomes including stem cell exosomes are produced and stored in a phosphate-buffered saline (PBS) or similar simple buffer, which can easily degrade the quality of exosome in a short time, as published in the Journal of Extracellular Vesicles by Dr. Samir Andaloussi et al. in 2022. Dr. Andaloussi discovered that exosomes are drastically fractured at all temperatures of +4 ~ −80 degrees in Celsius tested. This may be a reason why many liquid exosome products currently available on the market have limited or less efficacy in the field. ExoCoBio has been focused on developing its proprietary formulation for long-term stability.

Third, lyophilization is the best process for the long-term storage of exosomes at present. Combined with a specific formulation of storage buffer, lyophilization can extend and keep the quality of exosomes shelf stable for 2 years. Two different groups of scientists have proven that they could produce exosomes in compliance with the GMP procedure a few years ago [19, 20]. Liquid or frozen exosomes are stable only for a limited time or only in a special formulation. A challenge in clinical practice is the storage of exosomes in a cryo tank or a special freezer that generates temperatures of −80 degrees Celsius. If the cryo tank runs out of nitrogen, or the power is off during the weekend, the costly exosomes are no longer usable. Stability on the shelf at room temperature or in a standard refrigerator can help a clinic maintain safety standards more easily than with demanding specialized laboratory equipment.

Fourth, pure exosomes are efficacious, but the effects could be further improved. From our studies, exosomes are found to be significant "seeds" or triggers for regenerative or anti-inflammatory effects, because exosomes contain a huge number of growth factors, cytokines, short-chain RNAs, peptides, and lipids. However, for example, when we added specific amino acids or other small peptides, efficacy was better for regeneration as well immune modulation in our experiments. Furthermore, due to the high cost of pure exosomes, market acceptance has been limited. ExoCoBio has decided to change its product strategy and become the first company to develop a combination of formulation processes in order to stimulate the potency of stem cell-derived exosomes. In this way, we could provide quality products based on ASCE. ExoCoBio is very proud to help people suffering from a variety of problematic skin conditions in addition to regular cosmetic uses around the world.

5. A similar question for extraction. Did you try ultracentrifugation and then discard that method? Why?

Since the beginning of 2019, ExoCoBio has conducted various studies on the method of isolating exosomes. There are about 9 different methods to extract exosomes from conditioned media of stem cell culture. The most frequent way is ultracentrifugation, well known by many publications at that time [21].

We saw the advantages of ultracentrifugation for exosome isolation as follows:

- Easy to Use: Ultracentrifugation is one of the most effective methods for isolating exosomes from biological fluids and can provide high yields of pure exosomes.
- Versatility: Ultracentrifugation can be used to isolate exosomes from a wide range of biological fluids, including blood, urine, and saliva.
- Established protocol: Ultracentrifugation is a well-established technique for exosome isolation, with many published protocols and established best practices.
- Compatibility with downstream analysis: Exosomes isolated by ultracentrifugation are compatible with a wide range of downstream analyses, including Western blotting, ELISA, and electron microscopy.

However, the long-term goal of ExoCoBio was to provide high quality exosomes at an affordable price. From that point of view, there were these disadvantages of ultracentrifugation for mass manufacturing of exosomes as follows:

- Time-consuming: Ultracentrifugation can be a time-consuming process, especially when processing large volumes of the sample or separating exosomes from other vesicles with similar sedimentation rates.
- Expensive: Ultracentrifuges are expensive instruments that can require specialized training and maintenance, making them inaccessible to some researchers.
- Potentially damaging: Ultracentrifugation can potentially damage exosomes, especially if the conditions are not optimized for the specific sample being processed.
- Limited specificity: Ultracentrifugation can isolate a range of vesicles, including exosomes, but may also co-isolate other vesicles or non-vesicular components, reducing the specificity of the isolation method.

Therefore, ExoCoBio decided to utilize another technology and process, namely tangential flow filtration (TFF). This is a membrane-based separation technique used to separate and concentrate biological molecules and particles from a liquid sample. It involves passing the sample across a semipermeable membrane under pressure, allowing smaller molecules or particles to pass through the membrane while retaining larger molecules or particles on the membrane surface.

TFF could be used for a variety of applications that can process the large volume of stem cell conditioned media, including:

- Concentrating and purifying proteins, viruses, and other macromolecules.
- Removing impurities, such as salts, sugars, or detergents, from a sample.
- Clarifying cell culture media or biological fluids.

- Harvesting and concentrating cells or cell debris from a culture or fermentation broth.

Actually, at that time, ExoCoBio found that TFF was very similar to the serial filtration method used in the first publication of Dr. SK Lim about 15 years ago [2]. To find exosomes, Dr. Lim performed a series of filtration with different pore sizes to track down the paracrine effect of stem cell-derived exosomes.

TFF is a versatile and scalable technique, which can be easily adapted to process large or small volumes of a sample. It can be combined with other separation techniques, such as chromatography, to achieve a higher degree of separation or purification. TFF is widely used in bioprocessing, biopharmaceutical production, and research applications.

6. Now that you have your new facility, tell us what your company is currently doing

After 3 years and still ongoing about $20 million investment, ExoCoBio built the world's largest GMP mfg. facility of ASCE production, named ExoGMP™ in Osong, South Korea. The purpose of ExoGMP is to produce intravenously injectable grade exosomes that are fully GMP-compliant, for regenerative medicine and regenerative esthetics as well. Though neither KFDA nor FDA approval for this use has been

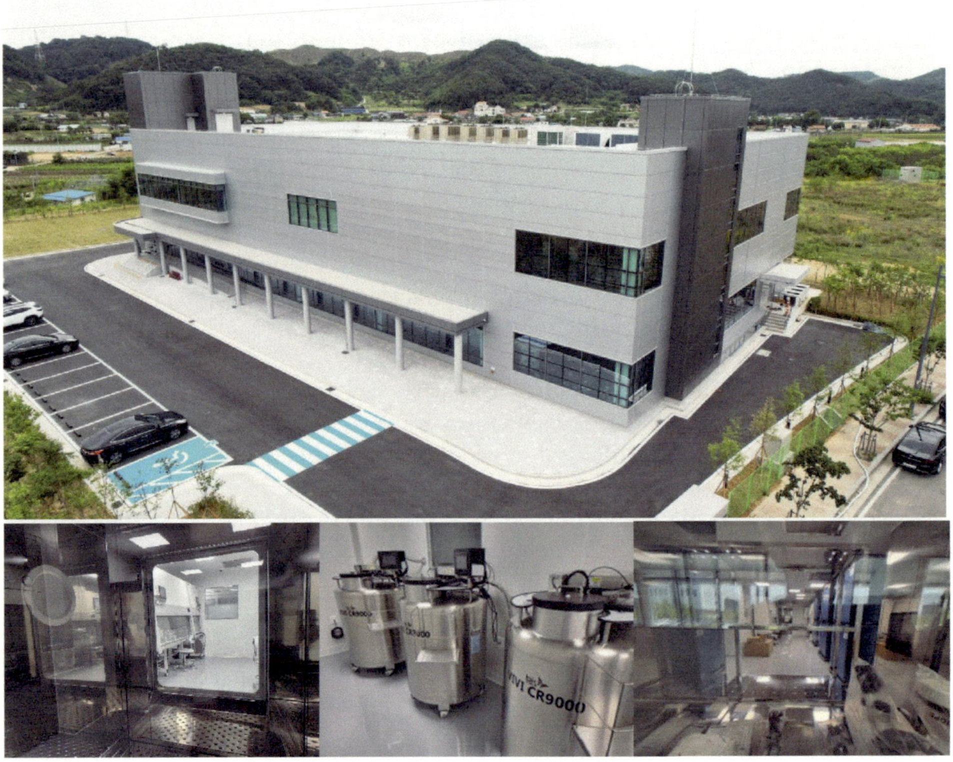

Figure 3.
ExoGMP™ in Osong, South Korea.

achieved, the company plans to be ready with this type of product once regulatory approval has been achieved (**Figure 3**).

ExoCoBio has installed more than 200 instruments and equipment, trying to establish about 300 standard operating procedures (SOP). Our team is committed to the production of quality exosomes and finalizing all the qualifications to hopefully produce the first batch of clinical-grade exosomes in the second quarter of 2023. ExoCoBio plans to initiate a Phase 1 clinical study in 2025.

The future of exosomes in esthetic medicine looks strong. However, regulatory issues are still a hurdle. Currently, there are no approved uses for exosomes, either in the medical or esthetic field. While the FDA does not regulate topical cosmetic use, a provider cannot claim to be using the product "off label" if injecting into patients. To stay safe, all exosome use should remain as a topical cosmetic product until full regulatory approval has been obtained.

Many postulations regarding future uses for exosomes have been made. From curing cancer to the reversal of genetic mutations and epigenetic cellular change, the potential for exosome therapies appears to be broad and strong. A current challenge is reading the "message" or contents of each exosome. Targeted or programmed exosomes would be able to direct recipient cells to behave in a certain way. Because of the popularity of the term, many products claiming to have exosomes either have none or have a minimal amount. While exosomes are not living cells, proteins in the contents will degrade over time, so without proper storage formulation, long-term shelf stability is not possible. Exosomes are merely a vehicle for the message they contain. Once we can safely and cost-effectively tailor the directions for cellular change that these tiny particles carry, we can potentially direct recipient cells to repair, reverse such processes as methylation or senescence, and reacquire lost metabolic functions.

7. Plant-derived extracellular vesicles

Plant exosomes, also known as extracellular vesicles, are small membrane-bound vesicles that are released by plant cells into the extracellular space. They are similar in structure and function to exosomes found in animals and other organisms. Plant exosomes contain various molecules such as proteins, lipids, and nucleic acids, which can be delivered to target cells and tissues to regulate various biological processes [22].

Research on plant exosomes is still relatively new. However, plant exosomes are involved in various physiological and developmental processes, such as cell-to-cell communication, stress response, and defense mechanisms. They have also been shown to play a role in inter-kingdom communication, where they can be taken up by other organisms such as fungi and bacteria [23]. In terms of anti-inflammation or immune modulation, edible *P. lobata*-derived exosomes promoted M2 macrophage polarization [24].

On Pubmed (pubmed.ncbi.nlm.nih.gov), we can find about 450 publications. One of the earliest publications is about multivesicular bodies (MVBs)-derived exosomes [23]. Further, one of the most recent publications is about the drug-delivery approach based on plant-derived exosomes for the treatment of inflammatory bowel disease and colitis-associated cancer [25]. In this publication, the isolation of plant-derived exosomes was done by ultracentrifugation mostly and it was found that the intake of plant miRNA may have a variety of effects on our bodies.

One of the R&D projects of ExoCoBio was to expand and apply ExoSCRT™ technology into plant- or microbial-derives extracellular vesicles or exosomes, to find new material. In that way, I was very interested in rose stem cell (Callus) – derived EVs (RSCE), because (1) roses have been the most popular plant and a cosmetic ingredient for humans, (2) there has still no scientific discovery on the contents of the rose stem cell-derived exosomes. ExoCoBio has been researching to isolate and characterize RSCE for the last 3 years and found a few biological functions as follows (As of now, all the data on RSCE are unpublished, to be submitted for publication soon.):

- Rose stem cell exosomes (RSCE) were obtained by separating and refining the RSC culture supernatant. The physical characteristics of the lipid membrane and the sizes of 30–200 nanometers were confirmed through Nano Tracking Analysis (NTA) and Transmission Electron Microscope (TEM) (**Figures 4** and 5).

- Preliminary miRNA analysis revealed that RSCE has more than 1000 kinds of miRNA which are mostly de novo sequences. Only about 30 kinds of them have been matched to human-derived miRNA sequences. Most of them are related to housekeeping functions.

- RSCE could increase the collagen production of human dermal fibroblasts by 40–120% in a dose-dependent manner and promote cellular migration by more than 20%.

- RSCE was found to have an anti-inflammatory function that the IL-6 production of macrophages was also reduced to 50–60%, depending on its concentration (**Figure 6**).

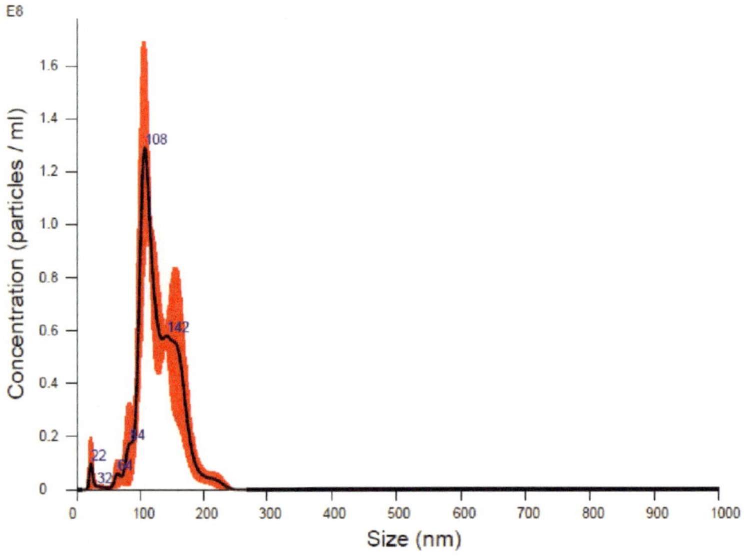

Figure 4.
RSCE NTA analysis. Source: ExoCoBio Inc. (unpublished data).

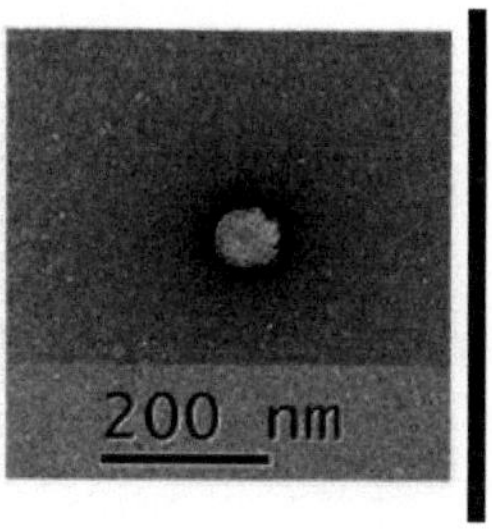

Figure 5.
RSCE TEM image. Source: ExoCoBio Inc. (unpublished data).

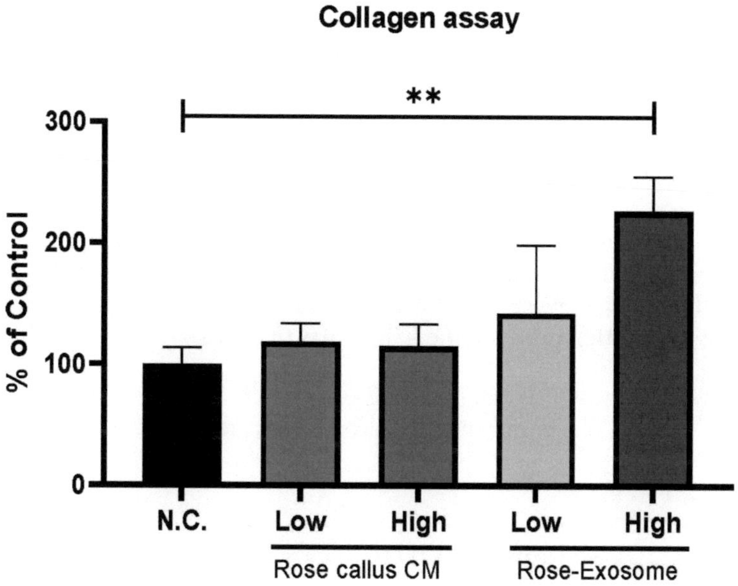

Figure 6.
*Collagen synthesis of RSCE in human dermal fibroblasts (HDF). *note: Rose callus CM is the supernatant of the stem cell (callus) culture of rose. Source: ExoCoBio Inc. (unpublished data).*

One disadvantage of plant-derived exosomes is that there is no universal quality standard yet. Many of the previous studies were done before the announcement of the minimal requirements established by the International Society of Extracellular Vesicles (ISEV). So, we need to be cautious in evaluating the data and results and make sure how to isolate and characterize plant-derived EVs. Moreover, the biogenesis pathways of plant-derived exosomes are also not well defined yet. Classifying plant-derived exosomes with the current terms used for animal EVs is still difficult due to a lack of current level of scientific discovery.

I believe that when we consider that microbes or bacteria are releasing extracellular vesicles and that kind of biology is universal across the kingdoms and species, it is very worth researching plant-derived EVs indeed for next-generation plant biology. ExoCoBio and other companies are trying to commercialize them as cosmetics or skincare products on the market.

8. Previous Writing

8.1 What is skin?

Our skin is a vital and complex organ that plays a crucial role in maintaining our overall health and well-being. Skin is the largest organ of the human body, and it is the outermost layer that covers and protects our entire body. It is a complex and multifunctional organ that serves many purposes. Some of the primary functions of the skin include:

- Protection: The skin acts as a barrier against harmful environmental factors such as UV radiation, pollution, and bacteria, which can cause damage or infection.
- Sensation: The skin contains a vast network of nerve endings that detect sensations such as touch, pressure, temperature, and pain.
- Thermoregulation: The skin helps to regulate body temperature by releasing sweat, which cools the body down, and constricting or dilating blood vessels to conserve or release heat.
- Hair: The skin plays an essential role in the growth and maintenance of hair. Hair is produced by hair follicles, which are small structures located in the dermis (the middle layer of the skin). The hair follicles contain specialized cells called keratinocytes, which produce the hair shafts that grow out of the follicle.
- Vitamin D synthesis: The skin produces vitamin D when exposed to sunlight, which is essential for maintaining healthy bones and teeth.

8.2 The structure of skin

The skin is the largest organ of the human body and has three main layers:

- Epidermis: This is the outermost layer of the skin and is made up of several layers of cells. The top layer of the epidermis is called the stratum corneum, which is composed of dead skin cells that have been shed from the skin surface. Further, we have a great skin barrier generated by a lipid layer of key lipid molecules like ceramides or dihydroceramides, or others. This skin barrier is critical for our skin health and aging. The epidermis also contains melanocytes, which are responsible for producing the pigment melanin that gives the skin its color.
- Dermis: This is the middle layer of the skin and contains various types of connective tissue, including collagen, elastin fibers, and hyaluronic acids. It also houses hair follicles, sweat glands, and sebaceous glands. The dermis is responsible for providing the skin with its strength and elasticity.
- Subcutaneous tissue: This is the innermost layer of the skin and is made up of adipose tissue (fat) and connective tissue. This layer contains the biggest number of stem cells in our body, which means that adipose stem cells and their exosomes are critical for skin health and aging, even though this is not well known previously. It helps to regulate body temperature and provides cushioning for the body's organs and bones.

8.3 The skin aging

Skin aging is a natural process that occurs as we age, and it is characterized by various changes in the skin's appearance, texture, and function. Some of the most common signs of skin aging include:

- Wrinkles and fine lines: As we age, the skin loses its elasticity, and wrinkles and fine lines begin to appear.

- Age spots: These are brown or black spots that appear on the skin, often on the face, hands, or arms, as a result of prolonged sun exposure.

- Dryness: As we age, the skin becomes drier and less able to retain moisture, leading to a rough, scaly texture.

- Thinning of the skin: The skin becomes thinner and more fragile as we age, making it more susceptible to injury.

- Loss of collagen and elastin: Collagen is a protein that gives the skin its strength and elasticity, and as we age, the production of collagen decreases, leading to sagging and loss of firmness.

9. Current trend in skin rejuvenation and exosomes

The trend in skin rejuvenation currently is towards non-invasive, minimally invasive, and more importantly, regenerative procedures that provide natural-looking results with little to no downtime. Patients are increasingly seeking out treatments that can address a variety of skin concerns, including wrinkles, fine lines, sun damage, and loss of volume, without the need for surgery or extensive recovery time. Some of the most popular non-invasive and minimally invasive treatments for skin rejuvenation include:

- Neurotoxins: Botulinum toxin injections, such as Botox® and Dysport®, can be used to temporarily reduce the appearance of wrinkles and fine lines caused by facial expressions.

- Dermal fillers: Injectable dermal fillers can be used to restore volume to the face, reduce the appearance of wrinkles and fine lines, and enhance facial features.

- Energy-based devices: Energy-based devices, such as lasers, radiofrequency, ultrasound, and light therapy, can be used to stimulate collagen production, tighten the skin, and reduce the appearance of wrinkles and fine lines.

- Chemical peels: Chemical peels use a solution to remove the outer layer of skin, revealing smoother, more youthful-looking skin.

- Microneedling: Microneedling involves using a device to create small punctures in the skin, stimulating collagen production and improving the texture and appearance of the skin.

- Platelet-rich plasma (PRP) therapy: PRP therapy involves injecting a concentrated solution of the patient's blood platelets into the skin, stimulating collagen production, and promoting tissue repair.

- Stem Cells: Stem cells have shown great promise in skin rejuvenation due to their ability to differentiate into various types of cells, including skin cells. In skin rejuvenation, stem cells can be used in various ways. Stem cells can be injected or applied topically to the skin, where they can release growth factors and cytokines that promote the growth of new cells, stimulate collagen production, and reduce inflammation. Another approach is to use stem cells to enhance the effects of other skin rejuvenation treatments, such as dermal fillers or energy-based devices. Stem cells can be mixed with dermal fillers or injected into the skin before or after energy-based treatments to improve their efficacy and enhance tissue repair.

- Exosomes: Exosomes are small vesicles that are released by cells, including stem cells. They contain various molecules, including proteins, lipids, and nucleic acids, that can regulate cellular functions and promote tissue repair and regeneration. Exosomes have emerged as a promising new approach to skin rejuvenation due to their ability to stimulate collagen production, promote tissue repair, and reduce inflammation. Exosomes can be obtained from various sources, including mesenchymal stem cells, and can be applied topically or injected into the skin. When applied to the skin, exosomes can penetrate the epidermis and dermis, where they can stimulate fibroblasts and other cells to produce collagen, elastin, and other extracellular matrix proteins that improve skin texture and reduce the appearance of fine lines and wrinkles. Exosomes can also promote tissue repair and reduce inflammation by modulating immune responses and promoting the growth of new blood vessels. This can help to improve skin health and reduce the risk of skin damage caused by environmental factors such as sun exposure and pollution. Clinical studies have shown promising results for the use of exosomes in skin rejuvenation.

10. Adipose stem cells and aging

Adipose stem cells, also known as adipose-derived stem cells (ASCs), are a type of stem cell found in adipose tissue (fat tissue). These cells have the ability to differentiate into various cell types, including adipocytes (fat cells), chondrocytes (cartilage cells), and osteocytes (bone cells). Adipose stem cells also have the strongest anti-inflammatory and regenerative properties, which make them valuable in the field of regenerative medicine.

During aging, there is a gradual loss of adipose stem cells in the body including facial skin and scalp, which can contribute to various age-related health problems. This loss of stem cells is thought to be due to a combination of factors, including decreased stem cell proliferation and increased cell death.

As the number of adipose stem cells decreases with age, the body's ability to regenerate and repair damaged tissues also declines. This can lead to a range of skin and health problems, including slower wound healing, more inflammation in the skin and other organs, decreased muscle mass, and decreased bone density.

Scientists have been actively researching ways to preserve and replenish adipose stem cells in the body, in order to promote better health and slow down the aging process. One promising approach involves the use of stem cell therapy, which involves the transplantation of stem cells into the body to replace damaged or depleted cells.

Recently, exosomes derived from adipose stem cells are being applied to treat a variety of diseases including dermatological and esthetic uses. Exosome esthetics refers to the use of exosomes in cosmetic procedures and treatments to improve the appearance of the skin, hair, and other parts of the body. In the field of esthetics, exosomes are used to stimulate the growth and regeneration of skin cells, reduce inflammation, and improve the overall appearance of the skin. Exosome-based treatments can be used to address a variety of cosmetic concerns, including fine lines and wrinkles, age spots, uneven skin tone, and acne scars. These treatments may involve the injection or topical application of exosomes directly to the skin or hair follicles. The exosomes can be derived from various sources, including mesenchymal stem cells, which are known to produce particularly potent exosomes with regenerative properties.

10.1 Exosomes for clinical applications

Exosomes are nano-sized vesicles of 30–200 nanometers that are released by cells and contain a variety of biomolecules, including proteins, lipids, and nucleic acids such as cytokines, growth factors, & microRNAs. Exosomes play important roles in cell-to-cell communication and have been found to have a wide range of potential clinical applications.

Here are some examples of the clinical applications of exosomes:

- Regenerative medicine: Exosomes have regenerative properties and can be used to promote tissue repair and regeneration. They have been studied for their potential use in treating various conditions, such as heart disease, liver disease, and neurodegenerative diseases.

- Anti-aging treatments: Exosomes have been studied for their potential use in anti-aging treatments. They contain growth factors and other molecules that can promote tissue repair and regeneration, which may help to slow down the aging process.

- Anti-inflammatory function: Stem cell exosomes, especially adipose stem cell-derived exosomes, have been found to have anti-inflammatory properties, which is one of the reasons they have potential therapeutic applications in various inflammatory diseases. For example, adipose stem cell exosomes have been found to inhibit the production of pro-inflammatory cytokines, such as TNF-alpha and IL-6, and promote the production of anti-inflammatory cytokines, such as IL-10. This can help to suppress the inflammatory response and promote tissue healing and regeneration like dermatitis or inflammatory bowel diseases.

- Drug delivery: Exosomes can be used as a vehicle for drug delivery, as they are capable of crossing biological barriers such as the blood-brain barrier. This makes them a promising tool for the targeted delivery of drugs to specific cells or tissues.

- Cancer treatment: Exosomes have been studied for their potential use in cancer treatment. They can be engineered to carry therapeutic agents, such as drugs or small interfering RNAs (siRNAs), to cancer cells. Additionally, exosomes can be used to stimulate the immune system to attack cancer cells.

- Diagnosis and monitoring of diseases: Exosomes contain biomolecules that can serve as biomarkers for various diseases. This makes them a potential tool for the diagnosis and monitoring of diseases, such as cancer and neurodegenerative diseases.

10.2 The differences and combination between exosomes and current technologies

Botulinum toxin is a neurotoxic protein produced by the bacterium *Clostridium botulinum*. This toxin is known to cause a severe form of food poisoning called botulism, which can be fatal in some cases. However, botulinum toxin has also been found to have therapeutic uses, particularly in the field of cosmetic and medical dermatology. In dermatology, botulinum toxin is used as a muscle relaxant to temporarily paralyze facial muscles and reduce the appearance of wrinkles and fine lines. The injection of botulinum toxin blocks the release of acetylcholine, a neurotransmitter that signals muscle contraction. This causes the targeted muscles to relax and reduces the appearance of wrinkles and fine lines.

Exosomes and botulinum toxins are two very different substances with distinct mechanisms of action and therapeutic applications. While both exosomes and botulinum toxins have potential applications in dermatology, they work through different mechanisms and have different therapeutic effects. Exosomes promote tissue repair and regeneration and have anti-inflammatory effects, while botulinum toxins are primarily used to reduce muscle activity and smooth wrinkles.

Dermal fillers are injectable substances used to restore volume and fullness to the face, reduce the appearance of wrinkles and fine lines, and enhance facial features. They are typically composed of a variety of materials, including hyaluronic acid, calcium hydroxylapatite, poly-L-lactic acid, and polymethylmethacrylate beads. Hyaluronic acid fillers are the most commonly used type of dermal filler. Hyaluronic acid is a naturally occurring substance found in the body that helps to hydrate and plump the skin. When injected into the skin, hyaluronic acid fillers can restore volume to the face, smooth out wrinkles and fine lines, and enhance facial features, such as the lips and cheeks. Mostly, dermal fillers are primarily used to restore volume to the face and reduce the appearance of wrinkles and fine lines. Only a few fillers have collagen-boosting effects, while exosomes can promote tissue repair and regeneration and have anti-inflammatory effects synergistically.

Energy-based devices for skin are non-invasive or minimally invasive devices that use various types of energy, such as light, radiofrequency, ultrasound, or laser, to improve the appearance of the skin. These devices can be used to address a range of skin concerns, including wrinkles, fine lines, sagging skin, hyperpigmentation, and acne scars. Some common types of energy-based devices for skin include:

- Laser: Lasers emit concentrated beams of light that are absorbed by the skin to stimulate collagen production and reduce the appearance of wrinkles, fine lines, and hyperpigmentation.

- Radiofrequency: Radiofrequency devices use electric energy waves to heat the skin and stimulate collagen production, resulting in tighter, firmer skin.

- Ultrasound: Ultrasound devices use sound waves to heat the skin and stimulate collagen production, resulting in tighter, firmer skin.

- Light therapy: Light therapy devices use different wavelengths of light to improve the appearance of the skin. For example, blue light therapy can help to kill acne-causing bacteria, while red light therapy can stimulate collagen production and reduce the appearance of fine lines and wrinkles.

Exosomes have been proven to work synergistically with these energy-based devices in dermatology. While exosomes give bio-stimulating signals to cells in the skin, energy-based devices provide manageable damage. Both mechanisms of action showed significant improvement to treat acne scars in combination with fractional CO2 laser and adipose stem cell exosomes recently.

11. Stromal vascular fraction (SVF), nanofat, and exosomes

SVF, Nanofat, and exosomes have shown promise in skin rejuvenation and other regenerative medicine applications. Stromal vascular fraction (SVF) and exosomes are both derived from stem cells and have been investigated for their potential applications in regenerative medicine and skin rejuvenation. However, there are some key differences between the three:

- SVF is a mixture of cells, including adipose-derived stem cells, as well as other cell types such as endothelial cells, smooth muscle cells, and immune cells. SVF also contains extracellular matrix proteins and growth factors that can promote tissue repair and regeneration.

- Nanofat is a minimally invasive cosmetic treatment that uses a small amount of the patient's fat to promote tissue regeneration and rejuvenation. The term "nanofat" refers to the small size of the fat particles that are injected, which are typically less than 500 microns in diameter. During the procedure, a small amount of fat is harvested from the patient using liposuction. The fat is then processed and emulsified to create a solution of small fat particles. The nanofat solution is then injected into the desired area of the body, such as the face or hands, using a fine-gauge needle.

- Exosomes, on the other hand, are tiny vesicles that are secreted by cells, including stem cells. Exosomes contain various molecules, including proteins, lipids, and nucleic acids, that can regulate cellular functions and promote tissue repair and regeneration. Stem cell exosomes are not or minimally immunogenic, which means that they are generally recognized as safe.

One key difference between SVF/Nanofat and exosomes is that SVF/Nanofat contains a mixture of cell types, while exosomes contain only the molecules that are secreted by stem cells. This means that exosomes are a more focused approach to stem cell-based therapies, as they target the specific molecules that are responsible for promoting tissue repair and regeneration. Another difference between SVF/Nanofat and exosomes is that SVF/Nanofat is typically obtained autologously by processing adipose tissue, while exosomes can be obtained from a variety of cell sources, including adipose-derived stem cells, bone marrow-derived stem cells, and mesenchymal stem cells. SVF/Nanofat is an autologous treatment while exosomes can be allogenic as "off-the-shelf products."

12. Key exosomes science and patents for dermatological use

Exosome research is a rapidly evolving field with many scientists and researchers contributing to its development. There are two famous scientists in exosome research:

- Dr. Jan Lötvall: He is a Swedish immunologist who is widely regarded as one of the pioneers of exosome research. He discovered the RNA transfer medicated by exosomes for the first time in the world in 2007 and his publication has the biggest citation number of 12,000 times in exosome science. He has made important contributions to the understanding of exosome biology and function, and his research has paved the way for the development of exosome-based therapies. He founded the International Society of Extracellular Vesicles (ISEV) and is the Chief Editor of the Journal of Extracellular Vesicles (JEV) at present. He has been doing a lot of jobs to set the standards of exosomes for years.

- Dr. Sai Kiang Lim: She is the first discoverer of stem cell-derived exosomes, which defined the "paracrine effect" of stem cells. Now she is a Senior Principal Investigator and Deputy Director at the Institute of Medical Biology at A*STAR in Singapore. Dr. Lim's research has focused on the use of stem cell-derived exosomes for tissue engineering and regenerative medicine applications. She has been developing stem cell exosomes as drugs for various inflammatory diseases.

In last years, lots of scientists and companies have created key patents for esthetic and dermatological uses based on exosomes. They are stem cell, plant, & microbe-derived, as follows:

- US Patent No. 10,071,050: This is the first patent on the skin rejuvenation effect of adipose stem cell exosomes in the world. It relates to a cosmetic composition for skin whitening, wrinkle improvement, or skin regeneration and includes, as an active ingredient, exosomes derived from stem cells comprising proliferating stem cells.

- US Patent No. 11,529,306: The lyophilized formulation of stem cell-derived exosomes and the anti-inflammatory composition including the same as an active ingredient is able to stabilize stem cell-derived exosomes and exhibit excellent anti-inflammatory effects, and particularly, exhibit remarkable anti-inflammatory effects as compared with not-lyophilized stem cell-derived exosomes isolated and purified from conditioned media of stem cells. Therefore, the lyophilized formulation of stem cell-derived exosomes and the anti-inflammatory composition including the same as an active ingredient is able to effectively prevent, suppress, alleviate, ameliorate, or treat inflammatory response or inflammatory diseases.

- US Patent No. 11,529,370: This patent is about composition for strengthening the skin barrier or improving skin barrier function that is able to improve objective indicators related to the protection of the skin barrier, the strengthening of the skin barrier, and/or the improvement of skin barrier function. The composition exhibits the effects of increasing the number of ceramides, dihydroceramides, and sphingoid bases, increasing the activities of enzymes that are involved in the synthesis thereof, and decreasing the activities of enzymes that are involved in the degradation thereof. In addition, the composition is able to restore skin barrier function by reducing TSLP, IL-4, and IL-13 which are closely associated with skin barrier damage, thus interrupting a vicious circle in which the lipids and proteins contributing to skin barrier decrease.

- US Patent No. 11,446,333: The present invention provides a composition for preventing, suppressing, alleviating, ameliorating, or treating pruritus comprising stem cell-derived exosomes as an active ingredient. The composition of the present invention is able to act against pruritus-inducing multiple cytokine targets, for example, IL-4, IL-31, and TSLP, and thus is able to be widely applied against pruritus caused by various factors and is able to effectively suppress and alleviate pruritus. In addition, when the composition of the present invention is applied directly to human skin, it is able to remarkably ameliorate pruritus-associated clinical scores, erythema, and the like. Thus, the composition of the present invention is able to be used as a pharmaceutical composition, a skin external preparation, and a cosmetic composition for preventing, suppressing, alleviating, ameliorating, or treating pruritus.

- US Patent No. 11,337,419: This patent relates to a method of lyophilizing exosomes using a cryoprotectant comprising methionine, mannitol, and trehalose is disclosed. The lyophilized exosome product shows a good appearance which maintains a porous sponge shape without forming ice crystals. In addition, the lyophilized exosome product can be applied to a pharmaceutical composition, a skin external preparation, and a cosmetic composition. For example, the lyophilized exosome product can be used as a solution obtained by simply mixing it with a diluent.

- WO 2020022731: This patent is the first plant stem cell-based in the world. The present invention provides a cosmetic composition comprising rose stem cell-derived exosomes as an effective ingredient for skin regeneration, skin elasticity improvement, or skin wrinkle reduction. The cosmetic composition of the present invention has excellent effects on skin regeneration, skin elasticity improvement, and/or skin wrinkle reduction.

- US Patent No. 11,534,392: This is a cosmetic composition including exosomes derived from Galactomyces as an active ingredient that is provided for skin regeneration, skin elasticity improvement, or skin wrinkle reduction. Cosmetic composition has excellent effects on skin regeneration, skin elasticity improvement, and/or skin wrinkle reduction.

13. Exosomes manufacturing and quality standards

Almost every cell is releasing exosomes so there are a huge number of types and sources of exosomes. So, it is very important to set up quality standards to produce exosomes for commercialization and clinical applications. There is currently no universally accepted quality standard for exosomes, as the field of exosome research is still evolving and the properties and characteristics of exosomes can vary depending on the source, isolation method, and intended use.

However, the ISEV has been trying to give minimal requirements on exosome standards from time to time. And there are generally accepted guidelines and best practices that have been proposed for the characterization and quality control of exosomes. These include:

- Size and morphology: Exosomes should be characterized by their size and morphology using techniques such as electron microscopy, dynamic light scattering, or nanoparticle tracking analysis. The size range of exosomes is typically between 30 and 200 nm, and they should exhibit a characteristic cup-shaped morphology.

- Protein markers: Exosomes should be analyzed for the presence of specific protein markers that are typically associated with exosomes, such as CD63, CD81, and CD9. The absence of contaminating proteins or markers from other cellular components should also be confirmed. Unfortunately, there are no generally accepted protein markers existing on or inside bacterial or plant exosomes, which needs vigorous research in the future.

- Nucleic acid content: Exosomes should be analyzed for their nucleic acid content, including DNA, RNA, and miRNA. The quantity and quality of nucleic acids can provide valuable information on the biological activity and potential therapeutic applications of exosomes.

- Purity and concentration: Exosomes should be purified to remove contaminants and characterized for their concentration using appropriate techniques such as Bradford assay, BCA assay, or nanodrop. Especially, blood-derived exosomes contain lots of lipoproteins or protein aggregates which are 100 times more than actual exosomes. A simple manufacturing process can not discriminate those impurities from exosomes due to their very similar size.

- Functional assays: Finally, exosomes should be tested for their biological activity using appropriate functional assays. For example, exosomes derived from stem cells should be evaluated for their ability to promote tissue regeneration or reduce inflammation, while exosomes intended for drug delivery should be evaluated for their efficacy and safety.

In particular, to get the best quality of exosomes, the manufacturing process must be Good Manufacturing Practices (GMP)-compliant. The ISEV and the International Society of Cellular Therapy (ISCT) gave a guideline for GMP manufacturing, for example, which requires the creation of master cell banks (MCB) and working cell banks (WCB) to get consistent stem cell quality. Those MCB or WCB are required to initiate stem cell therapy worldwide, while blood-derived exosomes are limited in terms of consistent quality due to a lack of cell bank establishment.

While these guidelines can help ensure the quality and consistency of exosome preparations, it is important to note that the field of exosome research is still evolving and there is ongoing debate and discussion around the best practices for exosome characterization and quality control.

13.1 Exosome stability and long-term storage

The stability of exosomes is an important factor that can affect their safety and efficacy. Exosomes are sensitive to environmental conditions such as temperature, pH, and oxidation, which can affect their structural integrity and functional activity. Therefore, proper storage and handling of exosomes are critical to maintaining their stability and potency.

Some factors that can affect exosome stability include:

- Lyophilization: The best storage condition for exosomes is considered lyophilization as published by 3 groups so far. Lyophilization removes water molecules from the exosome raw material and prevents protein or RNA degradation. Liquid- or frozen-exosomes are found to be very short-term stable around 3 ~ 6 months, depending on the storage temperature like −20 ~ −80°C.

- Temperature: Exosomes are sensitive to changes in temperature, and high temperature can damage their structure and function. Exosomes can be stored at a temperature between 2 and 8°C for long-term storage of up to 3 years after lyophilization, and, −20 ~ 80°C for short-term storage.

- pH: Changes in pH can also affect exosome stability. Exosomes should be stored in a buffer solution with a pH between 7 and 8 to maintain their stability.

- Oxidation: Exposure to oxygen can cause oxidative stress and damage to exosomes. Therefore, exosomes should be stored in an environment free from oxygen or under reduced oxygen conditions.

- Freezing and thawing: Repeated freezing and thawing can damage the structural integrity of exosomes. Therefore, it is important to avoid repeated freeze-thaw cycles and to store exosomes in small aliquots.

- Contamination: Exosomes can be sensitive to contamination from bacteria, viruses, and other contaminants. Therefore, it is important to maintain strict aseptic techniques when handling and storing exosomes.

Overall, proper storage and handling of exosomes are critical to maintaining their stability and potency.

13.2 Exosome-based aesthetic products

A huge number of exosome-based cosmetic products are available on the market worldwide. The regulatory requirements for exosome-based cosmetic products vary depending on the country or region where the products are intended to be marketed. In general, exosome-based cosmetic products may need to comply with the following regulatory requirements:

- Ingredient safety: Exosome-based cosmetic products must use ingredients that are safe for use in cosmetics. The safety of the ingredients must be supported by data from safety assessments, including toxicology studies, clinical studies, and other relevant data.

- Labeling: The labeling of exosome-based cosmetic products must provide accurate information about the product's ingredients, claims, and directions for use. The labeling must comply with the applicable regulations in the country or region where the product is intended to be marketed.

- Manufacturing: Exosome-based cosmetic products must be manufactured in compliance with Good Manufacturing Practices (GMP) to ensure product quality, safety, and consistency.

- Claim substantiation: The claims made about the product must be substantiated by scientific evidence. The evidence must be adequate to support the claims made in the labeling and advertising of the product.

- Registration/notification: Depending on the country or region where the product is intended to be marketed, exosome-based cosmetic products may need to be registered or notified to the regulatory authorities. The registration/notification requirements may vary depending on the product's intended use, claims, and ingredients.

In the United States, exosome-based cosmetic products are regulated by the Food and Drug Administration (FDA) or Personal Care Products Council (PCPC) as cosmetic products. The FDA does not require pre-market approval of cosmetic products.

To be a successful exosome product, it should be affordable with acceptable efficacy proved by non-clinical and clinical studies. The cost of exosome-based cosmetic products can vary depending on several factors, including the source of the exosomes, the manufacturing process, and the quality of the product. As exosome-based cosmetic products are still a relatively new technology, they may be more expensive than traditional cosmetic products. However, as the technology becomes more widely adopted, the cost of exosome-based cosmetic products may become more affordable.

It is important to note that affordability should not compromise safety and efficacy. Consumers should always choose exosome-based cosmetic products from reputable manufacturers, fully GMP-compliant and with lots of scientific publications, that have undergone rigorous safety and efficacy testing. The proven quality by a series of scientific publications and patents, rather than the simple number of exosomes, is the most important factor to choose products.

IN CONCLUSION, EXSOMES ARE NEW TECHNOLOGIES FOR ESTHETIC USE AND WE MUST CHOOSE SCIENTIFIC EVIDENCE-BASED EXSOME PRODUCTS.

Author details

Byong Seung Cho[1*] and Diane Irvine Duncan[2]

1 ExoCoBio Exosome Institute, South Korea

2 Plastic Surgical Associates, Fort Collins, CO, United States

*Address all correspondence to: ceo@exocobio.com

References

[1] Abels ER, Breakefield XO. Introduction to extracellular vesicles: Biogenesis, RNA cargo selection, content, release, and uptake. Cellular and Molecular Neurobiology. 2016;**36**(3):301-312

[2] Timmers L, Lim SK, Arslan F, Armstrong JS, Hoefer IE, Doevendans PA, et al. Reduction of myocardial infarct size by human mesenchymal stem cell conditioned medium. Stem Cell Research. 2007;**1**(2):129-137

[3] Xu R, Greening DW, Zhu HJ, Takahashi N, Simpson RJ. Extracellular vesicle isolation and characterization: Toward clinical application. The Journal of Clinical Investigation. 2016;**126**(4):1152-1162

[4] Basu J, Ludlow JW. Exosomes for repair, regeneration and rejuvenation. Expert Opinion on Biological Therapy. 2016;**16**(4):489-506

[5] Yu X, Odenthal M, Fries JW. Exosomes as miRNA carriers: Formation-function-future. International Journal of Molecular Sciences. 2016;**17**(12):2028

[6] Ohno S, Kuroda M. Exosome-mediated targeted delivery of miRNAs. Methods in Molecular Biology. 2016;**1448**:261-270

[7] Cho BS, Kim JO, Ha DH, Yi YW. Exosomes derived from human adipose tissue-derived mesenchymal stem cells alleviate atopic dermatitis. Stem Cell Research & Therapy. 2018;**9**(1):187

[8] Shin KO, Ha DH, Kim JO, Crumrine DA, Meyer JM, Wakefield JS, et al. Exosomes from human adipose tissue-derived mesenchymal stem cells promote epidermal barrier repair by inducing de novo synthesis of ceramides in atopic dermatitis. Cell. 2020;**9**(3):680

[9] Ha DH, Kim HK, Lee J, Kwon HH, Park GH, Yang SH, et al. Mesenchymal stem/stromal cell-derived exosomes for immunomodulatory therapeutics and skin regeneration. Cell. 2020;**9**(5):1157

[10] Cho BS, Lee J, Won Y, Duncan DI, Jin RC, Lee J, et al. Skin brightening efficacy of exosomes derived from human adipose tissue-derived stem/stromal cells: A prospective, Split-face, randomized placebo-controlled study. Cosmetics. 2020;**7**(4):90

[11] Kwon HH, Yang SH, Lee J, Park BC, Park KY, Jung JY, et al. Combination treatment with human adipose tissue stem cell-derived exosomes and fractional CO2 laser for acne scars: A 12-week prospective, double-blind, randomized, Split-face study. Acta Dermato-Venereologica. 2020;**100**(18):adv00310

[12] Ha DH, Kim SD, Lee J, Kwon HH, Park GH, Yang SH, et al. Toxicological evaluation of exosomes derived from human adipose tissue-derived mesenchymal stem/stromal cells. Regulatory Toxicology and Pharmacology. 2020;**115**:104686

[13] Hade MD, Suire CN, Suo Z. Mesenchymal stem cell-derived exosomes: Applications in regenerative medicine. Cell. 2021;**10**(8):1959

[14] Wang ZG, He ZY, Liang S, Yang Q, Cheng P, Chen AM. Comprehensive proteomic analysis of exosomes derived from human bone marrow, adipose tissue, and umbilical cord mesenchymal stem cells. Stem Cell Research & Therapy. 2020;**11**(1):511

[15] Bernstein DL, Jiang X, Rom S. Let-7 microRNAs: Their role in cerebral and cardiovascular diseases, inflammation, cancer, and their regulation. Biomedicine. 2021;**9**(6):606

[16] Grice EA, Segre JA. The skin microbiome. Nature Reviews. Microbiology. 2011;**9**(4):244-253

[17] Trounson A, McDonald C. Stem cell therapies in clinical trials: Progress and challenges. Cell Stem Cell. 2015;**17**(1):11-22

[18] Vizoso FJ, Eiro N, Cid S, Schneider J, Perez-Fernandez R. Mesenchymal stem cell Secretome: Toward cell-free therapeutic strategies in regenerative medicine. International Journal of Molecular Sciences. 2017;**18**(9):1852

[19] Bari E, Perteghella S, Di Silvestre D, Sorlini M, Catenacci L, Sorrenti M, et al. Pilot production of mesenchymal stem/stromal freeze-dried Secretome for cell-free regenerative Nanomedicine: A validated GMP-compliant process. Cell. 2018;**7**(11):190

[20] Bari E, Perteghella S, Catenacci L, Sorlini M, Croce S, Mantelli M, et al. Freeze-dried and GMP-compliant pharmaceuticals containing exosomes for acellular mesenchymal stromal cell immunomodulant therapy. Nanomedicine (London, England). 2019;**14**(6):753-765

[21] Sidhom K, Obi PO, Saleem A. A review of Exosomal isolation methods: Is size exclusion chromatography the best option? International Journal of Molecular Sciences. 2020;**21**(18):6466

[22] An Q, Hückelhoven R, Kogel K-H, van Bel AJE. Multivesicular bodies participate in a Cell Wall associated defense response in barley leaves attacked by the pathogenic powdery mildew fungus. Cellular Microbiology. 2006;**8**:1009-1019

[23] Mariana R, Marcela P, Mercedes E, Laura C. Apoplastic exosome-like vesicles a new way of protein secretion in plants? Plant Signaling & Behavior. 2012;**7**(5):544-546

[24] Cai Y, Zhang L, Zhang Y, Lu R. Plant-derived exosomes as a drug-delivery approach for the treatment of inflammatory bowel disease and colitis-associated cancer. Pharmaceutics. 2022;**14**:822

[25] Wu J, Ma X, Lu Y, Zhang T, Du Z, Xu J, et al. Edible Pueraria lobata-derived exosomes promote M2 macrophage polarization. Molecules. 2022;**27**:8184